Oral Surgery
for the General Dentist

Color Atlas of Dental Medicine

Editors: Klaus H. Rateitschak and Herbert F. Wolf

Oral Surgery for the General Dentist

Hermann F. Sailer and Gion F. Pajarola

Translated by
Thomas Hassell, D.D.S., Ph.D.
Seattle, WA, U.S.A.
with
Felix Stutz, D.D.S.
Winterthur, Switzerland

1649 Illustrations

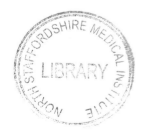

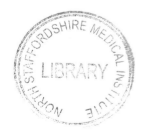

Thieme
Stuttgart · New York · 1999

Authors' Addresses

Hermann F. Sailer, D.D.S., M.D.
Dental Institute of the University of Zurich
Director of the Oral and Maxillofacial Section
Plattenstrasse 11, 8028 Zurich, Switzerland

Gion F. Pajarola, D.D.S.
Dental Institute of the University of Zurich
Head of the Oral and Maxillofacial Section
Plattenstrasse 11, 8028 Zurich, Switzerland

Editors' Addresses

Klaus H. Rateitschak, D.D.S., Ph.D.
Professor and Chairman, Department of
Cariology and Periodontology
Dental Institute, University of Basle
Petersplatz 14, 4051 Basle, Switzerland

Herbert F. Wolf, D.D.S.
Private Practitioner of Periodontics
Instructor, Dental Institute, University of Basle
Löwenstrasse 55, 8001 Zurich, Switzerland

Library of Congress Cataloging-in-Publication Data

Sailer, Hermann F. [Orale chirurgie. English] Oral surgery for the general dentist/ Hermann F. Sailer and Gion F. Pajarola : translated by Thomas Hassell and Felix Stutz.
p. cm.
– (Color atlas of dental medicine)
Includes bibliographical references and index.
ISBN 3-13-108241-0. –
ISBN 0-86577-707-1
1. Mouth–Surgery–Atlases. I. Pajarola, Gion F. II. Title. III. Series.
[DNLM: 1. Oral Surgical Procedures atlases. 2. Tooth Diseases–surgery atlases. WU 600.7S1320 1998a] RK529.S2513 1998
617.6'05–dc21 DNLM/DLC for
Library of Congress

Illustrations by
Joachim Hormann
Stuttgart, Germany

This book is an authorized translation of the German edition published and copyrighted 1996 by Georg Thieme Verlag, Stuttgart, Germany.
Title of the German edition:
Orale Chirurgie

© 1999 Georg Thieme Verlag, Rüdigerstr. 14, 70469 Stuttgart, Germany
Thieme New York
333 Seventh Avenue
New York, N.Y. 10001 U.S.A.

Typesetting by G. Müller, Heilbronn
Printed in Germany
by K. Grammlich, Pliezhausen

ISBN 3-13-108241-0 (GTV)
ISBN 0-86577-707-1 (TNY) 1 2 3

In the Series "Color Atlas of Dental Medicine"

K.H. & E.M. Rateitschak, H.F. Wolf, T.M. Hassell
● **Periodontology, 2nd edition**

A.H. Geering, M. Kundert, C. Kelsey
● **Complete Denture and Overdenture Prosthetics**

G. Graber
● **Removable Partial Dentures**

F.A. Pasler
● **Radiology**

T. Rakosi, I. Jonas, T.M. Graber
● **Orthodontic Diagnosis**

H. Spiekermann
● **Implantology**

H.F. Sailer, G. F. Pajarola
● **Oral Surgery for the General Dentist**

Preface

Our aim in the present volume has not been to create a textbook in the usual sense of the word, but rather a surgical manual that provides information mainly in visual form. The primary audience for this type of atlas is students, dental practitioners, and residents receiving training in oral and maxillofacial surgery. However, even experienced surgeons may find valuable information in the book, since many difficult procedures in oral surgery are illustrated step by step; in addition, the techniques developed in Zurich differ in many respects from those practiced elsewhere. The surgical procedures illustrated in this atlas are ones with which the authors have long-term clinical experience.

We have restricted ourselves in this book to dealing with surgical procedures in the oral cavity that can be carried out on an outpatient basis using local anesthesia—a narrower definition of "oral surgery." We are fully aware that there are some oral surgery procedures that can only be carried out under general anesthesia. All types of oral surgery demand appropriate training in dentistry; indeed, oral surgery is only one component of dentistry and maxillofacial surgery.

Our primary aim in this atlas has been to present cases and methods that will improve the quality of oral surgery procedures. Throughout the book, we have added many notes concerning "cautions" and "clinical tips" in an attempt to guide oral surgeons away from errors. In addition, we have added a new kind of guide providing a scale of severity and complexity—the simple/advanced/complex (SAC) index—which offers guidance on the degree of difficulty involved in each procedure.

A vast quantity of documentation has been gathered together for the atlas during the last five years, only about 5% of which has been included in the book. Without the willing assistance of many colleagues and co-workers, it would have been impossible to illustrate and describe the various surgical procedures adequately. We acknowledge special thanks to Dr. M. Makek, who provided the histological preparations, and Dr. P. Groscurth and his colleague, Dr. M. Manestar, who provided the cadaver specimens illustrating the facial nerves. We are also grateful to Dr. C. Schädle, who provided documentation for the three connective-tissue transplantations.

The superb professional photography in the atlas is the work of P. Halioua.

For untiring organizational efforts that resulted in outstanding documentation, we thank especially Ms. H. Ammann, Ms. E. Aziri, Ms. I. Sager and Ms. O. Stolz, as well as the entire team at our surgical outpatient clinic. Thanks are also due to our excellent librarian, Ms. H. Eschle, for her careful attention to the literature references. We gratefully acknowledge Dr. H. F. Wolf and Dr. C. Urbanowicz for their innumerable contributions during the preparation of the atlas. Our thanks go also to Dr. Thomas Hassell and Dr. Felix Stutz, as well as to Ms. Debbie Sorensen (Seattle), for their accurate work on this English edition.

H. F. Sailer, G. F. Pajarola

vi

Contents

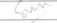

---

231 Dental Diseases of the Maxillary Sinus

---

241 Diseases of the Salivary Glands

Introduction

The traditional field of oral or dental surgery includes all surgical procedures within the oral cavity that can be performed under local anesthesia on an outpatient basis. Oral surgery is a specialized area of oral and maxillofacial surgery, and all of the basic principles of this medical discipline therefore also apply in oral surgery.

Oral surgery became a recognized medical specialty in the USA during the second half of the nineteenth century. James E. Garretson, who taught at the Dental College of Philadelphia, has been recognized as the first modern oral surgeon. He was both a physician and a dentist, and was therefore well qualified to perform intraoral surgical procedures. Significant steps in the development of oral surgery were the discovery of local anesthesia and the use of radiography for imaging structures. Professor Guido Fischer (Greifswald, Marburg, Hamburg) popularized the use of local anesthesia after 1906 through his tireless lecture tours in Europe and the USA. Fischer's success with local anesthesia was made possible by the earlier synthesis of epinephrine and procaine by the chemists Einhorn and Willstatter at the Hoechst company, around 1905, and the development of appropriate injection instruments by Cook (the carpule) and Fischer (the Fischer syringe). Surgical procedures still in use today in oral surgery were pioneered by a general surgeon, Dr. Partsch (apicoectomy 1896, cyst operations 1892, 1910). Partsch has been described as the man who "put the scalpel in the dentist's hand," not only for lancing abscesses, but also for targeted dental surgical treatments. Of course, innumerable other specialists have also made—and are continuing to make—substantial contributions in the field of oral surgery, developing and testing new methods.

The basic principles of surgery and wound healing in soft tissues and bone must always be observed when physicians or dentists use the scalpel. It should be remembered that each surgical procedure actually represents a physical injury, and that it is only the intention to bring about healing, with the patient's agreement, that protects us from legal consequences. It is therefore very important for surgeons to perform only those procedures that are justified by their training and experience. For this reason, we have attempted in this book to label all of the surgical procedures with an SAC score (see p. 2), as a form of quality control. This should in no way be interpreted as questioning surgeons' competence. Instead, the classification should serve to define simple procedures and distinguish them from those that are more difficult, indicating to dentists with less surgical experience where they should set their own limitations.

Classification of Procedures

The difficulties associated with various surgical procedures are often difficult to depict in an illustration. It seems reasonable, therefore, to classify the various procedures that are representative of a specific clinical situation according to the local risks and likelihood of postsurgical complications. This should allow each dentist to decide personally whether or not he or she is capable of carrying out a particular operation.

"SAC" Classification: Ⓢ = Simple, Ⓐ = Advanced, Ⓒ = Complex

Ⓢ = Simple
—Simple procedure without anatomically related risks
—Absence of surgical technical difficulties
—Lack of complications
—Can be performed by any well-trained dentist in a private dental office

Examples of simple operations with generally healthy patients:
- Tooth extractions
- Incision of abscesses in the alveolar process
- Flap procedures in the alveolar process
- Root resection in the anterior region
- Biopsy of mucosa
- Excision of benign pedunculated tumors of the vestibular oral mucosa
- Gingival resection and curettage

Ⓐ = Advanced
—Simple procedure, but with anatomically related risks
—Minor surgical technical difficulty
—Complications expected
—Can be performed by a surgically trained dentist in a standard dental practice

Examples of advanced procedures in patients with predictable systemic disorders (diabetes, hypertension, hypotension):
- Tooth extractions
- Removal of retained or impacted teeth
- Incision of abscess in the alveolar process
- Flap reflection on the alveolar process
- Apicoectomy
- Cystectomy, fenestration of cysts
- Correction of local defects on the alveolar processes
- Removal of peripheral sialoliths
- Mucosal biopsy

- Excision of benign tumors of the vestibular oral mucosa and the tongue
- Free gingival transplants
- Vestibuloplasty
- Gingival excision and curettage

Ⓒ = Complex
—More difficult procedures, with or without anatomically related risks
—Technically difficult surgically, and time-consuming
—Complications expected
—Can be performed by a surgically experienced dentist or oral surgeon under aseptic conditions on an outpatient basis

Complicated procedures in patients with systemic and local risk factors (diabetes, cardiac and circulatory problems, kidney or liver damage, hemorrhagic diathesis, breathing problems, allergies, immune suppression, following radiation therapy):
- All oral surgical procedures that can be performed under local anesthesia on outpatients in the presence of medical or technical risks or problems

Patient Examination

Diagnosis precedes treatment (Russell 1968).

Medical history and clinical findings will determine in each individual case whether there is a need for further examinations for diagnosis and treatment.

Medical History

Reasons for Presentation

The first meeting with the patient in the dental office starts with questions concerning the condition or problem that have led the patient to consult the physician or dentist. Data collection should include the medical condition and the patient's current problem, as they may be related. A thorough medical history must provide the attendant physician with a complete summary of previous medical or systemic conditions, which may be directly or indirectly related to the patient's current problem.

Health History

For psychological reasons, the term "health history" is preferable to "disease history." We therefore ask, "do you feel healthy?" or "is your health disturbed in any way?"

For patients with particular health risks, a thorough medical history is extremely important. The fact that patients have been able to reach the office without assistance has little to do with their actual health status. Targeted questioning must provide information that makes it possible to anticipate the effect of any therapeutic measure on the patient's systemic well-being (Schijatschky 1992).

A complete medical history will also include relevant information from the family history—for example, genetic disorders, tumors, deformities, and metabolic disturbances.

The Patient's Own Report

We start with the question, "Why have you come to see me? What problems are you experiencing?" The patient's own response to these questions will, in most cases, identify the main symptoms. This is important for the differential diagnosis, and can lead to a definitive diagnosis.

The physician now has a general idea about the patient's problem, and can expand the medical history using targeted questions.

Specific Questioning

No questionnaire, no matter how comprehensive it is, can replace a discussion between the physician and the patient (Dahmer and Dahmer 1992). At the start of the interview, the patient should be given the opportunity to speak freely. Do not interrupt. Do not ask several questions at the same time. Give the patient sufficient time to respond. While the medical history is being acquired, moralizing comments by the doctor are counterproductive and may cause the patient to withhold important information (Ingersoll 1987, Ringeling 1985, Schultz 1980). If only for medicolegal reasons, it is prudent to have an additional member of the medical staff in the vicinity while the patient is being questioned and examined; however, patients must also have the opportunity to speak in private with the examiner if they feel inhibited by the presence of a third person.

Cornerstones of Diagnosis

What symptoms or problems have you experienced to date?

How did the symptoms begin: were they sudden and acute, or gradual and chronic?

Have you had these symptoms for a long time, or is this an isolated occurrence?

What is the pattern of changes, e.g. their localization and accompanying symptoms?

What has happened so far, and what was the result of any previous treatment? Was there any improvement, or did the symptoms worsen?

Were there any outside factors that could have had an influence—e.g., smoking, alcohol, drugs, contact with sick persons, travel to foreign countries, dental treatment?

What is your personal opinion about the cause of the problem?

Practical Tips for Taking the Medical History

The discussion with a patient must take place in a calm atmosphere, and should not be disturbed by phone calls or interruptions by other office personnel.

Clinical Tip
Create an undisturbed atmosphere, avoid rushing the interview, win the patient's trust, be sympathetic.

Medical History Questionnaire

Standardized data collection using a medical history questionnaire has advantages, because the most important aspects are not forgotten, patients have to give written responses, and their shared responsibility is documented by the signature. Nevertheless, a doctor–patient discussion must follow any written questionnaire to clarify uncertainties and avoid misunderstandings. In addition, the initial medical history must be updated at subsequent appointments.

Implications for Treatment

On the basis of their knowledge and experience, physicians or dentists must be able to recognize all of the relevant information in the medical history, must understand the potential impact on subsequent therapy, and must incorporate such knowledge into the treatment plan.

Examples of Medical History Questions

1. Have you recently been hospitalized, or have you been treated by a physician? Why?
2. What is the name of your family doctor? Have you already visited a medical specialist?
3. Are you taking any medications on a regular basis? If so, which?
   —Painkillers
   —Antibiotics
   —Cortisone
   —Anticoagulants or hemodilution agents
   —Medicine for blood pressure or circulation
   —Anabolic drugs
   —Medication for diabetes
4. Do you use recreational drugs? Have you ever used marijuana or other drugs? (Tobacco, alcohol, hard or soft drugs; smoked, sniffed, injected? How much, how often?) How many cigarettes do you smoke a day? How many glasses of alcoholic beverages do you drink in the evening?
5. Do you have any heart problems, and do they affect your everyday life significantly? Can you climb two flights of stairs without having to stop?
6. Do you have high blood pressure?
7. Are you allergic to any foodstuffs or any other substances? Have you ever had an unusual reaction (e.g., allergy to injections, medications, or other substances)? Do you suffer from any of the following diseases:
   —Asthma
   —Hay fever
   —Diabetes
   —Epileptic seizures
   —Frequent headaches
   —Stomach or intestinal ulcer
   —Rheumatism
8. Do you have, or have you ever had, hepatitis or any other infectious diseases (tuberculosis, AIDS)?
9. Have you ever had any other serious disease? Have you ever been treated for a tumor?
10. Women patients: are you pregnant?

If pain is a significant part of the medical history, a special questionnaire is recommended (Cerbo et al. 1988, Isler 1984).

Clinical Tip
The medical history should be carefully documented. Tape recordings may only be made with the patient's permission. The more difficult or problematic the procedure, the more comprehensive the medical history details need to be.

Contact with the Patient's Family Physician

Before all surgical procedures, communication with the patient's family physician is imperative. Surgeons must never alter or reduce the dosages of a patient's medications on their own initiative; surgeons must consider the effects of their own procedures in terms of the possible consequences for the patient in terms of life and well-being. Communicating with the family physician is always important—not least for legal reasons.

Contact with the family physician should clarify the following questions:

—Can this patient be subjected to the stress of the planned surgical procedure?
—Do any other presurgical measures have to be undertaken, e.g., reduction of anticoagulant medications for a certain time? What is the current Quick's test value?
—Is antibiotic coverage necessary? If yes, who should prescribe?
—Does the patient's mental condition require any premedication?
—Should any medications be particularly avoided (possible interactions)?
—Which medications can be used to alleviate pain?
—Can the surgical procedure be performed on an outpatient basis?
—Can postoperative care be given at home?

Short Medical History

For dental emergency patients, pretreatment questioning can be limited to the critical areas. In every case, it must be determined whether the patient is at risk.

1. Have you been ill recently or under treatment by a physician? If yes, why?
2. Do you have circulatory or blood-pressure problems (for example, shortness of breath when climbing stairs)?
3. Do you have diabetes?
4. Are you taking any medications on a regular basis?
5. Have you ever had an unusual reaction to an injection by a physician or a dentist?
6. Do you have any allergies?
7. Have you ever had or do you now have a serious infectious disease (hepatitis, tuberculosis, sexually transmitted diseases, AIDS)?
8. Have you ever used marijuana or other recreational drugs?
9. Women patients: are you pregnant?

Documentation

The findings of the physical examination must be documented in addition to the medical history.

Case History

Most countries' health legislation makes it obligatory to record the medical data for every patient. Maintaining a medical file (medical history data, treatment rendered) also has a certain legal relevance. Therefore, a patient's medical record is a legal document, and must be a true and accurate record, with no omissions. After-the-fact alteration of medical records is not permitted; to do so borders on forgery or illegal falsification of documents. Patient records should be maintained for at least ten years, but this period varies in different countries and locales.

Data concerning the medical history and results of clinical examinations must be recorded in writing. Observations and diagnoses that result from such data, as well as the treatment planned and its performance, must also be documented chronologically. Information given to the patient (regarding potential complications, etc.) should be recorded in writing. Integral components of the complete patient record include all other patient records, such as radiographs, results from laboratory studies, and histopathological reports. Copies of all correspondence with the patient also belong in the permanent file. Photographs or dental study models may also be used to supplement the patient's records.

In principle, patients have the right to view their own medical records.

Personal Notes

The surgeon may record personal comments and observations on the case history and the treatment plan. Patients do not usually have right of access to such personal notes.

Surgical Report

A protocol must be created for every surgical operation. This must include the names of the surgeons, the assistants, the type of anesthesia, individual steps during the surgery, as well as any special circumstances (e.g., position and description of adjacent anatomical structures, nerves encountered, etc.).

Examination Methods

The dentist and the oral surgeon are trained in and knowledgeable about the anatomy, physiology, and pathology of the masticatory system, and should therefore be conversant with all of the appropriate methods of examination (Mitchell et al. 1971, Morris et al. 1983). It is advisable to use a regular routine for the various steps during patient examination, as this reduces the risk of overlooking any important findings. A distinction is made between the external examination of the face and neck, and the intraoral examination.

The physical examination may extend to other parts of the body if necessary, to clarify the relationships with known systemic disorders. In addition to information received from the patient's physician, dentists should also carry out their own thorough inspection. Whenever women patients are being examined, a female assistant should be present for legal reasons. This will preclude any subsequent accusations about inappropriate behavior during the physical examination.

1 Intraoral examination
Adequate illumination is critical for a thorough examination of the oral cavity. The light source should leave both hands free for manipulation of the oral mucosa.

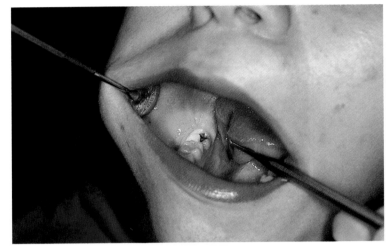

2 Instrumentarium for intra-oral examination
Two dental mirrors, lachrymal probe, pointed probe, graduated periodontal probe, anatomical and surgical forceps, scissors, suction tips, blunt probe, compass, and ruler.

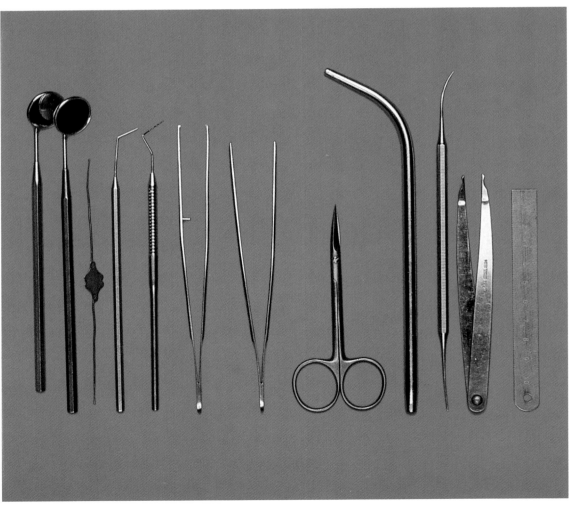

External Examination

The physical examination must detect pathological alterations, but should also include normal findings. These findings represent objective observations that can be perceived by the examiner.

Specific comments by the patient should precisely describe the duration, intensity, type, and location of a symptom (Dahmer 1994). How does the patient feel about a pathological change detected by the examiner? The answer to this question may provide information about the clinical significance of the observation in terms of possible aggravation or repression of any finding.

Inspection

The examination begins at the moment the patient walks into the consulting room.

Gait: assertive, lively, slow, timid. The patient's motor functions may indicate possible systemic disorders that warrant follow-up interrogation. In addition, the demeanor with which a patient presents gives the surgeon the information needed to conduct a compassionate dialogue.

The *handshake* varies considerably from person to person, but may provide tips on psychological peculiarities in the patient's current state of mind:
—Firm, strong, athletic
—Weak, despite a stocky build
—Moist, with apprehension or fear
—Shaky if under the influence of drugs

Constitutional Type

A patient's constitutional type may be of importance, as it may influence individual resistance, capacity, and adaptability. The patient's constitutional type also may be helpful for determining the reasonableness of a treatment plan. Physical and psychological characteristics define the four classic types.

Asthenic type: thin, short or tall person, with narrow shoulders, flat rib cage and a long, narrow head.

Athletic type: broad, well-developed shoulders, coarse facial features, pronounced chest, well-defined musculature, and a massive skeletal frame.

Pyknic type: stocky build, short neck, soft facial features, wide face, paunch, flat chest.

Dysplastic type: small stature, poorly developed, but without endocrine disturbance.

Closer Observation

Initial visual impressions may provide information about possible health problems.

Conspicuous external features:
—Facial form: symmetrical or asymmetrical, swelling or imperfections
—In the nasal region: external nares, shape, secretion
—Around the eyes: color of the conjunctiva and the sclera
—Perioral: color, pigmentation, shape, fissures, ulcerations, cracks
—Skin surface: reddening, blisters, telangiectasis, vascular abnormalities, pigmentations, efflorescence of all types, scars, surface consistency (wrinkled, fatty, slack, pasty, rigid)

Such external impressions cannot be recorded as objective findings. Nevertheless, such observations may provide an indication of problems that may exist, and can help the surgeon to focus and target the subsequent dialogue. Finally, any discrepancies between individual features or peculiarities will require further explanation.

Neurological Examination

Testing sensory perception in the facial region may provide clues to peripheral or central nervous system disturbances. This is highly important, partly for legal reasons.

Clinical Tip
Cranial nerve disturbance without obvious causes must be referred for diagnosis by a specialist.

Testing the Sense of Smell

Humans have a relatively weak olfactory sense, yet possess the ability to differentiate between thousands of scents. Testing the sense of smell can provide information about intact olfactory fibers or about any peripheral hindrance to olfaction. Testing is carried out by observing the patient's recognition of characteristically odoriferous substances, such as vinegar or eugenol.

Testing Motor Function

Cranial nerve VII (facial nerve). The seventh cranial nerve plays a major part in facial expression.

The mobility of the mimic musculature should be examined for bilateral symmetry:
—Forehead wrinkling
—Eye closure
—Pursing the lips (whistling)
—Baring the anterior teeth

Evidence of peripheral nerve damage includes paralysis of one side of the face, with a drooping corner of the mouth, lagophthalmos, and signs of Bell's palsy (eye looking upward, with failure of lid closure). If there is central paralysis of the facial nerve with only the inferior branch involved, the contralateral corner of the mouth will droop. Isolated loss of individual functions can also be caused by damage to any of the three peripheral branches of the facial nerve.

Cranial nerve III (oculomotor nerve), IV (trochlear nerve) and *VI (abducens nerve).* These cranial nerves control the movement of the eyeball.

Eyeball mobility is checked by asking the patient to follow a finger that is moved laterally. Double vision is a sign of reduced capacity for accommodation or incongruent movement, as well as positional differences between the eyes.

Reaction of the pupils to light, and abnormally dilated or constricted pupils, provide evidence of central disturbance, or may indicate drug abuse (narrow, constricted pupils). Unreactive pupils indicate severe central brain damage, e.g., prolonged oxygen deprivation, or may indicate lesions directly in the optic nerve. Both pupils normally react simultaneously even if light is shown unilaterally (indirect pupil reaction). Be alert for ocular prostheses or unilateral blindness.

Examination of Sensitivity and the Sense of Touch

Facial Skin Sensitivity

Cranial nerve V (trigeminal nerve). The sensory component of the trigeminal nerve is responsible for surface sensitivity of the face. Branches of the trigeminal nerve exit from the skull at the supraorbital, infraorbital, and mental foramina, and these sites should be examined individually (Schmidt 1985).

Sensitivity of the facial skin is tested by bilateral perception of an external irritant. With eyes closed, the patient should be able to distinguish between a sharp or a blunt challenge; this is easily accomplished by touching the skin alternately and irregularly with the point of a dental explorer and its curved section.

The threshold of perception is tested using a feather or a very fine artist's paintbrush. Reliable data can always be obtained by comparing contralateral sides of the face.

The quality of sensitivity is classified as:
—Normal sensitivity
—Reduced sensitivity
—Elevated sensitivity
—Lack of sensitivity (paresthesia or anesthesia)

Particularly important, especially with forensic questions, is two-point discrimination, in which the perceptible distance between two needle point placements is measured (in millimeters: 1–3 mm is normal for the tip of the tongue, and ca. 25 mm for the forehead) (Schmidt 1985).

Any spontaneous occurrence of abnormal sensations should be classified as paresthesia or dysesthesia.

Further specific tests, e.g., temperature sensitivity, threshold sensitivity, etc., are among the neurological examinations carried out by specialists.

Corneal Reflex

Approaching or actually touching the cornea—for example, with a piece of paper, causes the eyelid to close in a reflex reaction. If there is no reaction, it is a sign of central disturbance of the trigeminal nerve.

Functional Tests

Examination of the movement of the masticatory apparatus is often neglected. As with all other elements of data collection, however, this should be part of the overall oral examination. Functional disturbances of the masticatory system may account for otherwise unexplained pain phenomena in other regions (Jenni et al. 1988, Isler 1984, Krogh-Poulsen 1968, Schmid-Meier 1980, Wiehl 1983, Windecker et al. 1993).

Mobility of the Mandible

Ability to open the mouth is ascertained by measuring the distance between the incisal edges of the central incisors. The normal value is 35 mm, even in children.

Lateral and anterior motion is measured using the midline of the maxilla as a reference point.

Any inhibition of mandibular movement may become evident through restricted opening (trismus) or obstruction when closing the jaws.

Limited mandibular movement may be classified as:
—Resilient
—Elastic
—Rigid or blocked

Condylar Mobility

Sensitive palpation of the condylar region will identify freedom of mobility, mild interference, or clicking. Disturbances of movement caused by the articular disk can be described as initial, terminal, intermediate, or reciprocal, if the reverse motion is associated with a click at the same location. It is easier to analyze joint sounds when a stethoscope is used for auscultation. Often, the articular disk will be palpable in the lateral area of the joint during mandibular closure.

Occlusion

The patient's occlusion should be observed, and recorded as I–III under Angle's classification.

Any deviations in intercuspation that occur during spontaneous or guided mandibular closure should be recorded. When indicated, an articulation taper or occlusion wax should be used to record occlusal relationships or disharmonies. We recommend that study models and a bite registration be taken in every case.

Articulation

Interocclusal articulation represents the pattern of movement of the mandibular teeth in relation to their maxillary antagonists. This movement relationship can be depicted by various color markings on the teeth during intercuspation. Precise analysis of occlusion and articulation can only be carried out using study models mounted in an adjustable articulator.

Masticatory Musculature

Anterior component of the masseter muscle. The muscle is palpated between the thumb and forefinger to detect induration or painful areas.

Lateral pterygoid muscle. The forefinger or little finger of one hand is pressed between the ascending ramus of the mandible and the maxillary tuberosity in a cranial direction, to test for indurations or painful areas.

Origin of the masseter muscle. Finger pressure is applied to the outside of the cheeks on the right and left sides, proceeding cranially to detect induration or painful areas.

Temporal muscle. The fingertips are used to detect painful areas of the muscle surface on the skull and temples. This examination is performed as the patient opens and closes the mandible.

Hygiene During the Examination

It is imperative for gloves and masks to be worn during the examination. If the patient is suffering from an immune disorder (leukemia, HIV infection, immunosuppression) or infectious diseases (air transmission), a face mask is obligatory, as well as protective eyewear, as described in the International Dental Federation guidelines (FDI 1989).

Palpation of Lymph Nodes

The following lymph nodes are located in the orofacial region: temporal, submental, submandibular, cervical. Lymph nodes represent sites for the filtration of toxins, microorganisms, cellular fragments, etc. The lymph nodes play an important role in the genesis, proliferation, and differentiation of lymphocytes. Clinical examination of the lymph nodes can provide information about inflammatory, infectious, or malignant disorders.

3 Extraoral inspection
Left: Hair must be held away in order to observe facial skin and facial profile.

Center: Observation of left–right asymmetry from a cranial view.

Right: Frontal view with the patient's hair held back.

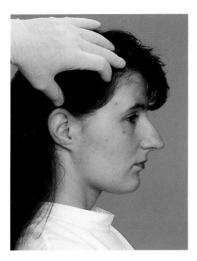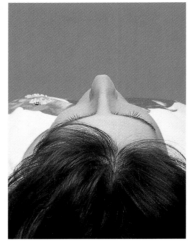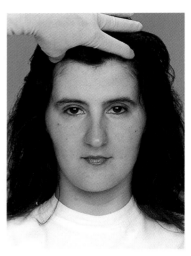

4 Checking for symmetry
Left: Use of a tongue blade makes it easier to identify facial asymmetries.

Middle and *right:* Determining the orientation of the occlusion plane in comparison with the plane of the two pupils.

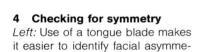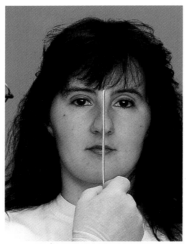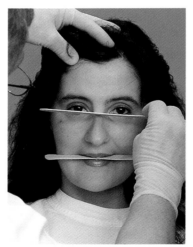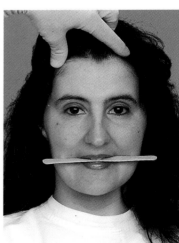

5 Checking motor function (facial nerve)
Left: Baring the teeth.

Center: Pursing the lips.

Right: Wrinkling the brow.

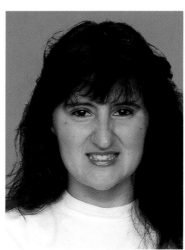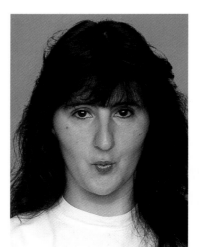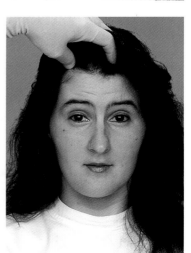

Palpation of the submandibular lymph nodes is performed using two fingers, comparing the left side to the right side. The temporal lymph nodes are located superficially, and are easily palpated. The facial and cervical lymph nodes are palpated by placing one hand on the patient's head and tilting it slightly forward. This relaxes the floor of the mouth and the musculature of the neck, allowing the examiner to use the other hand to palpate the submandibular, mental, and cervical lymph nodes to determine their size, consistency (soft/hard), and mobility.

Painful lymph nodes indicate an acute inflammation of the mucosa or the tonsils. Indolent lymph nodes are often detected after an inflammatory process has subsided, and they may persist for many months. They may, however, also be a symptom of tumor metastasis from the area drained from the lymphatic system. Enlargement of the lymph nodes may also occur with leukocytosis, lymphogranulomatosis, and in a number of viral diseases.

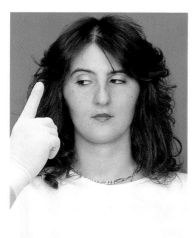 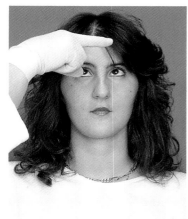 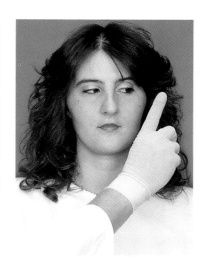

6 Examining eye movement (ocular nerve)
The eyes are tested for lateral and vertical movement and for the presence of double vision.

Palpation of Facial Contours

The contours of the face should be palpated bimanually, with left–right comparisons. Palpation should be performed without pressure on the fingertips. Any deviations from normal should be checked for consistency, mobility relative to underlying structures and skin surface, and associated pain.

Inspection of the Anterior Nasal Cavities

A thorough examination will include inspection of the nasal cavity using a speculum; this may detect abnormalities in the anterior segment of the alveolar process (cysts, abscesses, fistulas, odontogenic tumors) which may cause alterations in the floor of the nose. The examination is carried out by placing the beaks of the nasal speculum vertically, opening the nares, and examining the nasal cavity with appropriate illumination (Lehnhardt 1992).

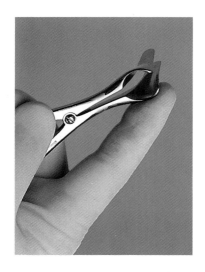 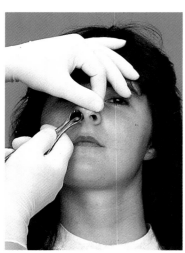 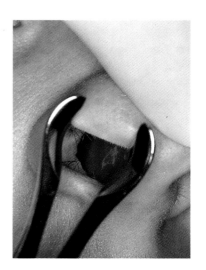

7 Inspection of the anterior nasal cavity
Left: Holding the nasal speculum.

Center: Placement of the nasal speculum for examination of the nasal entrance.

Right: Inspection of the anterior nasal cavity, with correct placement of the nasal speculum and sufficient illumination.

8   Palpation of the mid-face and forehead

Left: Bimanual and left–right comparative palpation of the supraorbital margin.

Center: Palpation of the infraorbital margin and the point of exit of the infraorbital nerve.

Right: Palpation of the mandibular contours.

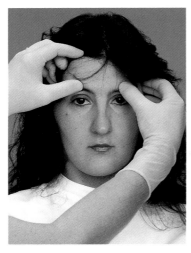 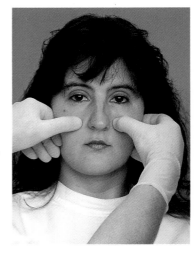 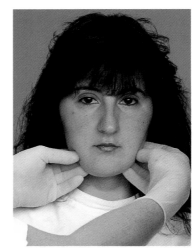

9   Palpation of the mandible and temporomandibular joints

Left: Testing the stability of the root of the nose on the frontal bone.

Center: Palpation of the chin contour.

Right: Palpating the temporomandibular joint regions bilaterally.

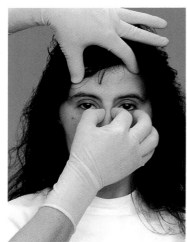 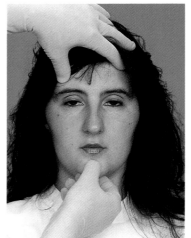 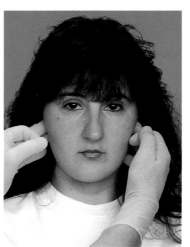

10   Palpation of the lymph nodes in the mandibular region

Left: The angular lymph nodes are palpated with the head in a relaxed position. Note that the free hand supports the patient's head.

Center: Palpation of the cervical lymph nodes along the sternocleidomastoid muscle to release tension. The patient's head is tilted slightly toward the opposite side and supported by the hand.

Right: Bimanual palpation of the sternocleidal lymph nodes.

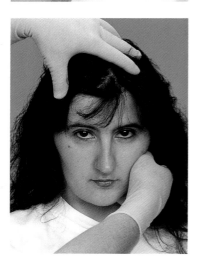 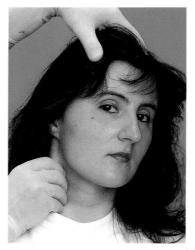 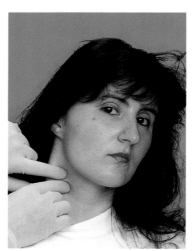

11   Palpation of the cervical lymph nodes

Left: With the patient's head tilted slightly forward, the occipital lymph nodes can be palpated.

Center: To relax the musculature of the floor of the mouth, one hand is used to support the head while the other hand palpates the submandibular lymph nodes.

Right: Bimanual palpation through the floor of the mouth for examination of the submental lymph nodes.

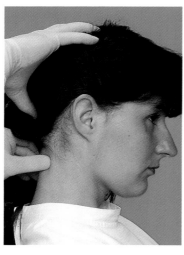 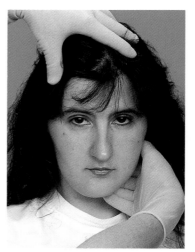 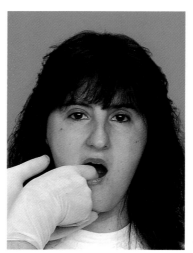

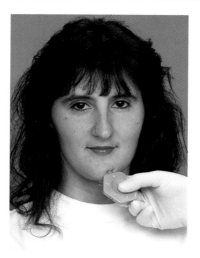 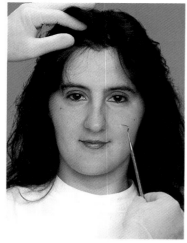 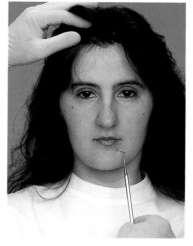

12 Sensitivity testing

Left: Two-point discrimination is a very precise method for testing skin sensitivity.

Center: Testing the superficial skin sensitivity in the region of the infra-orbital nerve using a pointed probe.

Right: Sensitivity testing in the region of the mental branch of the mandibular nerve.

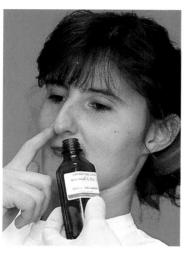 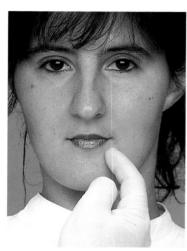 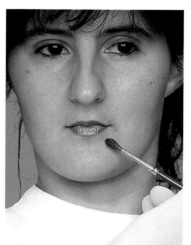

13 Sensory testing

Left: The sense of olfaction can be evaluated using volatile or perfumed substances.

Middle and *right:* Superficial skin sensitivity is evaluated by gently stroking the skin with the fingertips or with a soft brush.

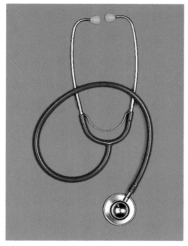 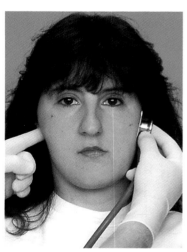 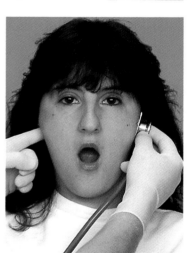

14 Auscultation

Left: The ordinary stethoscope is suitable for detecting sounds in the temporomandibular joint.

Middle and *right:* With the stethoscope applied with slight pressure over the joint region, the patient is asked to open and close the jaw. The characteristics of any unusual joint sounds are recorded, as well as the jaw position when such sounds are detected.

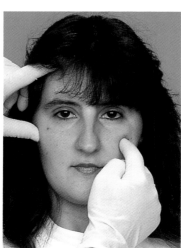 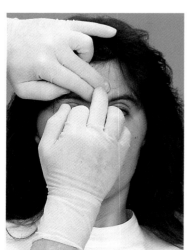 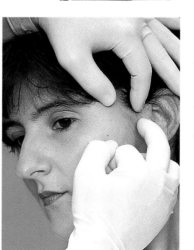

15 Percussion

Left: Percussion of the zygomatic bone for assessment of sensitivity to pain.

Center: Percussion of the anterior cranial sinuses.

Right: Percussion of the temporomandibular joint.

Oral Examination

The soft tissues within and surrounding the oral cavity are an intimate area. The clinician should therefore be considerate during examination of this region (Ingersoll 1987, Mitchell et al. 1971, Morris et al. 1983).

Inspecting the Dentition
Fully dentulous. With 28 teeth present, the patient is considered fully dentulous; the third molars are not considered, although their presence or absence should be noted.

Partial edentia. All missing teeth must be identified; a printed chart makes the survey easier. The four quadrants are designated numerically, one through four, beginning with the maxillary right quadrant (1) and ending with the mandibular right quadrant (4). The deciduous dentition is also identified using quadrant numbers (5–8).

Example: The first permanent molar in the maxillary right quadrant is tooth number 16 (one/six).

Apparent edentia must be confirmed by radiography.

Overview of Dentition
Healthy. No untreated caries or defective restorations, no periodontal pockets larger than 3 mm.

Unhealthy. Open carious lesions, multiple missing teeth, suppurating periodontal pockets larger than 3 mm, defective restorations.

Notes should be made concerning the condition and viability of crowns, bridges, and prostheses.

Testing the Vitality of the Teeth
For thermal testing, CO_2 can be used to apply cold (Obwegeser and Steinhäuser 1963), and warm gutta percha can be used to apply heat.

These temperature sensitivity tests provide information about the condition of the dental pulp:
—Vitality
—Inflammation (hyperemia)
—Pulpal necrosis

Caution
The failure of a tooth to react to the application of cold does not constitute proof that the tooth is not vital.

The sensitivity of a tooth may be inhibited despite intact vitality of its pulp, due to peripheral or central nerve damage.

Periodontal Condition
Various indices can be used to standardize and objectify the collection of periodontal data (Ciancio 1986, Lang et al. 1990, Mühlemann and Son 1971, Rateitschak et al. 1996):
—Gingival erythema
—Gingival bleeding
—Gingival enlargement
—Gingival ulceration
—Gingival recession
—Periodontal pocket formation
—Tooth mobility

Reference may be made to Rateitschak, Wolf and Hassell, *Periodontology* (third edition, New York: Thieme, 1999).

Caution
Periodontal data collection elicits systemic bacteremia. Patients who are at risk for focal infections (endocarditis, immunosuppression) must receive antibiotic coverage prior to periodontal examination.

Evaluation of Tongue Mobility
This test consists simply of asking the patient to stick out the tongue and move it from side to side. Deviations from normal should be noted. Is the patient able to move the tongue in such a way that the maxillary and mandibular vestibula can be approached? Any anatomical hindrances, e.g., a short lingual frenum, should be noted.

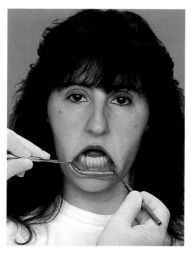 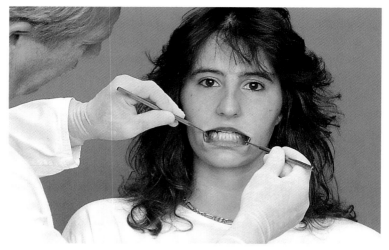

16   Oral inspection—overview
Inspection of the cheek mucosa.

Left: Inspection using two mirrors provides good visual access for examining the oral labial areas.

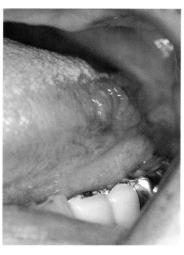 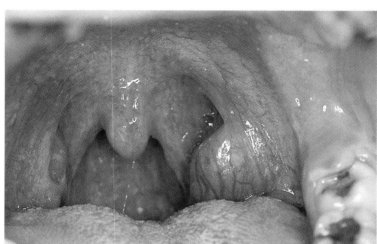

17   Base of the tongue and tonsillar ring
Examination of the floor of the mouth and the tonsillar ring.

Left: This examination should include the base of the tongue as well as the retromolar region.

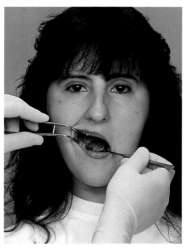 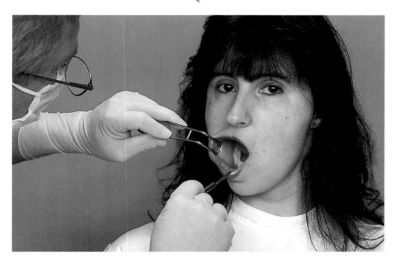

18   Buccal mucosa
A simple wire cheek retractor allows unrestricted examination of the buccal mucosa.

Left: Examination of the lingual and palatal areas is possible using a mirror.

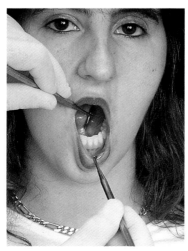 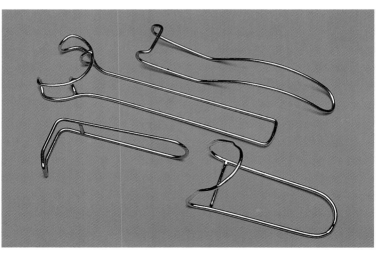

19   Cheek retractors
Various sizes and shapes of cheek retractors are commercially available.

Left: A dental mirror can be used to deflect the tongue, allowing improved visual access for examining the lateral floor of the mouth.

20 Compression test
A transparent spatula can be used to examine bluish, engorged areas. If pressure is applied and the mucosa loses its color, a diagnosis of hemangioma can be made.

Right: A retention cyst does not disappear when pressure is applied.

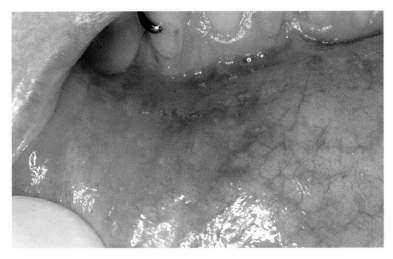 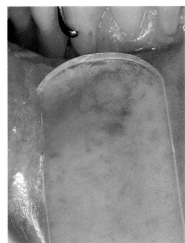

21 Lichen test, Nikolsky's sign
If vesicular lesions exist, rubbing them gently and with minimal pressure on the mucosa may elicit a blister; this represents a positive Nikolsky's sign.

Right: A similar response can be produced with the air syringe.

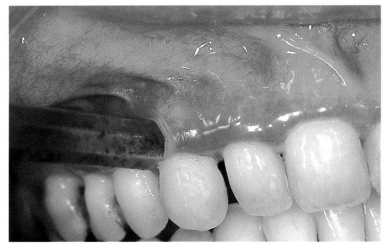 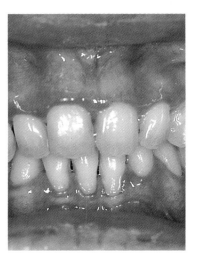

22 Vitality testing of the teeth
The most reliable results can be achieved by testing with CO_2.

Right: Modern carbon dioxide systems are equipped with an electronic valve.

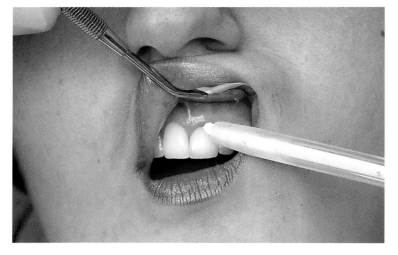 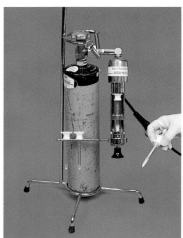

23 Periodontal examination
Tooth mobility can be measured objectively using the Periotest instrument.

Right: Periodontal pockets are measured using a graduated probe.

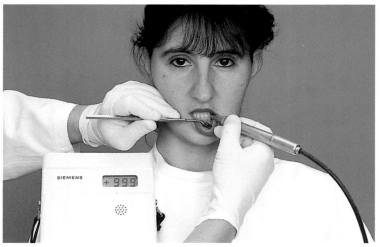 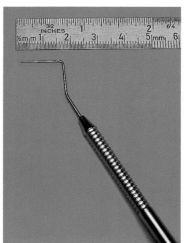

Mucosal Examination

The anatomical classification of oral mucosa is based primarily on its microscopic structure. However, a more functional definition describes oral mucosa as covering, masticatory, or sensory (Bork et al. 1993, Mitchell et al. 1971, Pindborg 1993, Schroeder 1992, Strassburg and Knolle 1991).

An active search should be made for pathological alterations in the oral mucosa. Patients are seldom aware of these, and even malignant alterations may not produce any subjective symptoms for a considerable time.

Particular attention should be given to the predilection sites for carcinoma during the intraoral inspection: floor of the mouth, ventral surface of the tongue, lateral border of the tongue, retromolar trigone, and the palatal arch.

It is advisable to use a regular sequence for this inspection to ensure that no area is overlooked: 1. lips, 2. buccal and labial mucosa, 3. hard and soft palate, 4. surface of the tongue, 5. base of the tongue, 6. oropharynx, 7. ventral surface of the tongue, 8. lateral and anterior floor of the mouth (Pajarola and Sailer 1995, Sonis et al. 1995, Strassburg and Knolle 1993)

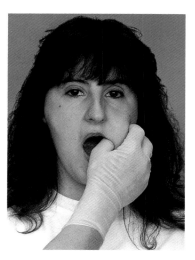
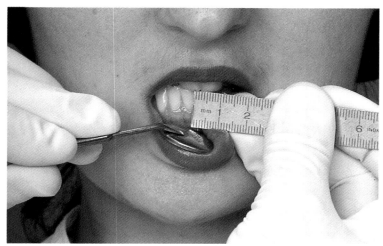

24 Functional tests
Maximum jaw opening should be measured in centimeters, as well as the interincisal distance and the extent of mandibular excursive movements.

Left: All accessible masticatory musculature should be palpated using two fingers at both the origin and insertion. Indurations or points causing pain should be noted.

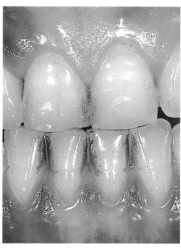
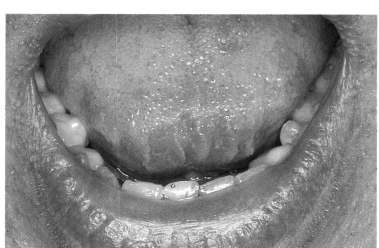

25 Parafunctions
Patients with a chronic tongue-thrusting habit will have impressions of the teeth on the surface of the lingual border.

Left: Spontaneous and guided mandibular movement will identify dental abrasion that has resulted from clenching or bruxism.

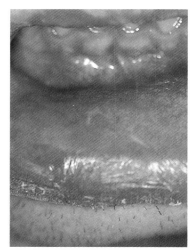
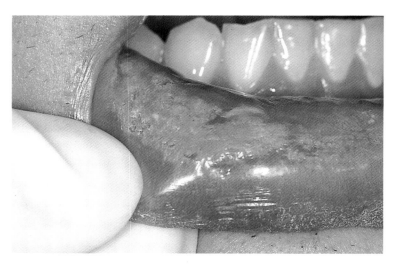

26 Mucosal alteration
Hyperkeratosis or fibrosis of the oral mucosa may also be signs of parafunction. Clinical signs of this type must be observed and recorded before the appropriate diagnosis is reached. This is exemplified in the case depicted here, of a 23-year-old man.

Left: Ten days after the patient ceased his lip-biting habit, the clinical symptoms disappeared.

Palpation of the Oral Cavity

Manual or digital palpation of the oral cavity provides information about the consistency, surface configuration, and extent of tissue alteration, as well as its relationship to neighboring structures.

Palpation of the Floor of the Mouth

Using the index finger of the right hand, the soft tissues of the floor of the mouth are pressed against the fingers of the left hand positioned beneath the mandible. This will reveal any induration of the floor of the mouth as well as any discomfort elicited by pressure.

It is important to ascertain the size, consistency, and shape of the submandibular gland. Stroking the submandibular duct or applying pressure to the submandibular gland, allows the quality of the saliva to be appraised: clear, cloudy, thin, or viscous.

Palpation of the Tongue

The tongue is grasped with a gauze square, pulled forward, and palpated with two fingers of the other hand. While the tongue is held between the thumb and middle finger, the index finger is used to palpate the dorsum.

The examiner should be aware of consistency, any asymmetry, swelling, induration, pain on pressure, and surface configuration.

Caution
Gag reflex. A mask and eye protection should always be worn.

Additional Examinations

Testing the Sense of Taste
This test is carried out with bilateral comparison in the various regions of the tongue, the palate, the cheek, and the inner surface of the lips, testing for sensitivity to "sweet," "sour," "salt," and "bitter." Appropriate solutions to be prepared: concentrated sugar and salt solutions, lemon in water, and lidocaine solution (Altner 1985). The anterior two-thirds of the tongue are innervated by the trigeminal nerve (lingual nerve); the tip of the tongue senses "sweet," while the lateral tongue borders sense "salty," and "sour." The posterior third of the tongue is served by the glossopharyngeal nerve, and this area of the tongue senses "bitter." For this reason, damage to the lingual nerve does not inhibit the patient from tasting bitter substances.

These simple tests, however, do not provide a completely objective evaluation. The methods stem from

Palpation of the Parapharyngeal Space

An index finger is used to palpate the anterior palatal vault:
—Parapharyngeal soft tissues (firm?)
—Palatal tonsils
—Styloid process in the tonsillar region

Examination of the Soft Palate

Ask the patient to say "aah," and observe the movement of the soft palate and the position of the uvula in its midline position.

Lateral cephalometric radiographs taken in rest position and during phonation can provide additional information about the adequacy or inadequacy of the palatal and pharyngeal region.

Nose-Blowing Test

A positive response to this test indicates the presence of a patent oroantral communication. The patient is asked to hold the nose closed and to exhale vigorously (nose-blowing) with the mouth open. The examiner can detect any air that is expelled via an alveolus or fistula. This procedure does not always provide a positive result even when there is an oroantral communication. Perforation into a maxillary sinus may be closed loosely by a flap of mucosa (valve defect). On the other hand, asking the patient to attempt to express air with the lips closed can provide positive evidence of a connection to the nose or sinuses (Lehnhardt 1992).

descriptions by Hänig in 1901, and have been used fairly uncritically ever since. Collings (1974) pointed out that the sensory areas of the tongue are individually distributed and that the accepted classification is probably based on an error of interpretation. More recent investigations (Bartoshuk 1993, Bartoshuk and Beauchamp 1994) have shown that the sense of taste in individuals can vary between "super-tasters," representing about 20% of the population, "medium tasters" (60%), and "nontasters" (20%).

Sensitivity to taste qualities is distributed over the entire tongue surface. The dorsum of the tongue contains practically no taste buds. Females are more sensitive to "sweet" and "bitter."

These more recent discoveries have to be taken into consideration when testing the sensory function of the tongue, especially when damage to the lingual nerve is suspected.

Diagnosis of Focal Infection

Definition

A focus of infection is defined as any pathological alteration in the jaw region recognized as a source of acute or chronic infection.

Active Focal Infection

Any condition that represents an infectious alteration must be regarded as an active focus.

Acute infection. Abscesses, empyema, bacterial and viral stomatitis, ulcerations.

Chronic infection. Exudative periodontal pockets, fistula formations, necrotic teeth or root fragments, inflammatory osteolysis, infected cysts, root fragments, impacted teeth, and foreign bodies with clinical or radiographic signs of inflammation, generalized gingivitis, sialolithiasis.

Potential Focal Infections

Any condition that may in the future develop into an infectious process represents a potential focus of infection.

Such conditions include: teeth with extensive restorations or carious lesions that may develop pulpitis, impacted but symptom-free teeth and foreign bodies, all endodontically treated teeth, deep periodontal pockets, dental cysts, sialoliths.

Assessment and Therapeutic Implications

The assessment of potentially dangerous effects of potential or manifest foci of infection, and the therapeutic implications, depend on the type of treatment that is planned (Sonis et al. 1995)—for example, whether a patient is to undergo radiotherapy or chemotherapy, immunosuppression following organ transplantation, or a surgical procedure with a risk of endocarditis (e.g., a heart-valve replacement). This assessment requires extensive clinical experience.

Dental Risks of Radiotherapy

All potential and patent foci of infection must be eliminated. A comprehensive and extensive examination must be conducted. The expected increase in caries activity, greater susceptibility to radiation osteomyelitis in the mandible than in the maxilla, and the patient's oral hygiene have to be taken into account, as well as general state of health and immune-defense status. In most cases, more radical treatment is indicated in the irradiated area.

Dental Risks in Immunosuppression and Chemotherapy

Insidious as well as chronic but symptom-free sources of infection should be regarded as danger zones.

All dentogenic infectious foci must be eliminated, so that no new foci are created:
—Comprehensive periodontal treatment
—Osteoplasty and apicoectomy
—Endodontic treatment
—Tooth extraction and removal of foreign bodies

All dental treatment must be completed before organ transplantation and institution of immunosuppression or chemotherapy. Any dental treatment performed thereafter requires the utmost caution. The patient's general state of health and the justification for the dental treatment must be discussed with the physician.

Focal Infection in Patients with a Risk of Endocarditis, Polyarthritis, and Other Rheumatic Diseases

All dental foci must be eliminated so that no new foci can develop:
—Comprehensive periodontal treatment
—Osteoplasty and apicoectomy
—Endodontic therapy
—Tooth extraction and removal of foreign bodies

In consultation with the physician, the justification for the planned dental treatment as well as more limited alternative forms of therapy should be considered. Antibiotic coverage should always be given.

With certain rheumatological, dermatological, and ophthalmic diseases, it is advisable to identify all patent foci and all impacted or endodontically treated teeth. The treatment sequence should be selectively prioritized, and discussion with the referring physician is recommended.

Clinical Tip
Particularly if the dental procedure is irreversible, the patient must be fully informed that elimination of the questionable focus may have no influence on the overall disease process.

Diagnosis of Focal Infection

Thoroughly informing the patient about the purpose and goals of the planned examination is an important element in diagnosing focal infection. Only motivated patients will be able to grasp the need for the often radical measures needed. The patient's emotional condition must also be considered sympathetically; patients undergoing therapy for tumors are often depressive. There is also the fact that patients usually have no dental discomfort, and therefore regard dental and oral surgical treatment as being unnecessary. Periodontal examination using a probe can cause bac-

teremia (Jokinen 1970). If this is to be prevented, antibiotic coverage should be prescribed (American Dental Association 1991, Barco 1991, Dajani et al. 1990).

27 Data collection form for diagnosing focal infection
All clinical findings are entered schematically. Observations should differentiate between active and potential foci. Treatment is dictated by the pattern of disease or the goal of focal diagnosis. For patients who are to undergo radiotherapy, all foci, both active and potential, must be eliminated.

Regarding:....................................

Dear colleague,

Thank you very much for referring the above patient
for clarification of a potential **dental focus of infection.**

Your diagnosis:....................................

Our findings on: .... (date)
Clinical oral examination:
Dental status:

8 7 6 5 4 3 2 1	8 7 6 5 4 3 2 1
8 7 6 5 4 3 2 1	8 7 6 5 4 3 2 1

/ = lacking, + = vital, − = nonvital, V = periodontal involvement, R = root fragment, F = fistula

Mucosa:
Occlusion/articulation:
Other observations:
Radiographic exam:
Panoramic/periapical:

8 7 6 5 4 3 2 1	8 7 6 5 4 3 2 1
8 7 6 5 4 3 2 1	8 7 6 5 4 3 2 1

RF = root filling, O = osteolysis, FB = foreign body, R = retained/impacted, C = cyst

Conclusion: Focus of infection

Active:

Potential:

Treatment recommendation:

8 7 6 5 4 3 2 1	8 7 6 5 4 3 2 1
8 7 6 5 4 3 2 1	8 7 6 5 4 3 2 1

X = extraction, ET = endodontic therapy, P = periodontal therapy, Re = resection/surgical treatment

Procedure we performed on:............................(date)

Suggested additional therapy:...........................

Elimination of the focal infection will be be carried out at our clinic according to the recommended procedures. The general dentist will carry out any additional dental treatment.

Yours sincerely,

Data Collection

Clinical Tip
Immunosuppressed patients and those at risk for endocarditis must receive antibiotic coverage before clinical examination.

An examination to detect focal infection consists of comprehensive clinical and radiographic data collection for the entire oral cavity and adjacent structures. Clinical observations include symptom-free nonvital teeth and dormant periodontal pockets, as well as inflammatory mucosal alterations and ulcerations.

A panoramic radiograph will assist in the search for inflammatory processes, impacted teeth, foreign bodies, and cysts in the alveolar bone. Any tooth that reacts negatively to the CO_2 test should be viewed using a periapical radiograph to detect apical pathology or inspect the quality of a root canal filling. The Waters projection (half-axial maxillary radiograph) provides information about inflammatory processes within the maxillary sinuses.

A special data collection form (Fig. 27) should be used in these cases.

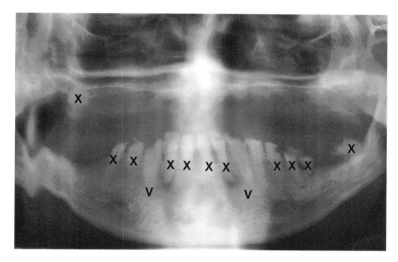

28 Diagnosis of focal infection
To assist in the diagnosis, the clinician requires a panoramic radiograph as well as all clinical data, including pocket probing depths, evaluation of tooth mobility, and tooth vitality determinations.

X = Extraction
V = Root treatment

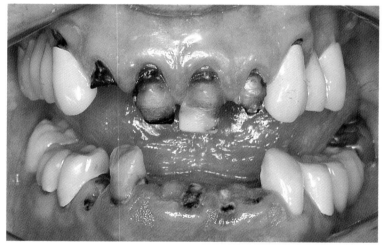

29 Dental sequelae of radiotherapy
In spite of systematic publicity and encouragement to maintain oral hygiene, ideal plaque control is often difficult to maintain due to xerostomia and mucosal inflammation. A common consequence of this is generalized smooth surface caries.

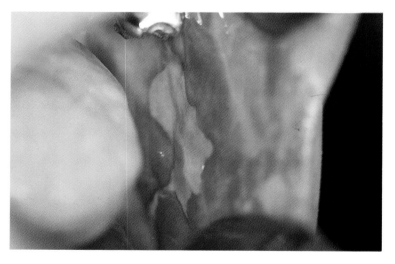

30 Effects of radiotherapy on the oral mucosa
Irradiation also directly affects the oral mucosa. The resulting radiation stomatitis, as shown here, is often very painful, inhibiting adequate oral hygiene by the patient. For this reason, such patients should be provided with individual instruction and regular follow-up visits, including professional tooth-cleaning procedures during and after radiation treatment.

Additional Clinical Examination Methods

These include puncture biopsy, cytological smear, vital staining, investigative anesthesia, tissue biopsy, fine-needle puncture, and ultrasound examination.

The puncture method is helpful when examining exudations of accumulated fluids (maxillary sinuses, cysts, abscesses, empyema in the maxillary sinus or temporal mandibular joint), and for collecting material to analyze causative agents and test bacterial resistance. Vital staining of the mucosa (e.g., with toluidine blue) can demonstrate epithelial activity in hyperkeratotic lesions and suggest the most appro-priate biopsy location (Mashberg and Samit 1989).

Smears of secretions or pus can provide bacteriological information (e.g., using Microstix to detect *Candida*). For cytological examination to detect tumors in the oral cavity, we prefer a targeted biopsy above a cytological smear.

Clinical Tip
The transport medium for material collected during puncture or smear must be appropriate for cultivation of anaerobes (e.g., Portagerm), because otherwise only a portion of the bacteriological spectrum can be examined.

31 Simple test for candidiasis
A smear is taken on an appropriate culture medium, and incubated for 24 hours at 37 °C.

The Microstix system is used to reveal *Candida:* the smear shown here clearly reveals punctate black staining.

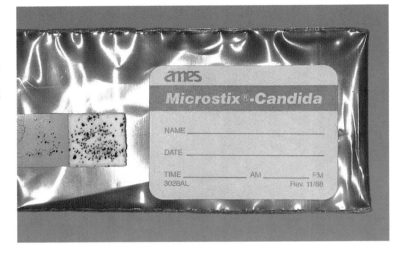

32 Incubator
A simple incubator is satisfactory if it incorporates a thermostat for maintaining temperature at 37 °C.

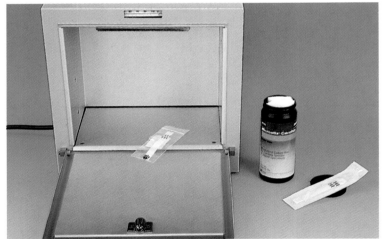

33 Bacteriological smear
The sample has to be taken using sterile techniques.

Right: Identification of anaerobic bacteria is only possible using an appropriate transport medium (e.g., Portagerm).

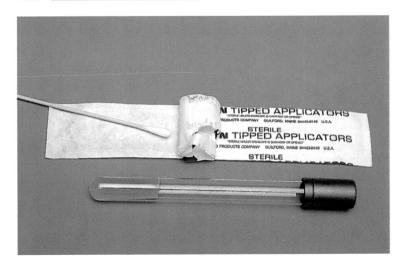
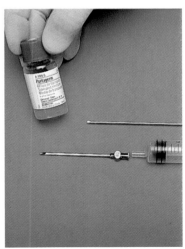

Surgical Principles

Course of Treatment and Operating Room

Organization

A surgical procedure requires planning. Not only must the course of the operation and the goals of the procedure be established, the requisite personnel and necessary armamentarium have to be defined before beginning the operation. The armamentarium and replacement instruments have to be sterile and ready to hand; correct functioning of all items of equipment must be checked. Perioperative measures also have to be checked. Will a stent be required? Is any osseous replacement material going to be used? Are any untoward consequences expected—for example, hemorrhage?

A minimum surgical team consists of the surgeon, a chairside assistant, and an operating nurse. One other person should be on hand or available in case of unanticipated circumstances requiring additional equipment or supplies.

Operating Room Hygiene

The operating room must be easy to clean. Smooth surfaces on cabinets, floor, and walls simplify disinfection procedures.

There must be sufficient space to give the surgical team freedom of movement, and to allow for additional instruments or apparatus that may be required. A crowded operating room carries a risk of contamination in the surgical operating field.

In addition, there should also be sufficient space to allow resuscitation equipment to be brought in and used if necessary.

Hygienic Zones

In order to clearly define the freedom of movement of the surgeon and surgical team within the operating room, it is advisable to designate specific zones clearly.

Sterile zone. This comprises the immediate surgical field, with sterile drapes and sterile clothing for personnel. All instruments and equipment within this zone are either sterilized or packaged in a sterile manner.

All other areas in the operating room are considered *hygienic zones.* This means that only personnel with fresh, clean clinic clothing can enter these, and all instruments, apparatus, and surfaces are disinfected.

Hygienic Requirements

It is impossible to achieve aseptic conditions in the oral cavity; however, contamination from foreign sources can be prevented.

One absolute prerequisite for this is that contamination by microorganisms not associated with the patient must be prevented (Bössmann and Bönning 1989, Fischer 1991, Greenspan et al. 1987, Wiehl and Guggenheim 1993, Heeg and Setz 1994).

Clothing. This must consist of sterilized fabric or dis-posable garments, including a gown, cap, face mask, protective eyewear, and gloves. All disposable articles must be waterproof.

Hand disinfection. Handwashing in preparation for a surgical procedure must also include attention to the fingernails.

Even though rubber gloves are worn, hand disinfection still deserves careful attention. If gloves are damaged during a procedure, there is a possibility of contaminating the surgical field.

34 Operating room
Surgical procedures demand suffi-cient space within the operating area; there must be space for the surgical team, for their equipment, and also for resuscitation equip-ment if it is required.

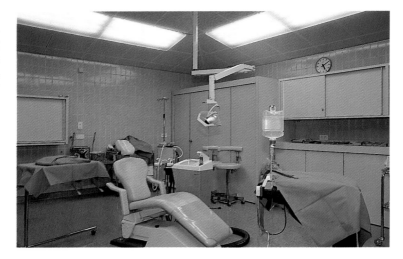

35 Hygiene zones
Aseptic work is made possible by dividing the room into a sterile zone and a hygienic zone.

1 Entrance for the patient
2 Entrance from the sterilization room
3 Hygienic zone
4 Surgical nurse
5 Mobile cabinet
6 Surgical assistant
7 Surgeon

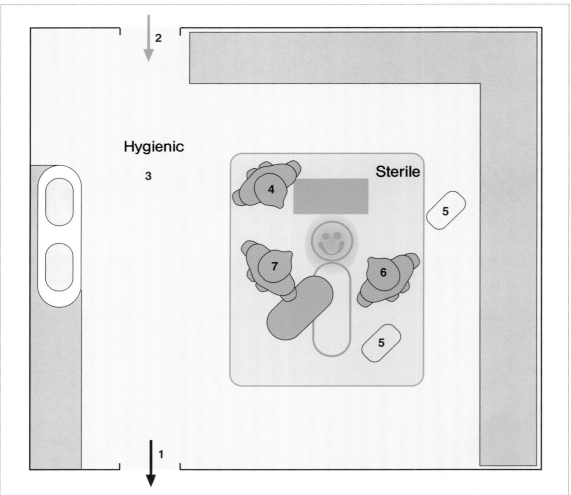

Preoperative Measures with the Patient

Hygienic Procedures

In addition to the preoperative information that is provided, the patient must also be prepared for the procedure hygienically (Heeg and Setz 1994).

If the patient's oral hygiene is inadequate, prophylactic measures should be carried out by a dental hygienist before the operation. Immediately preceding any surgical procedure, the patient should rinse for two minutes with a 0.2% chlorhexidine solution. This dramatically reduces the numbers of intraoral microbes.

The perioral region is disinfected using a solution that is not irritating to the skin, such as Betadine or 3% hydrogen peroxide.

For most oral surgical procedures, the patient is seated upright in a treatment chair. Two large, sterile drapes are used to cover the patient; the first covers the patient's chest and shoulders, while the second is folded in a triangular form, covers the head and face, and is affixed to the other drape using a towel clamp. This technique keeps the patient's hair out of the surgical field.

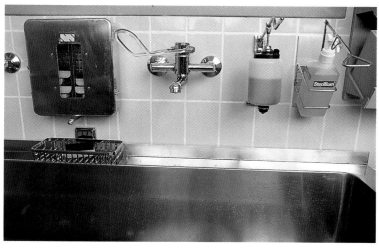

36 Scrub sink arrangement
Adequate space must also be available for hand washing and disinfection for all members of the surgical team.

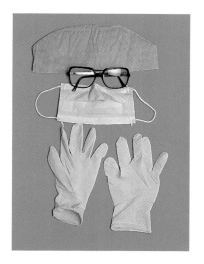

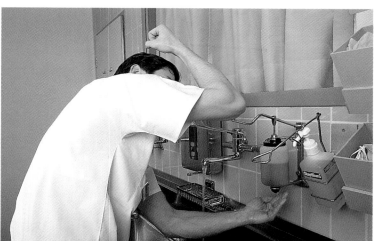

37 Hand disinfection
Hand washing and disinfection must be carried out before every surgical procedure.

Left: Personal protection is provided by a surgical cap, protective glasses, a face mask, and gloves.

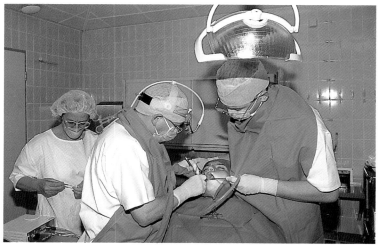

38 Surgical team
Every oral surgical procedure requires a surgeon, a primary assistant, a surgical nurse, and an additional person in the background to supply unanticipated equipment or supplies.

Premedication

The best type of "premedication" is to give the patient an explanation of the procedures before the day of surgery, and establish trust. These simple measures guarantee that the patient will be cooperative. Any preoperative medication should be discussed in advance with the patient's physician; a responsible adult must accompany the patient on the day of surgery. Sedatives that can be administered orally include barbiturates (phenobarbital) or diazepam (Valium). Local anesthetic dose must be adjusted accordingly.

Medical Monitoring

Most situations in oral surgery permit direct observation of the patient, so it is not necessary to monitor vital functions in healthy patients.

In special cases, it may be advisable to monitor a patient's vital functions throughout the procedure—even when using only local anesthesia—using a pulse oximeter, electrocardiography, and a blood pressure cuff. The surgeon may choose to have an anesthetist standing by (Fast 1993, Rothlin and Babotai 1988, Meier et al. 1994), or to have an indwelling intravenous catheter placed to ensure access to a vein.

39 Preparing the patient
Before drapes are placed, the immediate perioral region is swabbed with a disinfectant. Most of the face is subsequently covered with sterile drapes.

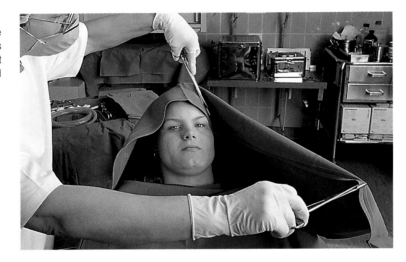

40 Sterile drapes
Sterilized cloth serves as surgical drape material.

Right: Disposable surgical drape.

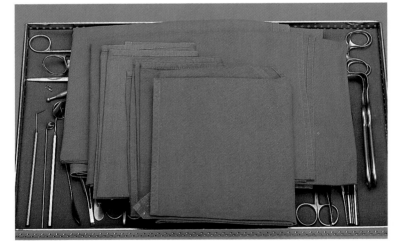 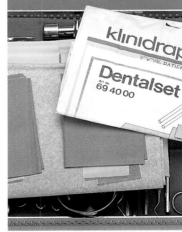

41 Surgical field
The patient's torso and head are draped in such a way that the surgical team cannot come into contact with nonsterile areas during the procedure.

Disposable sterile drapes are a useful alternative to sterilizable cloth drapes for infrequent use, but are more expensive.

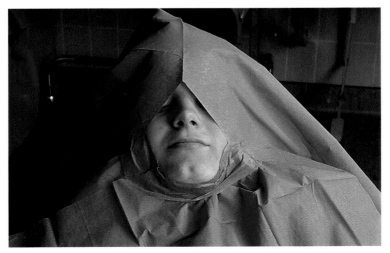

Armamentarium

The basic oral surgery armamentarium has only undergone minor changes and modernization for decades. Today, oral surgical instruments are manufactured using high-quality, corrosion-resistant steel. Many of the simple and frequently-used instruments are now available as sterile disposable items. The most commonly used of these are instruments for carrying out injections, incisions, or rinsing.

There is a wide range of instrument shapes and sizes; many well-known surgeons have contributed to the continuing development and evolution of instruments for oral surgery. Reference may be made to the comprehensive discussion of surgical instruments by Ghanremani and Arndt (1994). The following description is confined to those instruments routinely employed in our clinic.

Instrument Sets

Every surgeon develops a set of personally preferred instruments for routine or special procedures. We start with a basic set, which can be modified or enhanced depending on the procedure being performed. This reduces the time and effort involved in preparation and repackaging, and also cuts down on wear.

Instruments for Soft-Tissue Surgery

In oral surgery, the straight-handled scalpel with a no. 15 blade is the most commonly used instrument. The blade is generally oriented perpendicular to the underlying bone. The pre-planned incision is made with a continuous stroke in one direction. Repeatedly retracing the initial incision invariably leads to irregular wound margins, increased postoperative pain due to edema, and may favor infection.

The pointed no. 11 blade is particularly indicated for delicate mucosal incisions or excisions.

Angled scalpels are used for incisions in hard-to-reach areas (tuberosity, anterior palate).

Pointed or blunt scissors work well for trimming and shaping soft tissues.

When incisions have to be made in highly vascularized tissues, the electrotome has distinct advantages. The various electrosurgical tips can also be used for gingivoplasty, e.g., using electrosurgical loops.

Accurate incisions in soft tissues can also be achieved using lasers. However, the equipment is still extremely expensive, and for routine outpatient procedures, the cost is not justified by the advantages. The same is true of some ultrasound instruments.

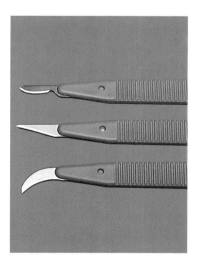
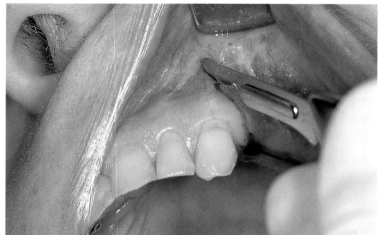

42 Instruments for soft-tissue incisions
The scalpel is used for all mucosal incisions. For typical flap reflection, a single clean stroke separates the mucosa and periosteum. Disposable scalpels are little used in oral surgery. Special scalpels with various shapes can be used to advantage in specific situations.

Left: The classical instrument for incisions is a scalpel with a disposable no. 15 blade (top).

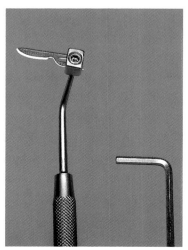
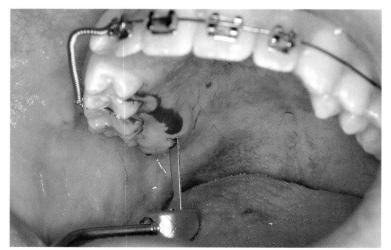

43 Angled scalpel
These angled scalpels are particularly suitable for precise incisions in the posterior segments.

Left: This scalpel handle takes a normal disposable blade, which can be set at various positions to create special incisions in the oral cavity.

44 Mechanical mucotome
The Möhrmann powered mechanical mucotome has distinct advantages for harvesting mucosa for transplantation.

Right: The blade is replaceable, and the head can be adjusted to suit the situation.

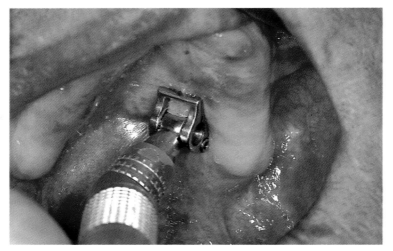 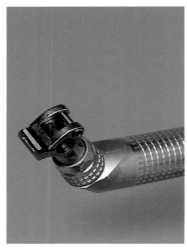

45 Manual mucotome
Experienced surgeons may still prefer the manual mucotome. The thickness of the harvested transplant is determined by the angulation of the blade.

Right: The manual mucotome is available in various widths.

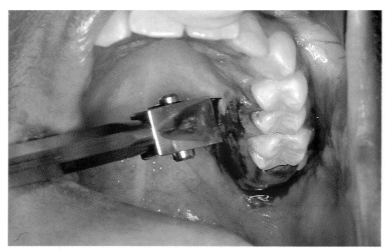 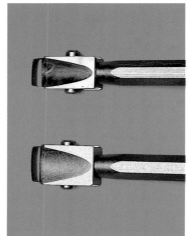

46 Scissors
Blunt scissors are indicated for separating the mucosa from subjacent tissues.

Right: Many different shapes and sizes of scissors are available for various applications in oral surgery.

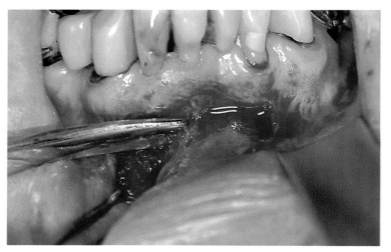 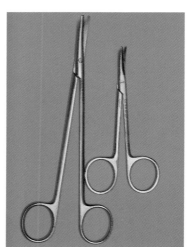

47 Electrotome
The high-frequency electrosurgical loop is indicated for gingivoplasty and for excising hemorrhagic tumors.

Right: The electrosurgical loop is useful for removing papillomatous tissue, while the needle electrode is indicated for plastic surgery at the gingival margin.

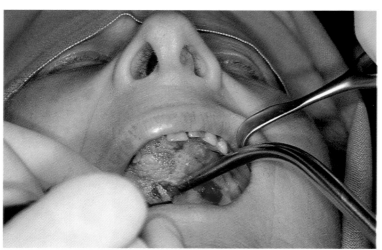 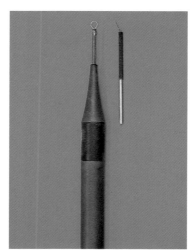

Cryosurgery

Treatment for expansive but superficial mucosal alterations can be readily performed using cryosurgery. Even
small hemangiomas and salivary retention cysts can be
treated in this way.

Cryosurgery is defined as the necrotization of tissue
by freezing. Temperatures ranging from –70 to –180 °C
are required. These temperatures freeze the cell cyto-
plasm, leading to irreversible cessation of cellular
function. Several different effects of ultracold temperatures account for such cellular death (Hausamen
1973, Leopard 1975):

—Cell wall rupture.
—Dehydration and electrolyte disturbance.
—Enzyme inhibition.
—Protein denaturation.
—Effects of thawing.

An indirect effect of cold is damage to capillaries.
Such an effect takes hours to occur, but is of clinical
significance, because the damage leads to localized
ischemic necrosis.

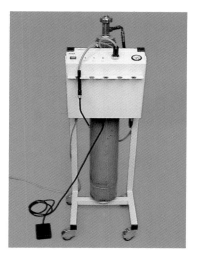 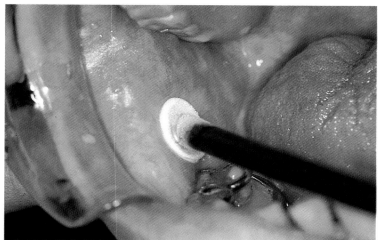

48 Cryosurgery—nitrous oxide
Focal freezing causes tissue
necrosis, which is followed by
reepithelialization. Using nitrous
oxide, a temperature of –75 °C can
be achieved. This is adequate for
freezing thin, superficial lesions.

Left: The apparatus consists of a
tank of nitrous oxide and a probe
that is cooled using the Thompson
effect.

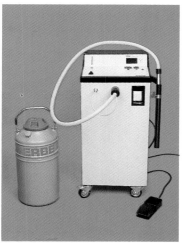 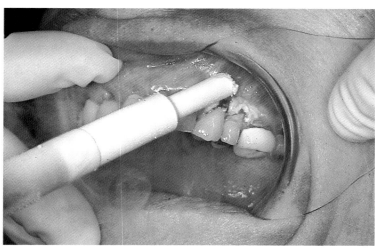

**49 Cryosurgery—liquid
nitrogen**
With liquid nitrogen, a temperature
of about –180 °C is achieved, but
this requires rather complicated
equipment. However, this degree
of cooling is adequate for freezing
firm lesions up to 2 mm thick.

Left: The apparatus regulates the
temperature automatically. Tissue
freezing is accomplished by direct
contact with the liquid nitrogen,
which is delivered through the
probe.

For the application of ultracold temperatures in the oral
cavity, only closed cryprobes are indicated. Two phenomena of physics are exploited:
—Cold due to evaporation, as the liquid nitrogen eva-
porates (–180 °C).
—The Joule-Thomson effect, which elicits a pressure
drop as nitrous oxide escapes (–70 °C).

When applying the cyroprobe, keep in mind that the
zone of cooling radiates circumferentially from the
probe tip, and that the temperature is higher further
from the tip. Blood flow in the vicinity dissipates the
cold, thus creating a selflimiting zone of freezing. This

zone encompasses a few millimeters in the oral
mucosa. The colder the temperature, the deeper will be
the depth of penetration into the mucosa.

Indication
Cryosurgery finds its special indication for treatment
expansive hyperkeratotic lesions of the oral mucosa,
and for small hemangiomas in the mouth.

Cryosurgery is not indicated for treatment of malignant lesions. It is possible to excise tissue for histological evaluation immediately after cryosurgery. See
also the chapter "Plastic Corrections of Soft Tissues"
and "Tumors."

Instruments for Osseous Surgery

Operating on calcified tissues requires force to be used. The energy that is applied is transformed into material deformation and heat. Rotating instruments, in particular, can generate significant heat, which is injurious to vital hard tissues. At a temperature of 47 °C, irreversible damage occurs in bone. Heat necrosis of bone is related directly to the temperature, and this is a factor of the revolutions per minute (r.p.m.), the burr shape, the cooling system, and the amount of pressure applied (Fuchsberger 1987, Grunder and Strub 1986). At speeds of 500–1000 r.p.m., thermal injury is minimal,

and osseous healing without sequestration can be expected. For drilling in bone, fissure burrs are indicated. At all times, the burr must be continuously cooled using physiological saline or Ringer's solution.

50 Bone cutters
Osseous surgery is performed very carefully, using surgical cutters. Very fine-bladed devices should be avoided because they tend to clog, leading to overheating of the bone. The typical oral surgery set-up includes various cutters for different applications.

Right: A contra-angled handpiece expands the range of applicability of rotating instruments in the oral cavity.

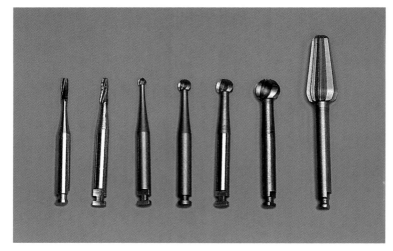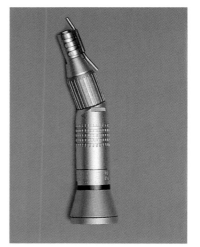

51 Osteotomy
Working in bone with rotating instruments requires continuous cooling. This necessitates a reliable fluid-dispensing system that can be controlled simultaneously with the drill motor. For osteotomy, fissure burrs are indicated, or the Lindemann bone cutters that were developed specifically for osseous surgery. The sharp teeth of these cutters can entrap and traumatize adjacent soft tissues, and they should therefore be used only by experienced surgeons.

Right: Lindemann bone cutters

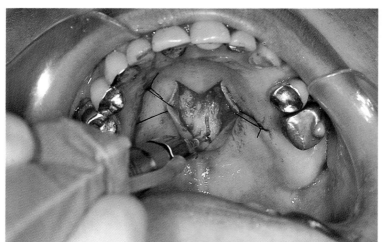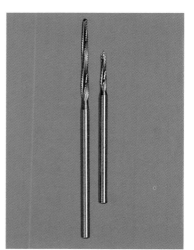

52 Trephine drill
The hollow trephine drill is particularly suitable for harvesting bone specimens for histopathological examination.

Right: Hollow trephine drills are available in various diameters.

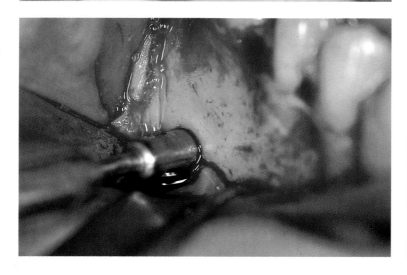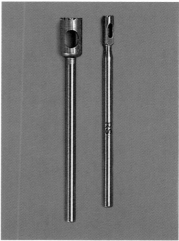

Internal or External Cooling?

To prevent thermal injury during osseous surgery with rotating instruments, a system for internal cooling of burrs has been developed (Kirschner and Meyer 1975). This cooling system is capable of significantly reducing temperature development during drilling, but only if the cooling solution is released without obstruction (Bolz and Kalweit 1976). When deep drilling into bone is being carried out, the excess heat that is created must be dissipated through the surface.

Ostectomy should be performed slowly and intermittently, preferably with larger cutters; this ensures that friction and heat are kept at acceptable levels (Schmitt et al. 1988).

Although there is no risk from heat generation when chisels and bone rongeurs are used, experience is required, and these instruments cannot be used as substitutes for drilling in most circumstances.

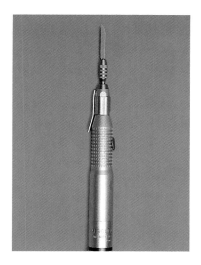
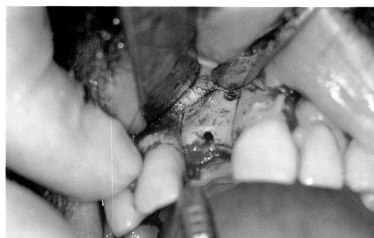

53 Oscillating cutter
The oscillating cutter is well suited for osteotomy of the maxillary ridge.

Left: This elegant model is excellent for creating fine osteotomy incisions.

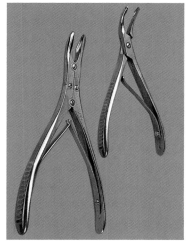
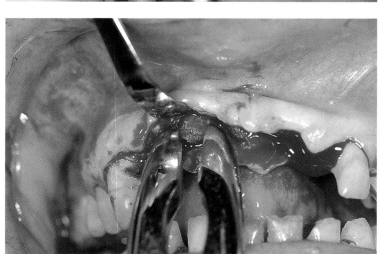

54 Luer forceps (rongeurs)
This hand instrument can be used when less precise bone remodeling is required.

Left: Various models are available for different applications in osseous surgery.

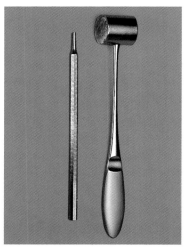
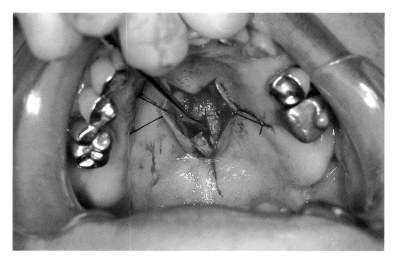

55 Mallet and chisel
These ancient surgical instruments are still used even in today's armamentarium, and are suitable for removing bone or pathological processes attached to bone (ankylosed teeth, tumors). Patients need to be reassured before the procedure, as these instruments can be perceived as rather brutal.

Left: Many different sizes and shapes of mallets and chisels are available for oral surgical applications.

Sterilization and Operating Room Hygiene

Macrohygiene

The spatial arrangements in a well-organized operating room must meet the following requirements:

Clean zone: office environment, common use rooms.

Hygienic zone: the dental or surgical operating room.

Sterile zone: the chairside surgical environment.

Microhygiene

This term applies to all of the methods and materials used for disinfection and sterilization.

It is of the utmost importance that the operating room and office lay-out should make it impossible for sterilized instruments to be contaminated by used instruments. This can be guaranteed by the spatial organization of the sterilization area into infected, hygienic (clean) and sterile zones.

56 Hygiene zones
The sterilization room should be arranged to receive and dispense instruments without cross-contamination. The room must have identifiable infected, hygienic, and sterile zones.

1 Receiving area for contaminated materials
2 Gross cleansing and disinfection
3 Preparation of clean instruments
4 Sterilization
5 Sterile storage
6 Entrance to operating room

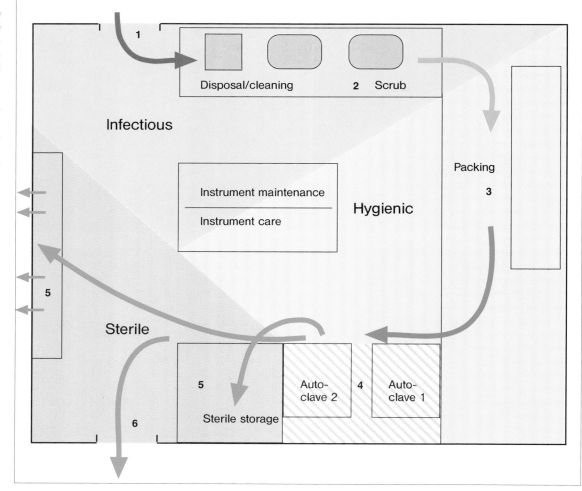

57 Sharps disposal
Appropriate containers must be at hand for disposal of used sharp instruments that are not reusable.

Right: Blades should be removed from the scalpel handle using a forceps or hemostat, in order to avoid personal injury.

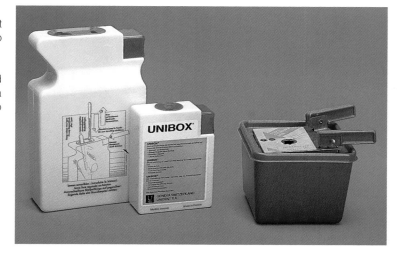
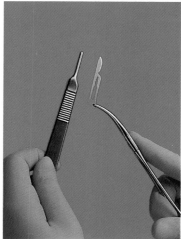

Hygiene Plan

In some regions, there are official written regulations for operating-room hygiene. The hygiene plan lays down procedures that ensure that hygiene measures are implemented. The plan specifies the agents and procedures to be used for disinfection and sterilization, and where each is to be applied. Guidelines and materials arranged in tabular form are easy to follow, and provide an overview. Similarly, checklists for individual areas, e.g., for equipment and for room disinfection, assist the personnel responsible for each procedure. The hygiene measures should also include guidelines for regulating patient appointments: treatment of infectious patients should be scheduled at the end of the day.

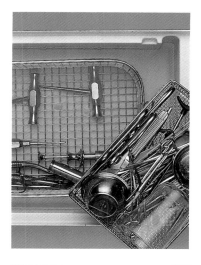
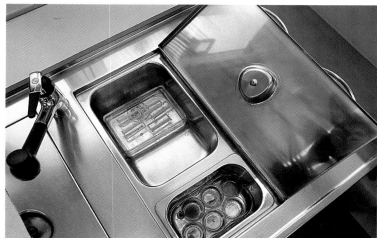

58 Disinfection
Even before they are washed and sorted, instruments must be disinfected, either in a disinfectant bath or using machines for this purpose. This considerably reduces the risk of infection if an injury occurs during subsequent preparatory procedures.

Right: A disinfection bath such as this can be added to any sterilization room.

Left: Instruments go into the disinfection bath immediately after disposable items have been removed from the instrument tray.

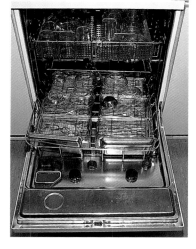
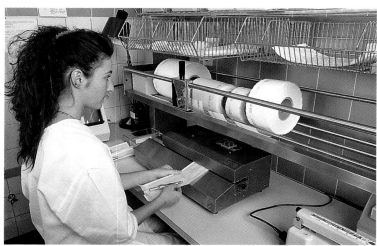
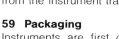

59 Packaging
Instruments are first checked for functioning and completeness, and then packaged and dated.

Left: Automatic washing machine for cleaning pre-disinfected instruments. This machine also provides a thermal disinfection cycle.

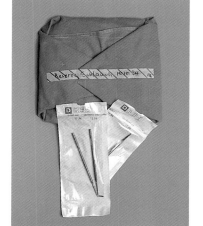
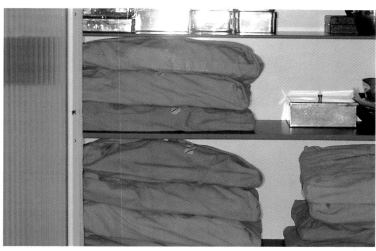

60 Storage
All sterile materials, such as tray set-up packs, should be stored in lockable cabinets.

Left: Instruments are sealed in sterilization bags or double-wrapped in drapes and closed with indicator tape. Each pack should have the date of sterilization on it, along with the signature or initials of the person who prepared it.

Surgical Procedures in Detail

Mucoperiosteal Flaps

Flap reflection consists of lifting the mucosa, together with the periosteum, away from the bone surface. A flap that maintains the integrity of the periosteum is less traumatic, it can be repositioned perfectly, and it provides direct vision of the alveolar bone in the surgical field.

Buccally reflected flap. This type of flap is almost universally used in oral surgery to reveal the alveolar process. It can be made as wide as necessary, it provides perfect direct visualization of the field, and it can be repositioned precisely.

Variations include the *paramarginally reflected flap* and the *coronally reflected flap.* These are indicated for providing access to small areas of the alveolar bone surface, and provide somewhat limited visual access. Repositioning can be difficult, and subsequent scar formation can be a problem.

61 Flap reflection
Following the initial incision through the mucosa and periosteum, an elevator is used to create the flap and expose the underlying bone. The integrity of the periosteum should be maintained.

Right: Elevators with rounded, sharpened ends are ideal.

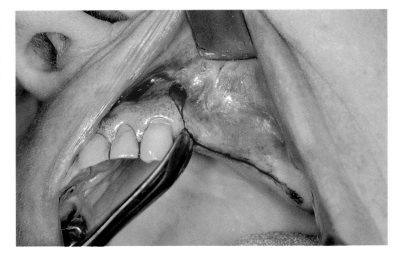
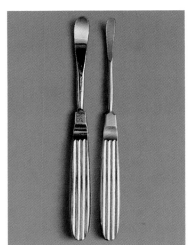

62 Surgical forceps ("pick-ups")
These small tweezers are ideal for holding the reflected flap and for removing debris from the field. Their use should be limited, however, because the sharp beaks do cause minor injuries to the mucosa.

Right: Various sizes and shapes of surgical forceps are available.

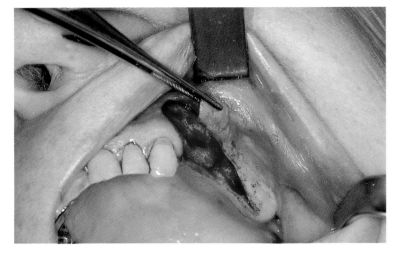
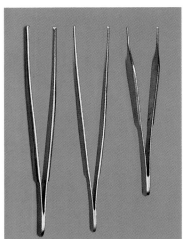

63 Tissue retractor
This instrument provides an excellent method for holding back a mucoperiosteal flap, causing very little tissue trauma.

Right: A double-ended tissue retractor is also available for holding broad flaps.

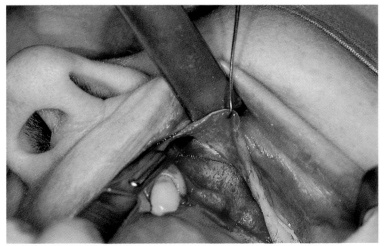
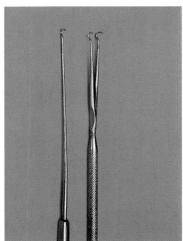

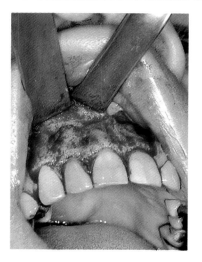

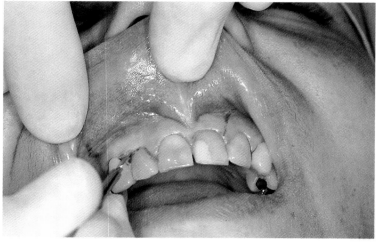

64 Trapezoidal flaps
This is a universal flap form for creating access to the labial aspect of the alveolar process.

Advantages: visual access, secure repositioning, scar-free healing.

Disadvantages: if periodontal pockets are deep, gingival recession and exposed root surfaces may ensue.

Left: Perfect visual access to the apical region.

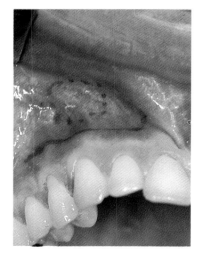

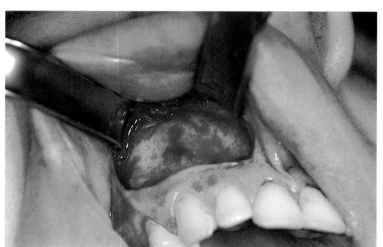

65 Primary incision
The point of divergence of the releasing incisions at the gingival margin is important; note how the interdental papillae are kept intact.

66 Vestibular flaps
If it is necessary to avoid involving the marginal periodontium, the primary incision can be made at the mucogingival junction, followed by apical flap reflection. An angled releasing incision makes flap repositioning easier.

Advantages: the marginal gingiva remains intact.

Disadvantages: limited visual access, scar formation during healing, possible osseous defect directly beneath the soft-tissue margin.

Left: The primary incision is made at the transition line between the attached gingiva and mobile mucosa.

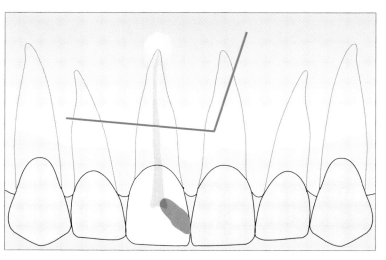

67 Primary incision
Either a triangular flap or a trapezoidal flap can be created. A clear, sharp angle at the divergence of the releasing incision simplifies flap repositioning.

Mucosal Flaps

In this procedure, the periosteum is not reflected with the flap. The tissue is separated immediately above and adjacent to the periosteum, or within the submucosal soft tissue. Mucosal flaps can be created using the no. 15 scalpel angled obliquely, or with fine-pointed scissors or blunt scissors.

It is the flap of choice for vestibuloplasty with secondary epithelialization, or for submucosal vestibuloplasty, for free gingival grafting, and for correction of labial or buccal frena.

Indication

The mucosal flap is used to harvest soft tissue for covering defects elsewhere, or to create a deepened vestibulum in dentulous or edentulous arch segments.

68 Mucosal preparation
If only the mucosa is to be released, blunt scissors can be used for supraperiosteal reflection.

Right: Reflection to deeper levels can include submucosal connective tissue for example, during a submucosal vestibuloplasty.

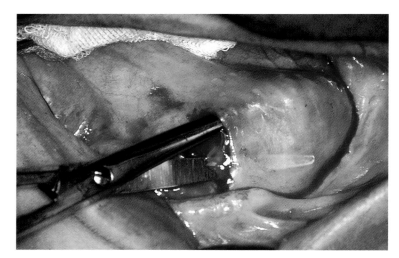 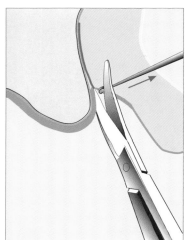

69 Supraperiosteal preparation
By positioning the scalpel more parallel to the mucosal surface, it is possible to create a mucosal flap without approaching the periosteum.

Right: Care must be taken to avoid injuring adjacent structures, e.g., the lingual nerve.

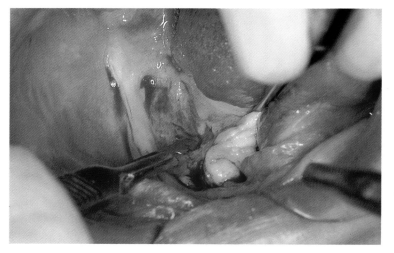 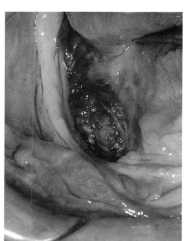

70 Flap extension
Horizontal incisions through the periosteum allow lengthening of a mucoperiosteal flap for example, to create a soft-tissue flap to cover an oroantral opening.

Right: The flap can be relocated far toward the palatal aspect.

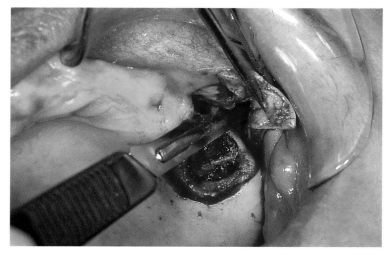 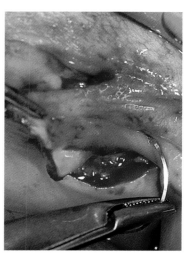

Flap Extension

The oral mucosa of the vestibular region is elastic and extensible; however, a mucoperiosteal flap cannot be stretched, because the underlying periosteum is non-elastic. A tissue flap can be extended only after the periosteum is cut perpendicular to the direction of reflection.

Laterally Repositioned Flap

This technique can be used to cover an existing mucosal defect. However, the procedure creates an undesir-

ed denudation wound, which heals by secondary intention, or may be covered if the mucosa is sufficiently extensible. Defining a flap for repositioning demands precise geometric planning, as well as careful attention to preserving an adequate blood supply to the tissue segment destined for repositioning.

Indication

It is generally necessary to section through the periosteum for coverage of the alveolar process after tooth extraction, or for closure of an oroantral communication using a vestibular flap.

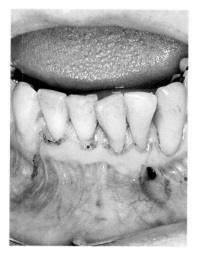
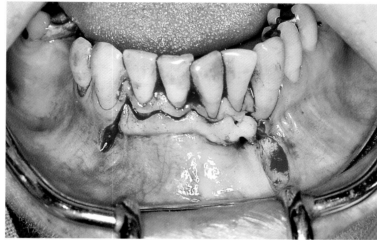

71 Laterally repositioned flap—primary incision
Indicated for covering mucosal defects on the alveolar process. Note here the fistula above an osseous defect near tooth 32. The delineated flap extends over four teeth.

Left: Marking the flap borders before making the primary incision for a flap to repair a mucosal fistula.

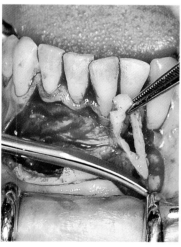
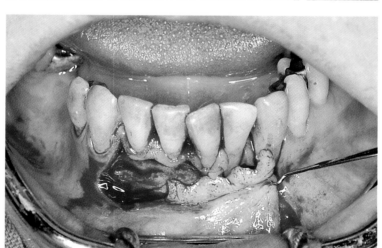

72 Flap reflection
The flap is laterally repositioned by about one tooth width to cover the defect.

Left: The tissue surrounding the defect is excised, and the flap is positioned laterally to cover the wound site.

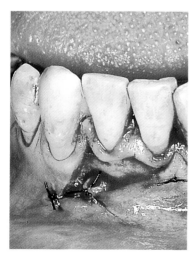
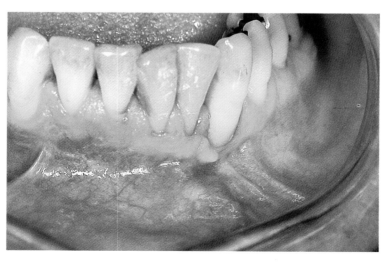

73 Postoperative course
The clinical situation one year after the operation.

Left: The denudation near tooth 42 was partially covered by stretching the flap; the residual defect healed by secondary epithelialization.

Routine Procedures during Surgical Intervention

Wound Management

A distinction is made between "open" and "closed" wound healing. Postoperative care is determined by the type of healing that is anticipated.

Closed Wound Management

This is achieved by adaptation and fixation of the wound margins with sutures or, in certain special situations, using tissue adhesives. Primary wound closure and healing is enhanced not only by precise flap reflec-

tion and repositioning, but also by use of an adequate suturing technique. The quality and consistency of the mucosa must be taken into account when sutures are placed. In most cases, mucosal wound margins are closed by means of individual, interrupted sutures. The mattress suture technique provides particularly tight wound margin adaptation. Continuous sutures are indicated only if the mucosa is in immediate contact with underlying bone (e.g., gingiva).

If antibiotic coverage is not initiated, a closed wound that is contaminated will quickly become infected.

74 Armamentarium for suture placement
Needle holder (Gillies), surgical forceps, anatomic forceps, tissue hook (Gillies).

Right: Suture material. Monofilament thread (e.g., Supramid 5) is preferable. Resorbable materials (catgut, Dexon, etc.) can be used for submucosal suturing, or in situations in which subsequent suture removal may be difficult.

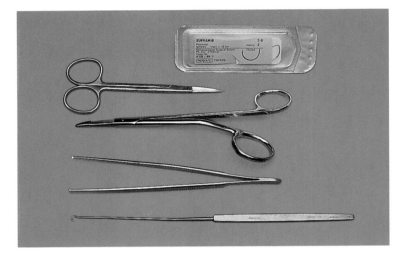
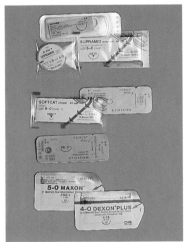

75 Suture needles
For suture placement in the oral cavity, the 5/8 needle with a flat profile and a honed tip is preferred. Other shapes are available for special situations.

Right: Modified forms of the Gillies needle holder; the elegant shape simplifies suture placement in the oral cavity, where space and visual access are often limited.

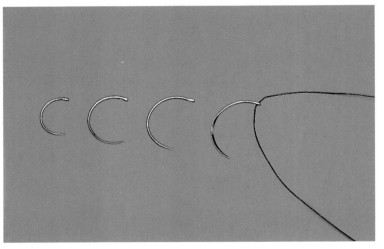
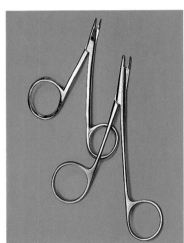

76 Needle holder
The Gillies needle holder fits the hand well. In contrast to scissors, only the thumb is actually inserted into the handle.

Right: Some needle holders have locking devices; these may restrict freedom of movement.

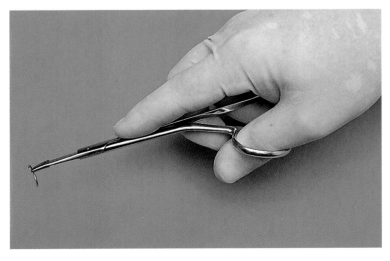
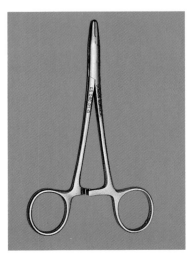

Suture Material

Nonresorbable. For suturing the oral mucosa, the monofilament, nonexpansile materials are ideal (polyamide, Supramid).

Resorbable. Catgut (collagen), Dexon or Vicryl (polyglycolic acid) are used for subcutaneous sutures or in areas where suture removal is difficult or impossible (e.g., fixation of mucosa to periosteum during vestibuloplasty). Maxon or Dexon (polyglactin) are indicated for suturing in mucosal areas where access is limited.

Size. For normal mucosa: 3–0 = 3 = 0.3 mm. For extremely fine sutures: 4–0 = 2 = 0.2 mm.

Needles

Because of the limited access, curved 5/8 needles with a honed tip and a flat profile are indicated for the oral cavity. Needles with a round profile can turn in the needle holder, preventing precise positioning of the suture.

Caution

Braided and resorbable suture materials are not indicated for use in the oral cavity because of the wick effect, which can contaminate the base of the wound with saliva.

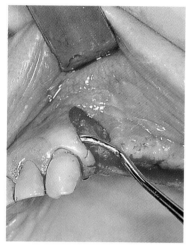
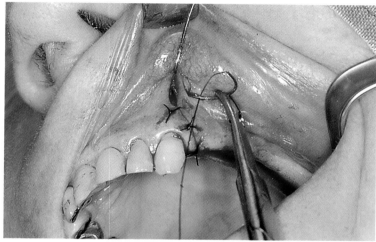

77 Suturing—interrupted sutures
Precise repositioning of the muco-periosteal flap is a prerequisite for healing without scar formation. The distance between interrupted sutures is 3 mm.

Left: For better adaptation, a fine elevator can be used to mobilize adjacent tissue.

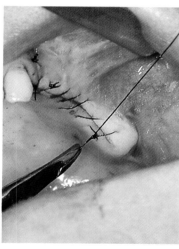
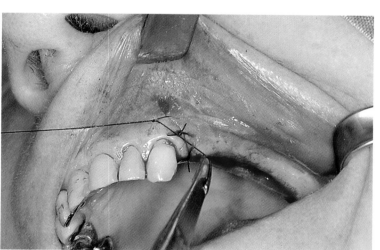

78 Suturing—continuous sutures
The releasing incision is closed using interrupted sutures.

Left: Along the alveolar process, with keratinized gingiva, continuous sutures can achieve excellent wound margin closure.

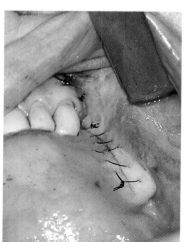
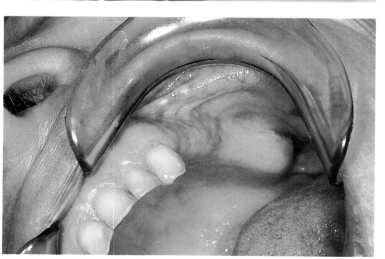

79 Postoperative course
The clinical view reveals scar-free healing three months postsurgically.

Left: Suture placement completed.

80 Mattress sutures
This technique is indicated when especially tight closure of an oral wound is necessary, as here during closure of an oroantral communication. All sutures are placed in advance, to allow manipulation of the tissue flaps.

Left: The tissue flap adjacent to tooth 26 is completely sutured into place.

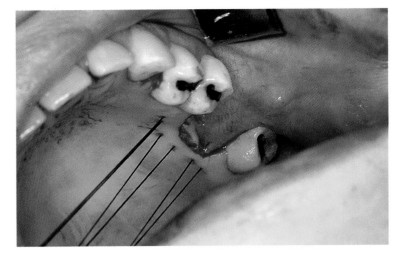

81 Resorbable suture material
This material is used in situations in which postoperative suture removal would not be possible, as in this case, where the mucosa is being attached to the periosteum.

Right: The mucosal flap is sutured to the periosteum near tooth 16.

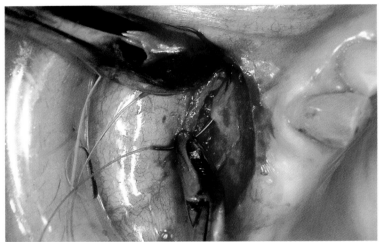
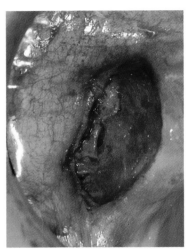

82 Subcutaneous suture technique
Spreading the wound margins and approximating the subcutaneous connective tissue using resorbable suture material.

Right: The suture is placed precisely in the subcutaneous tissues on each side of the wound.

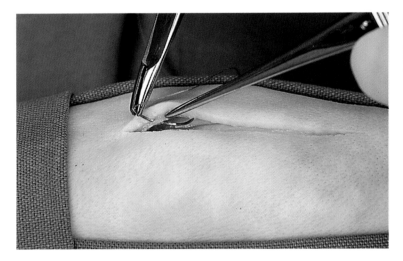
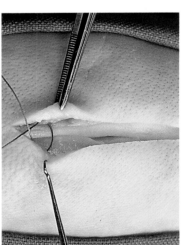

83 Horizontal reverse suture
This is useful for tight adaptation of wound margins. The margins are everted slightly. This type of suture can also be placed continuously.

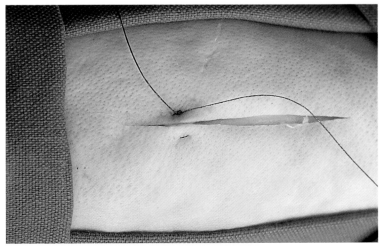

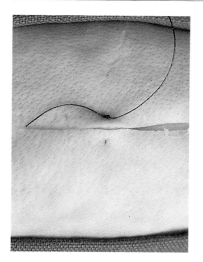

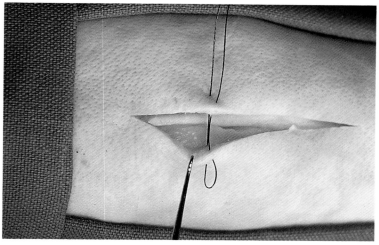

84 Vertical mattress suture
The suture is placed through both wound margins in direct approximation.

Left: This suturing technique provides tightly apposed wound margins. It can be used in special situations as when the tissue edges are not ideal.

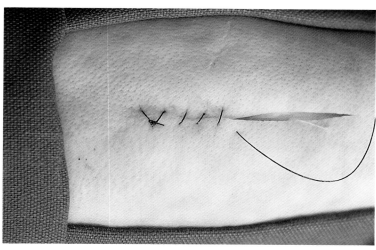

85 Continuous suture
This can be used to close wounds in especially taut tissues. It also provides excellent hemostasis.

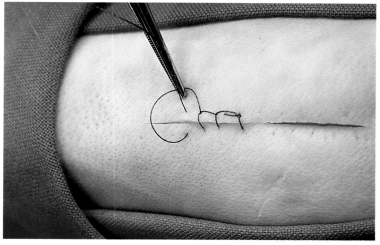

86 Margin suture
This suture is very useful for hemostasis.

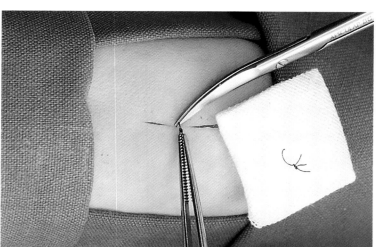

87 Suture removal
The suture is grasped with a fine anatomic forceps, and then cut using pointed scissors. If the suture is entrapped in a scab, application of hydrogen peroxide or NaCl solution will make removal easier. If pieces of suture are left embedded in the tissue, complications such as infection or granuloma formation can ensue.

Open Wound Management

Healing by secondary intention is the goal—i.e., the wound is left open to allow the formation of granulation tissue when it is left open. Secondary epithelialization of the wound follows. In open wound healing, the exposed tissue can be covered with a surgical dressing, or the wound surface can be exposed to the oral cavity. In either case, a fibrin layer covers the wound within a few hours. The goal of this type of treatment is to maintain this fibrin layer. Because the wound remains open, infection of the surgical site is avoided. Although the wound surface may be contaminated, clinical infection does not ensue because self-cleaning mechanisms in the oral cavity are sufficient to clean the wound. The phase of healing until complete epithelialization general lasts three or four weeks.

Open wound treatment is indicated if there is a high risk of infection—for example, after extraction of mandibular third molars, surgery in acutely infected tissues, and in extensive mucosal defects (vestibuloplasty with secondary epithelialization). In severely traumatized soft-tissue wounds, healing by secondary intention is advisable to prevent infection.

88 Wound dressing
Extensive mucosal defects can be left to secondary healing by applying a nonadhesive wound dressing (iodoform–Vaseline gauze).

Right: The wound dressing is held in place by means of a palatal acrylic stent.

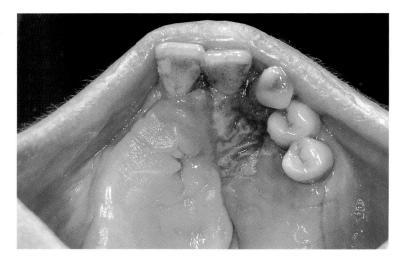
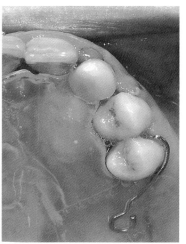

89 Preparing the iodoform dressing
Sterile Vaseline (white soft paraffin) is placed in a flat vessel. The iodoform gauze is laid on top of this, and the vessel is placed in a warm environment to liquefy the Vaseline. The excess Vaseline is then removed, and the vessel is sealed. These operations must be carried out in sterile conditions.

Right: Placing the iodoform gauze on the liquid Vaseline.

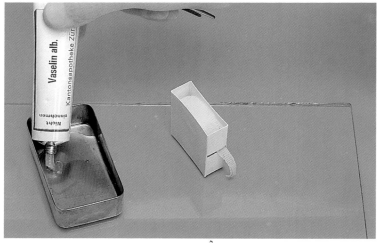
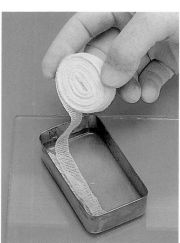

90 Shelf life
The sterile dressing is stored in a closed vessel. It can be stored for approximately eight weeks, after which the gauze starts to discolor due to oxidation. The dressing should then no longer be used.

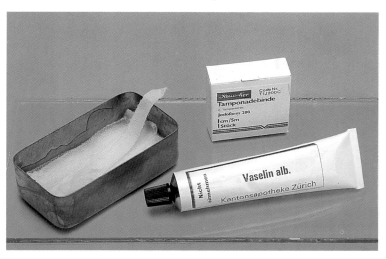

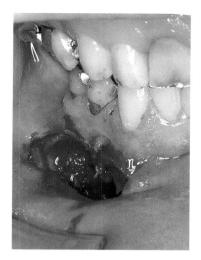
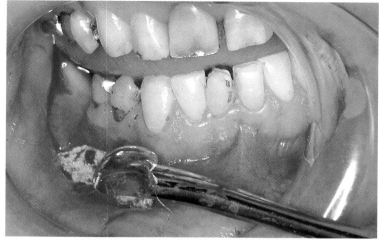

91 Wound closure using an acetone adhesive
When it is necessary to fill a defect, an acetone tissue adhesive can be used to close the area off, preventing the intrusion of saliva.

Left: Clinical view after enucleation of a radicular cyst in the right mandible, from the buccal aspect.

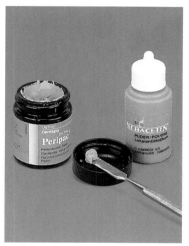
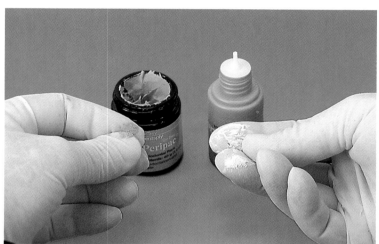

92 Preparation of a gingival dressing
Tissue dressings (periodontal pack) have a putty-like consistency, but harden when in contact with moisture. To prevent colonization by oral microbiota, an antibiotic powder (e.g., Nebacetin) can be mixed into the dressing before application.

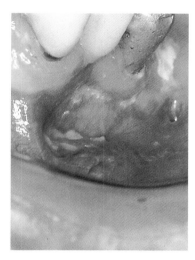
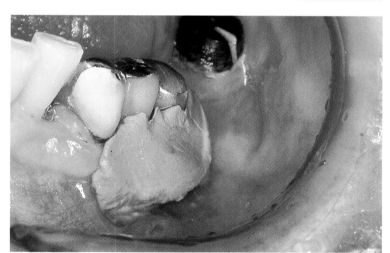

93 Gingival (periodontal) dressing
A periodontal dressing (Peripac) is being used here to protect a free gingival graft near tooth 34. This photograph was taken three days after the surgery, and the transplant has remained in the proper position.

Left: Ten days after removing the dressing. The transplanted tissue has a reddish-pink color, indicating successful revascularization.

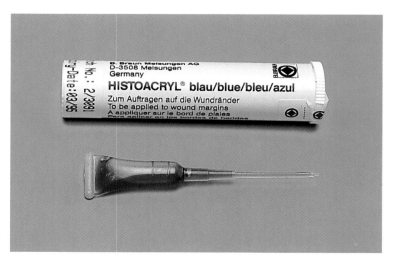

94 Tissue adhesive
Tissue adhesives are composed of acrylics, which harden when exposed to moisture. In special situations for example, when it is not possible to place sutures or when suturing is not indicated, these tissue adhesives provide an alternative. A disadvantage is that most of the agents are toxic to tissues.

95 Making a protective wound dressing plate

Heated clear acrylic is drawn down onto a plaster model, then trimmed appropriately. If necessary, this type of plate can be reinforced using self-polymerizing resin. The plate should be easy to remove, so that the patient can carry out oral hygiene.

Right: Scissors, knives and files can be used to trim the plate.

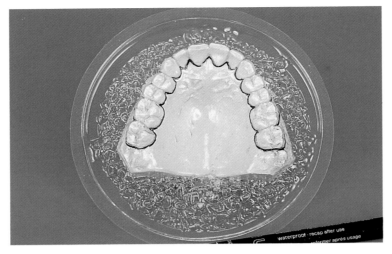 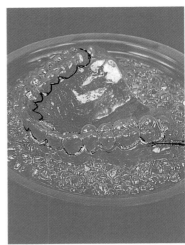

96 Finished plate

The finished plate is transparent; the wound can be visualized through it.

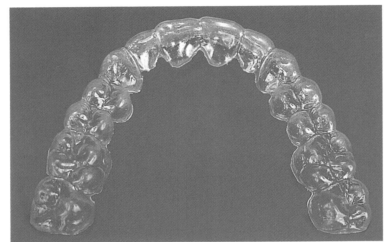

97 External bandage

Skin wounds are covered with sterile gauze, and then secured with an adhesive plaster dressing.

Right: Fresh sutures after an excision on the right side of the chin.

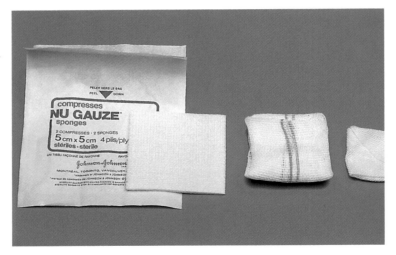 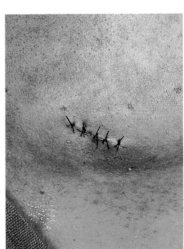

98 Adhesive strips

Fine adaptation of sutured wound margins can be ensured by using adhesive strips (e.g., Steri-Strip).

Right: Adhesive strips applied to a sutured incision wound.

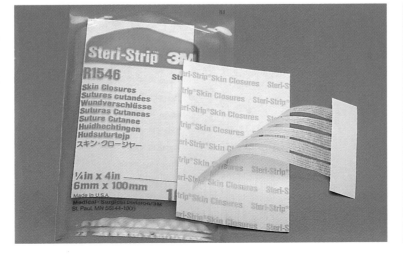 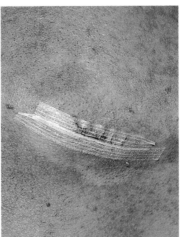

Hemostasis

The source and type of hemorrhage have to be determined by carefully and systematically suctioning and sponging the surgical field. Differentiation must be made between bleeding from soft tissue or from bone, and between diffuse and arterial hemorrhage. Countermeasures include compress application, ligation, cauterization (electrosurgery) or tamponade. Application of bone wax is an alternative possibility. Topical application of concentrated epinephrine is a countermeasure that we avoid because of the risk of systemic shock. If the patient has a coagulation dis-

order, the use of fibrin adhesives may be considered (p. 47).

Caution
Regardless of the technique used to stop bleeding, the local anatomy should always be borne in mind in order to avoid ligating or cauterizing a nerve.

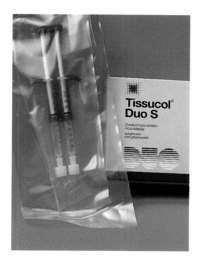
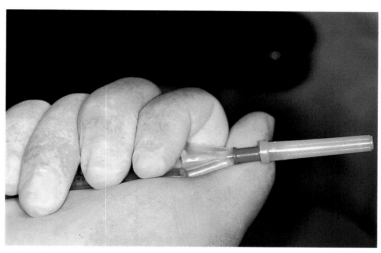

99 Tissue adhesive
In special circumstances, such as when there are problems with hemorrhage, a fibrin-based tissue adhesive (e.g., Tissucol) can be applied to arrest postsurgical bleeding and to cover wound margins. The procedure is very simple: the double syringe is thawed, and the adhesive is applied directly.

Left: The two components of the tissue adhesive are provided in a combination syringe.

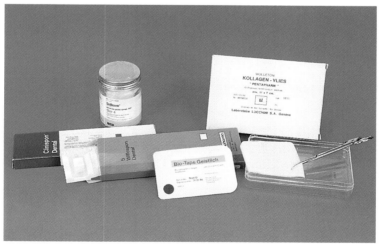

100 Carrier substances
For application to osseous wounds, the fibrin adhesive can be combined with a carrier substance, such as collagen.

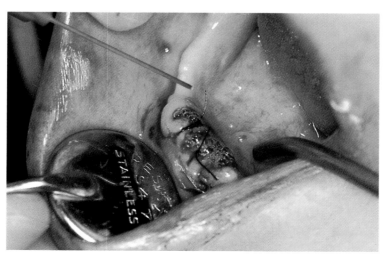

101 Wound coverage
The fibrin adhesive is simply injected onto the sutured wound; the setting reaction is virtually instantaneous.

Instrument Preparation

Disinfection. Contaminated instruments should first be disinfected before personnel attempt to deal with them. This substantially reduces the risk of infection if an inadvertent injury occurs. The danger can be reduced even further by first running the contaminated instruments through a thermal disinfection cycle before they are further handled.

Washing. Disinfected instruments are washed by hand using a brush and cold water, and then dried.

Preparation and inspection. Clean instruments are properly arranged, and then checked for proper functioning and for any damage or excessive wear. Nonfunctional instruments are discarded, and moving parts are lubricated with special oil.

Packaging. Instruments are arranged into sets or kits, and then wrapped in a double layer of heat-resistant drape. The pack is closed with an indicator tape; individual instruments can be packaged in special sterilization bags. Materials intended for sterilization should be dated and initialed by the person responsible.

Sterilization. Surgical instruments are sterilized in the autoclave. Sensitive instruments or equipment can be gas-sterilized. The manufacturer's instructions for the sterilizers must be strictly observed.

Storage. Sterilized instruments and kits should be stored in locked cabinets or drawers. With proper storage, sterility can be maintained for three months.

102 Basic instrument set
The instruments shown here represent a basic oral surgical set in combination with the standard dental set-up: scalpel handle, blades, preparation scissors, narrow and wide elevators, sharp spoon excavator, Black excavator, scaler, curette, fine suction tips, irrigation tip, vessel for rinsing solution, cheek retractors with short handles, artery clamp, towel clamp, needle holder, tissue retractor, sponges.

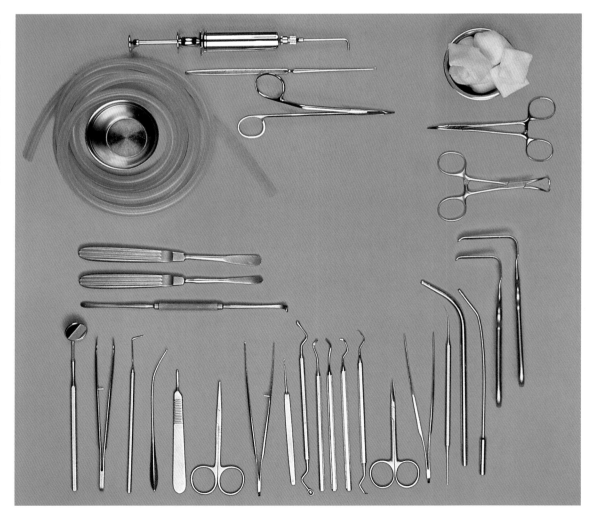

Medical Principles

Blood Clotting

In addition to tissue regeneration (wound healing), blood clotting is a critical prerequisite for surviving all types of physical injuries.

The body's capacity to close off severed blood vessels spontaneously and to coagulate blood that has escaped is a very complex biological phenomenon. Blood clotting occurs as a step-wise process. An important feature of this process is the prevention of spontaneous thrombus formation within healthy tissues.

Normal Course

Thrombogenesis
Thrombogenesis is a multifactorial, three-phase biological process:
—Vascular contraction.
—Thrombocyte aggregation or thrombus formation (conversion of prothrombin to thrombin, conversion of thrombin to fibrin).
—Retraction of the fibrin clot into a thrombus.

Fibrinolysis
Fibrinolysis occurs as a three-phase biological process:
—Activation of lysokinases (tissue reaction).
—Conversion of plasminogen to plasmin.
—Proteolysis of fibrin into fibrinopeptides.

Disturbances of Blood Clotting

Hemorrhagic diathesis, absent factors:
—Hemophilia.
—Von Willebrand's disease.
—Liver disorders.

Effects of medicaments:
—Targeted (anticoagulation).
—Medicament abuse (aspirin).

Thrombocytopenia:
—Werlhof's disease.

Thrombosis tendency:
—Surgical interventions.
—Tumors.
—Corticoids.
—Abrupt cessation of anticoagulant therapy

Clinical Tip
If the decision is made at the outset not to provide substitution for coagulation factors that are absent, using fibrin adhesives provides a potential method of hemostasis and wound treatment, in combination with careful suturing.

Wound Healing

Normal Course

Goal. The aim is to prevent a tissue defect by reapproximating separated tissue segments and replacing mucosal soft tissue via spontaneous physical reactions.

Regeneration. The healing process results in replacement of lost tissue by identical new tissue.

Repair. Lost tissue is replaced by dissimilar tissue (connective tissue, scar).

Wound healing is influenced by the body's capacity for regeneration, and the nature of the tissue destruction. The excellent vascularity of tissues in the orofacial region, as well as the local host response capacity of the oral mucosa, provide optimal conditions for rapid wound healing. Disturbances of wound healing are extremely uncommon, and usually indicate some related systemic disorder.

The nature of the injury can affect the course of wound healing.

Mechanical injury:
—Incisions, surgical wound (scalpel).
—Tearing or crushing injury.
—Abrasion.
—Impact wound.
—Bone injuries: fractures.

Thermal injury:
—Burns, electrosurgery, laser, freezing.
—Cryosurgery.

Chemical injury:
—Chemical burns, caustic burns

Radiation injury:
—Radiotherapy

Phases of Wound Healing

Phase I: exudation.
Phase II: proliferation.
Phase III: regeneration.

Primary Wound Healing

The Latin term is *sanitatio per primam intentionem.* This is characterized by an undisturbed course of healing, with perfect adaptation of the wound margins, and minimal inflammatory reaction. An example is the healing of a surgical incision wound that has been closed with primary sutures.

Secondary Wound Healing

The Latin term is *sanitatio per secundam intentionem.* This is characterized by delayed wound healing, in which all three phases are extended due to necrosis of the wounded tissue and an exaggerated inflammatory response.

Examples include extraction wounds, unstirred wounds, and complications resulting from suture dehiscence.

Disturbances of Wound Healing

Dehiscence of sutured wounds may result from:
—Inadequate suture technique (inverted wound margins).
—Incorrect positioning of the wound margins (insufficient mobilization).
—Tension within the tissue flaps.

Infection of wounds can occur due to:
—Hematoma formation.
—Foreign body or contamination of the wound.
—Nonsterile wound treatment.
—Tears or compression leading to necrosis.

Postoperative Care

Wound healing is always associated with a local inflammatory reaction. This means that the postoperative period will be characterized by swelling and pain in the surgical area. These symptoms of inflammation can be kept within tolerable limits by appropriate physical and medicinal ancillary treatment. Excessive swelling may lead to suture failure and delay of wound healing, while postoperative pain will have a negative impact on the patient's everyday life. The most important prerequisites for a normal course of healing include careful use of all surgical instruments, precise incisions, and gentle use of wound retraction instruments to avoid tissue damage.

Suture Removal

Sutures should be removed from skin wounds in the facial region three to six days postoperatively, and from intraoral mucosal wounds after 7–12 days, depending on the complexity of the procedure, the condition of the tissues, and the anatomical location, e.g.:
—Nonirritated gingival margin: seven days.
—Atrophic mucosa of the vestibule: 10 days.
—Retromolar area (mobile mucosa): 12 days.

Suture removal is carried out using pointed scissors and an anatomical forceps. Each suture should be carefully examined to ensure complete removal. Residual suture material within tissues can lead to infection or granuloma formation.

Anti-Inflammatory and Analgesic Medications

The clinical signs of inflammation result mainly from vascular reactions. It is therefore advisable to minimize such reactions immediately postoperatively by appropriate measures.

Nonsteroidal anti-inflammatory drugs are ideal for the elimination of pain and the reduction of inflammatory symptoms. Administration of these medications should be limited to the three-day postoperative period.

Antibiotics

It is not necessary to prescribe antibiotics routinely to prevent infection after routine oral surgical procedures. Targeted antibiotic treatment is indicated, however, if postoperative complications are expected due to a previously existing infection, e.g., after transplantation into an infected area, with open fractures, if osteitis is present in the region of a fracture, or if the oral surgical procedure has been preceded by radiation therapy.

The use of antibiotics may also by indicated if the patient's host response is impaired or absent—for example, in cases of poorly controlled diabetes, immunosuppression, AIDS, or in elderly patients. Where there is a danger of focal infection (e.g., endocarditis, rheumatoid arthritis), preoperative antibiotic coverage is obligatory (Pallasch and Slots 1991).

Topical Disinfection

If a patient's normal oral hygiene regimen is liable to be affected by the surgical procedure, oral rinses with 0.2% chlorhexidine solution should be prescribed. Patients should also be advised to avoid foodstuffs that encourage plaque accumulation.

Topical Therapy

Cold
Cold packs should be applied externally during the first two to six hours postsurgically. This will reduce any reactive hyperemia and edema formation, reducing pain and lessening the tension within the mucosa. Reduced tension considerably reduces the danger of wound margin dehiscence. We recommend waterproof ice bags or commercially available cold packs for external application as soon as surgery is completed.

Heat
Applying heat enhances the circulation of the blood, but simultaneously also accelerates the inflammatory process. An important effect of heat is to enhance the healing of inflammations without any tendency toward the development of infections, in addition to producing more rapid tissue consolidation subsequent to chronic infection. External heat should not be applied during the first few postoperative days, as this could lead to an exaggeration of swelling. Low-grade superficial infections without actual abscess formation can be favorably affected by applying heat, making subsequent surgical therapy (incision and drainage) easier.

Moist heat has a softening and hyperemic effect. This can be used to soften indurated lesions with inflammatory infiltrates following abscesses, and to accelerate inflammatory processes.

Ultraviolet and Infrared Light

Light with a short wavelength (ultraviolet) or long wavelength (infrared) produces heat, and may have some positive effects on the healing process. Ultraviolet light is also damaging to bacteria and therefore has a disinfectant property, although only very superficially.

This type of treatment may be helpful during chronic inflammatory processes.

Ultrasound and Microwaves

Ultrasound waves penetrate tissue more deeply, and cause warming. This stimulates blood circulation and healing processes. In inflammatory processes with infection, the formation of abscesses is enhanced.

> **Clinical Tip**
> The topical application of heat to an anesthetized region of the face can lead to burns. Any equipment for applying heat must be connected with a time-limiting switch.

Physiotherapy

Passive movement of the musculature can release tension.

Targeted directional massage can produce favorable responses in inflamed soft tissues.

In particular, massaging the lymphatic system can accelerate the draining of interstitial fluids. This can release previously blocked interstitial regions, allowing inflow of nutritive fluids, which will accelerate regenerative processes.

Some reports have suggested that massaging specific reflex zones may help to reduce pain. However, we do not regard these effects as having been clearly demonstrated, and there is a lack of successful experience.

Complementary Methods

Low-Level Laser Therapy

Low-energy laser beams (up to 120 MW) can directly cause bioactivation of cellular processes, and therefore may enhance the healing process. However, it has not yet been possible to demonstrate a reliable clinical therapeutic effect.

Acupuncture

Acupuncture is based on discoveries made in Chinese medicine, in which balanced corporeal functions and the interrelationship between the body's organs are significant via regulated pathways (meridians). Stimulating certain points along the meridians can influence some functions. Given a certain depth of knowledge, acupuncture can have a reasonable place in treatment. For example, acupuncture can be used to influence certain healing processes and condition the body for the planned surgical procedure. Clinical experiments have demonstrated that endogenous morphine-like substances are released by acupuncture treatment (Bahr 1989).

Electrotherapy

For posttraumatic conditions in which there is pain and disturbed muscle function, appropriate and targeted individual electrotherapy can often achieve analgesia in addition to accelerating the reinstatement of motor functions. The physiotherapist should be provided with information about the diagnosis, the location of the functional disturbance, intensity of treatment, and treatment intervals. Electrotherapy generally consists of galvanic current and various impulse currents.

Homeopathic Medicine

Homeopathic medicine is a relatively noninvasive healing procedure that can also be used to advantage in dentistry, and which enjoys a high level of acceptance by patients. For practitioners with little experience in this field, the indications for using homeopathic medicine will be limited. In the present book, limitations of space preclude any more extensive discussion of this interesting medical specialty.

High-Risk Patients

Circulatory Disturbances

Oral surgical procedures in patients with cardiac or circulatory diseases always involve a risk of acute cardiovascular complications, such as attacks of angina pectoris. Other complications may also occur later, particularly in patients with preexisting endocarditis. The oral surgeon must therefore gather full information concerning existing risks by taking a thorough medical history and consulting the patient's physician. Preoperative laboratory studies are not often necessary or helpful (Wagner and Moore 1991), and these should always be performed by the physician. Extreme care should be exercised when administering local anesthetics (aspiration to preclude intravascular injection, slow injection, reduction of vasoconstrictive additives), possible premedication (bromazepam, 1.5 mg), monitoring circulatory and pulmonary functions (pulse oximetry), and infection prophylaxis if there is a risk of endocarditis (antibiotic coverage) (Rothlin and Babotai 1988). If the patient has a cardiac pacemaker, it may be necessary to restrict the use of any instruments that create an electromagnetic field (Jaquiéry and Burkart 1993). In general, all patients presenting medical risks must be scrutinized for their suitability for outpatient treatment, as well as the necessity for postoperative observation or concurrent treatment (Fast 1993).

Bleeding Tendency

There are numerous conditions that require prophylaxis for possible thrombosis—for example, patients who have had a myocardial infarction, dialysis patients, those with constrictions of the cardiac vessels, those who have recently undergone surgery, etc. The type of treatment determines the tendency toward excessive hemorrhage or coagulation disturbances after the procedure. For the most part, these patients carry documentation stating their medication and its dosage, as well as the actual clotting defects. The Quick's test value is usually also provided as a criterion for the coagulation disturbance that may be expected. If the situation is in any way unclear, contacting the patient's physician is mandatory (Mäglin 1974, Mounce 1990).

Drug or Medicament Abuse

A great number of medicines are available without prescriptions (analgesics, sleeping pills), and many patients have medications from previous conditions (antibiotics, tranquilizers); therefore, only a precise medical history with targeted questioning can provide information about a patient's actual use of drugs.

The use of drugs containing acetylsalicylic acid for several days can lead to a coagulation disturbance with the risk of hemorrhage. Uncontrolled self-medication with antibiotics can create a clinical picture that mimics infection.

The use of tranquilizers or other sedatives can influence the effectiveness of local anesthesia.

Infection

Patients with an increased risk for infection, or for whom infection presents special dangers (e.g., patients with endocarditis, immunosuppression, AIDS, radiotherapy, leukemia at certain stages, etc.) should only be treated after antibiotic coverage has been provided; these patients may require hospitalization for oral surgical procedures. All surgical procedures involve a risk of bacteremia.

Prophylaxis for endocarditis should be prescribed according to the appropriate guidelines (e.g., American Heart Association).

Risk of Endocarditis

Bacterial endocarditis is an infection of the heart valves or the cardiac endothelium. Dental treatment is considered to be the most frequent cause of bacteremia, which can lead to endocarditis. Previously damaged endothelial structures of the heart are particularly susceptible—for example, valvular damage following rheumatic fever, preexisting endocarditis, inherited or congenital heart valve defects, and especially patients with heart valve replacements.

Bacteria that are commonly found in the oral cavity are often responsible: alpha-hemolytic streptococci, enterococci, pneumococci, and staphylococci. Heimdahl et al. (1990) used serotyping to demonstrate that microorganisms in the blood of endocarditis patients were identical to the strains found in dental plaque. The risk of bacteremia from the oral cavity depends on the extent of soft tissue injury, and the severity of the preexisting infection. In these patients, intraoral examination should only be performed with antibiotic coverage, because even periodontal pocket probing can elicit bacteremia.

Radiotherapy

As is also the case with skin, irradiation of the oral mucosa is associated with early and late reactions. Even at a radiation dose of 5 Gy, erythema is observed, followed by mucositis, atrophy, and finally ulceration of the oral mucosa. The soft palate, hypopharynx, and floor of the mouth are particularly sensitive, followed by the more resistant keratinized zones of the gingiva, hard palate, and dorsum of the tongue. Tissue reactions that develop later include mucosa atrophy, edema, scarring, and the development of candidiasis.

Another consequence of radiotherapy is susceptibility to dental caries, which is enhanced by xerostomia, accelerated decalcification of enamel, and inadequate oral hygiene.

Irradiation provokes degeneration of salivary gland tissue, resulting in hyposalivation. The quality (composition) of saliva is also altered. Following irradiation, the saliva becomes more acidic and more viscous. The buffer capacity is reduced; sodium, calcium, chloride, and magnesium ions increase, as well as the protein content. Such alterations persist over long periods of time. A relationship to dental caries activity is easy to ascertain.

The intraoral microbial flora shows an increase in *Streptococcus mutans*, lactobacilli, fungi, and *Actinomyces naeslundii*. Other bacteria, such as *Neisseria* species, *Streptococcus sanguinis,* and fusobacteria decrease.

The resulting clinical symptoms include a burning sensation, hypersensitivity, and alterations in taste perception. These can be attributed to xerostomia, mainly because the breakdown of foodstuffs is decreased and therefore the sensory mechanisms on the tongue and other mucosal areas are not triggered.

The most important effect of radiation therapy is vascular damage. This has direct effects on the reactive capacities of all types of tissue, particularly bone. The determining factors for the development of radiation osteonecrosis or radiation osteomyelitis are the nature and the duration of the irradiation, the expanse of the jaw segment that is irradiated, the size of the tumor of the jaw, and the condition of the remaining dentition. Radiation osteonecrosis can be expected after a total dose of over 66 Gy (Glanzmann and Grätz 1995). Particularly in the mandible, a fear of osseous damage is the primary incentive for detecting and eliminating foci of infection before radiation therapy is instituted.

Immunosuppression

Medications may have direct effects. For example, cyclosporine can cause gingival enlargement, especially in younger patients. Clinically obvious manifestations of gingival overgrowth will be observed within four to six months after the immunosuppressive regimen is started. In addition, there is an increased risk of infection because of the inhibition of cellular functions in the bone marrow. Chronic but quiescent dental infections, such as deep periodontal pockets or apical osteitis, may be exacerbated. Due to the anti-inflammatory effects of immunosuppressive drugs, the cardinal symptoms of infection are restricted to pain with fever and possible radiographic signs. Infections of the oral mucosa quickly ulcerate, but the typical reddening of the ulcer margin is not observed because of the reduced reaction. Mucosal ulcerations represent entry points for general infections when no other source of an identified sepsis is found.

Chemotherapy for Malignancy

Patient-related problems. Forty percent of patients who receive chemotherapy develop symptoms in the oral cavity. These effects are strictly age-related. With young patients (under 12 years), intraoral symptoms can be expected in 90% of cases (mucositis, ulceration). The malignancy itself may have an accessory role through its direct effect on the oral mucosa, as in hematological diseases. Patients with poor oral hygiene and preexisting endodontic and periodontal infections have a higher risk of developing oral infections during chemotherapy. On the other hand, an inflammation-free oral cavity is at much lower risk of developing any infectious problems during chemotherapy.

Treatment-related problems. Not all of the chemotherapeutic agents are equally stomatotoxic, nor do they all have identical effects on the oral mucosa. The antimetabolites, which inhibit DNA synthesis, are more likely to cause mucositis. Alkyl derivatives have a similar effect. The temporal sequence of administration also influences the side effects. A specific amount given as a single dose can have much more serious effects than the same dosage administered over a longer period of time. All effects of chemotherapeutic drugs on the oral mucosa are potentiated if radiotherapy is administered to the head and neck region at the same time.

Tooth Extraction

Every dentist uses a favorite technique as a routine procedure. The aim of this section will therefore only be to provide some very basic principles and suggestions regarding the removal of teeth. The most common method is extraction using a forceps. Before applying the forceps, however, a desmotome is first used to sever the marginal periodontal tissues. The beaks of the forceps are then positioned along the long axis of the tooth, between the gingiva, periodontium, and alveolar margin, to grasp the tooth firmly. Using forceful push/pull maneuvers in the axial direction, with luxating movements determined by the shape of the root or roots, the deeper periodontal fibers can be severed, and the tooth can be removed.

This procedure usually expands the alveolar walls, which may also be fractured in some locations (Partsch 1917, Frenkel 1989a). Every tooth that is removed must be carefully inspected to ensure that no root fragments have been left behind. The medicolegal consequences of unremoved fragments can be significant (Freyberger 1971). The number and variety of instruments for tooth extraction is so large that the present discussion will concentrate only on the most important, universally used instruments.

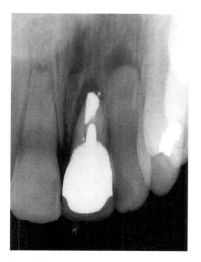 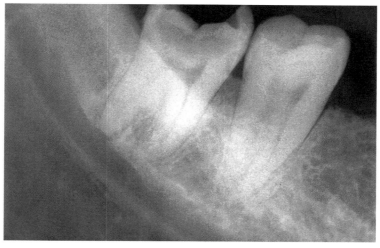

103 Indications for tooth extraction—deep caries
The radiograph shows a severely damaged tooth 47 with a widened periodontal ligament space at the apical region.

Left: This endodontically treated tooth shows persistent apical osteolysis, a classic symptom of chronic infection.

Indications

Teeth have to be extracted when they cannot be saved by conservative, periodontal, prosthetic, orthodontic, or surgical measures, or when their retention is not reasonable in view of the patient's systemic condition, the overall oral situation, and the local conditions.

Some indications for tooth extraction include:
—Deep caries, an unfavorable cost–benefit ratio, and reasonable certainty that a patient cannot be motivated to implement adequate oral hygiene.
—Apical osteitis, particularly when endodontic or surgical intervention does not appear promising.
—Root fractures.
—Extremely deep periodontal pockets.
—Acute local infection, if extraction will prevent the spread of infection and the tooth does not appear to be worth saving. Teeth can be extracted at any stage of the infectious process. Waiting for swelling to subside only causes an unnecessary delay in the healing of an infection. "There is an erroneous idea … that it is improper practice to remove a tooth when the face is swollen" (Winter 1943). The only exception to this rule is pericoronitis of the mandibular third molars.

104 Indications for tooth extraction—root fractures, internal periodontal infection
Root fracture in tooth 25: this tooth cannot be saved.

Right: Periodontal breakdown and apical osteolysis of tooth 31; the internal periodontal infection cannot be successfully treated due to the advanced tissue loss.

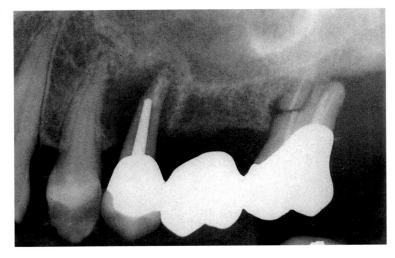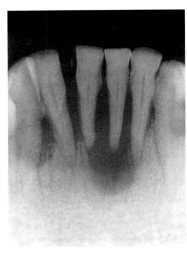

105 Acute infections
Acute infection of a nonvital tooth 26. The lesion is widespread, and the condition of the remaining dentition requires a radical approach to be taken to eliminate the cause.

Right: Clinical view of an abscess formation on the buccal aspect of tooth 26.

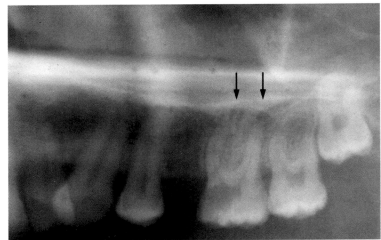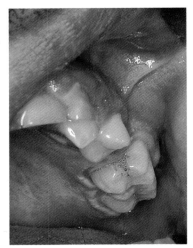

106 Oroantral connection
At the apical aspect of tooth 18, there is a patent connection with the maxillary sinus near the denuded root of the adjacent tooth. Complete closure of this defect by osseous regeneration will only be possible after extraction of tooth 17.

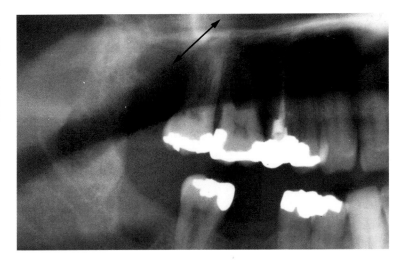

107 Inadequate space
Tooth removal may be indicated when space along the arch is inadequate, or if there is functional disturbance, as with this young adult in whom orthodontic treatment was carried out and tooth 23 represented a risk for the remaining dentition in terms of oral hygiene and periodontal considerations.

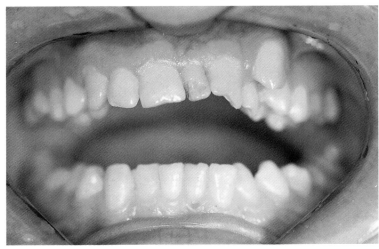

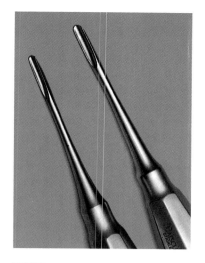

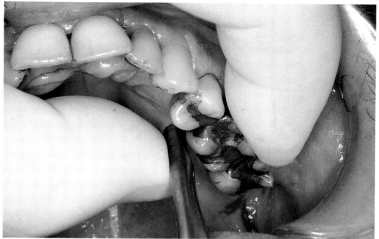

118 Luxation of the tooth—use of the straight elevator

Using minimum pressure and rotatory movements within the periodontal ligament space, the tooth is moved within its alveolus in such a way that any remaining connective-tissue fibers are severed.

Left: The size of the elevator should be determined by the size and cross-sectional profile of the tooth root.

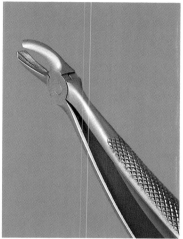

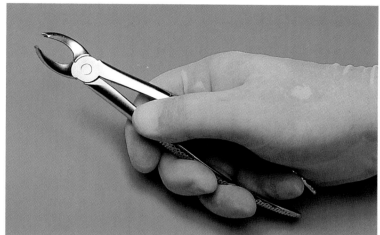

119 Extraction of the tooth—use of the forceps

Specific forceps are indicated for left or right maxillary molars, based on the shape of the roots. These forceps allow forceful manipulation with secure guidance.

Left: Forceps for extracting right maxillary molars.

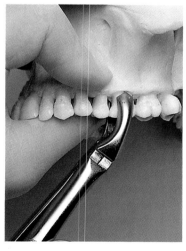

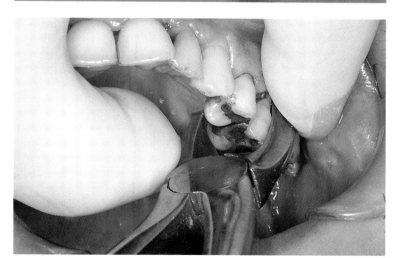

120 Use of the forceps

Use of a forceps in the maxillary left posterior segment. Note that the beaks grasp the tooth at the transition from crown to root.

Left: Actual luxation of the tooth is effected by sagittal movements and suitable force, but with simultaneous protection of the alveolar process using the fingers of the other hand. Often, a "controlled" fracture of the buccal alveolar wall occurs.

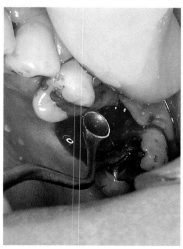

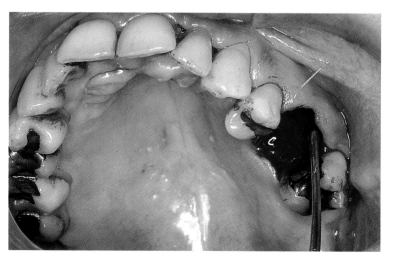

121 Curettage of the alveolus

A blunt probe is used to explore the bottom of the alveolus to reveal any perforation of the maxillary sinus. The popular technique of having a patient hold the nose and blow is not always a reliable sign of an oroantral connection.

Left: After removal of the tooth, the alveolus is curetted with a spoon excavator to removal any inflamed tissue.

122 Removing individual roots

The removal of molars that are severely damaged, or have extremely curved roots, is best achieved by sectioning the tooth and removing the individual roots.

Right: A groove drilled into the tooth permits access for an elevator to separate the crown from the roots.

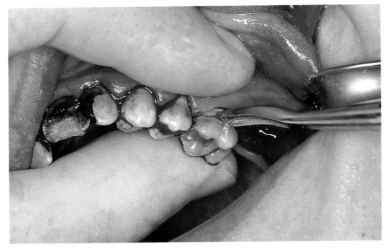
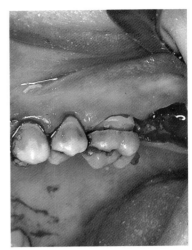

123 Separating the roots

After the crown has been removed, the roots are separated using a carbide fissure burr.

Right: The maxillary molar shown here has been sectioned according to the anatomical locations of its three roots.

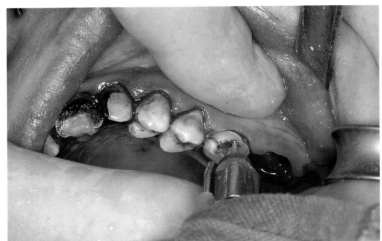
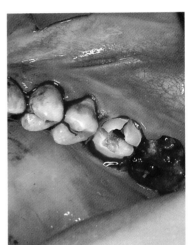

124 Use of the straight elevator

Light rotatory movements of the straight elevator are used to dislodge the separated roots. Any pressure applied in the apical region involves a risk of forcing a root tip into the maxillary sinus.

Right: Use of a straight elevator.

1 Luxation of the root with slight pressure and mainly rotatory movement of the elevator.
2 Luxation of the root as in 1, but with additional distal tipping.

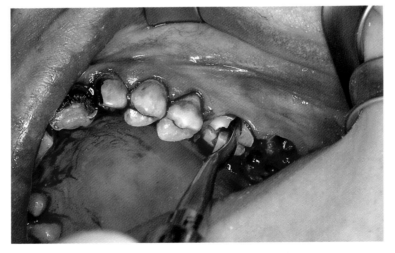
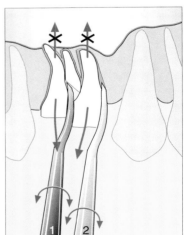

125 Root forceps

Roots that have been freed from the supporting tissues can be removed using a pointed root forceps, preferably with diamond-coated beaks.

Right: Root forceps for use in the maxilla.

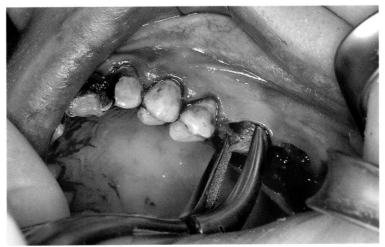
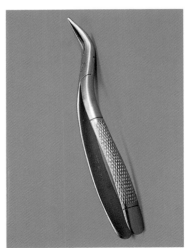

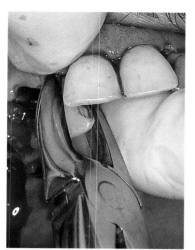
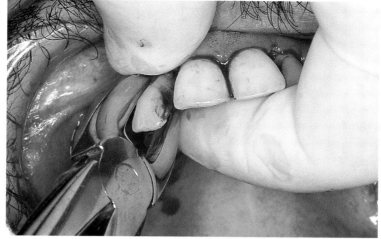

126 Extraction of maxillary premolars and anterior teeth
With due consideration for root shape, the teeth are extracted using a combination of tipping and rotatory forces. The alveolus is subsequently compressed.

Left: Tooth 12 is being luxated with palatal displacement.

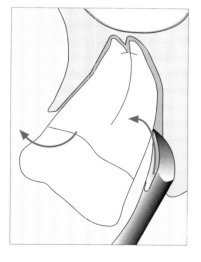
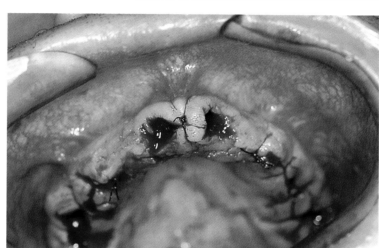

127 Wound closure
In multiple extractions, the gingival margins should be readapted using interrupted sutures. Care should be taken to maintain the gingival papillae. Cross-suturing of interrupted papillae may create aesthetic difficulties with subsequent fixed prosthetic restorations.

Left: Excessive gingival tissue is carefully removed.

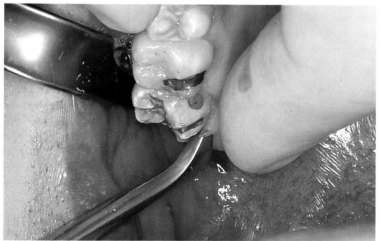

128 Maxillary third molars
These teeth are usually easy to remove toward the buccal aspect, using a cross-handle bar elevator such as the Seldin's elevator applied palatally.

Left: Seldin's elevator being used from the palatal aspect.

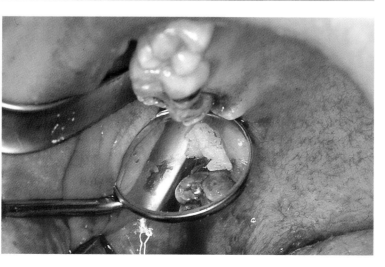

129 Wound treatment
A light tamponade can be placed if a blood coagulum does not form. If inadvertent opening into the maxillary sinus has occurred, a decision must be made on whether to carry out a complete and secure tissue closure, or use a superficial bandage and closure with acetone adhesive to await spontaneous natural closure (small perforation, large alveolus).

Multiple Extractions

When extracting numerous adjacent teeth, the following measures should be noted:
—Maintenance of the alveolar ridge through careful extraction of individual roots, with separation of molar roots.
—Osteoplasty of the alveolar ridge to remove sharp bony segments, using Luer forceps or a large round burr. Removing interradicular septa allows the lateral alveolar walls to be compressed (see also bone recontouring, p. 297).

—Application of papillary sutures to adapt the wound margins in the anterior segment and to maintain gingival contour, and use of alternate papillae sutures in the posterior segments to enhance rapid healing.

130 Multiple extractions— alveolar ridge contouring
When serial extractions are performed, sharp bony edges should be smoothed.

Right: The Luer forceps is ideal for evening out osseous contours.

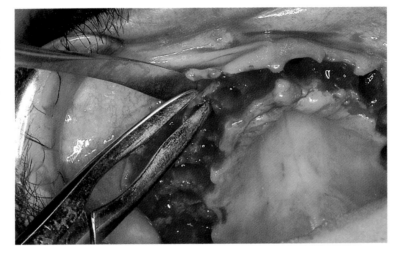
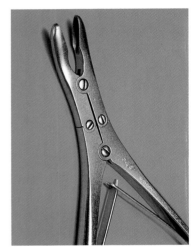

Ⓢ

131 Wound closure
After a complete arch extraction, every effort should be made to close the osseous wound completely.

Right: If the maxillary sinus has been opened, the buccal flap can be extended to cover the osseous defect, and sutured into place.

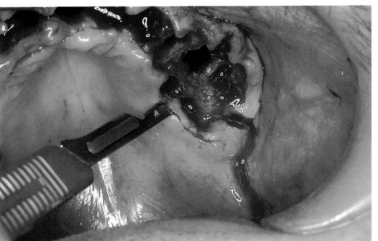
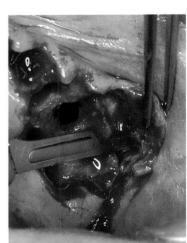

132 Wound closure
Continuous sutures over the alveolar ridge and a mattress suture in the area of tooth 26 provide adequate closure of an open maxillary sinus.

Right: The previously prepared immediate denture is modified and adapted, and then seated immediately.

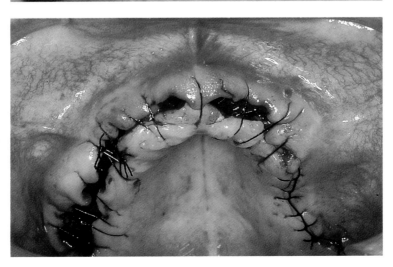
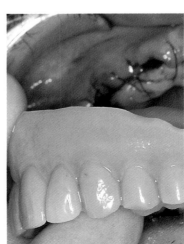

Extractions in the Mandible

The density of the osseous structure of the mandible is much greater than that of the maxilla, and therefore more often requires sectioning of multirooted teeth before extraction.

The position of the mandibular canal must always be considered when curetting alveoli in the posterior segment.

Because of its massive compact bony structure and the relatively poor blood circulatory system, the healing potential in the mandible is poorer than in the maxilla. Tooth extraction that is accompanied by osseous crushing by the manipulation of elevators, and even routine removal of teeth, often lead to disturbances of healing or postextraction pain. Complications of this type can be prevented by placing a wound dressing that incorporates iodoform–Vaseline strips.

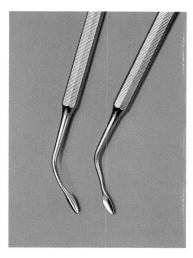
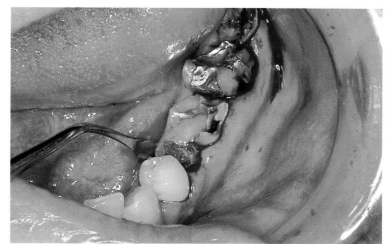

133   Removal of mandibular molars
Severing the periodontal attachment fibers using the desmotome.

Left: Desmotomes with various angulations are available for use in the mandible.

Ⓢ

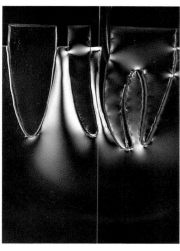
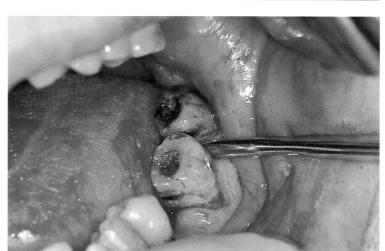

134   Use of the straight elevator
When luxating a tooth using a straight elevator, the force being applied to the adjacent teeth must be borne in mind. Remember that the forces are reciprocal if the elevator is used inappropriately.

Left: Polarized light demonstrates the forces that have to be absorbed by neighboring teeth.

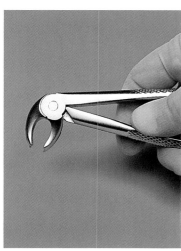
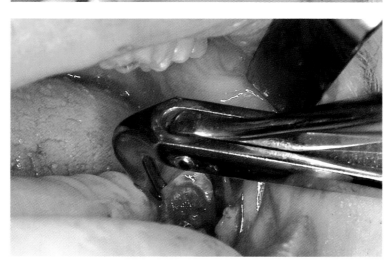

135   Use of the forceps
Actual removal of a tooth that has been prepared for extraction using an elevator is accomplished with a forceps.

Left: Forceps for use in the mandible are angled appropriately, and have pointed beaks, providing a good purchase on mandibular teeth.

136 Extraction of mandibular molars using the "cowhorn" forceps

This special forceps allows removal of mandibular molars that have an open furcation.

Right: The beaks of this forceps grasp the tooth at the furcations and lift it out of its alveolus.

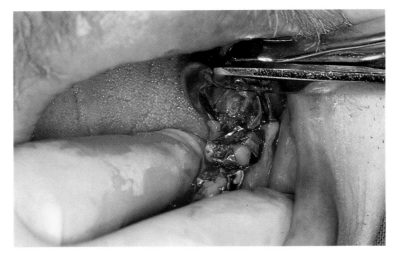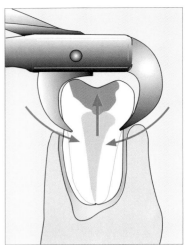

Ⓢ

137 Removal of individual roots—segmenting the roots

Severely damaged molars, and those with roots that are severely dilacerated, are usually sectioned at the furcation, and the roots are removed individually.

Right: Use of the straight elevator to separate and remove the individual roots.

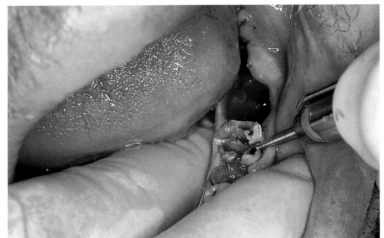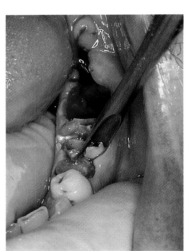

138 Cryer elevator

After one root has been removed, the remaining root can be luxated via access from the empty alveolus.

Right: Use of a Cryer elevator.

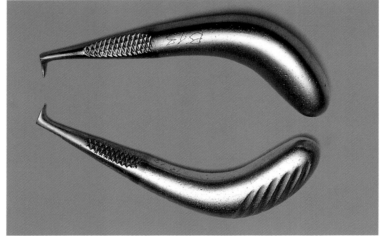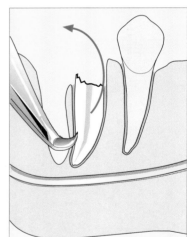

139 Hand position when using the Cryer elevator

Depending on how the elevator is grasped, more or less force can be applied.

Right: Holding the Cryer elevator in the fist makes it possible to exert strong forces that are highly targeted.

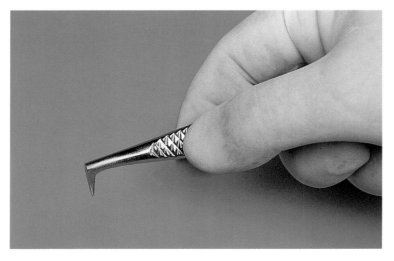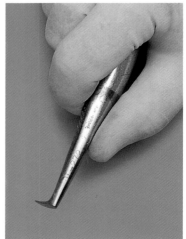

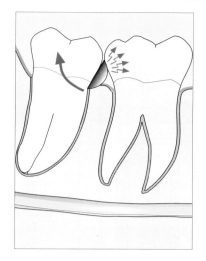

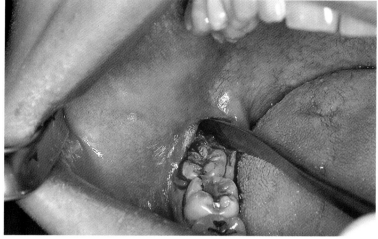

140 Removal of mandibular third molars—use of the Seldin elevator

More or less normally positioned teeth that do not have an unfavorable root form can be removed in a distobuccal direction using the Seldin elevator. There must be enough space distal to the crown to allow luxating movements by the elevator.

Left: Use of the Seldin elevator. Note the reciprocal force on the adjacent tooth.

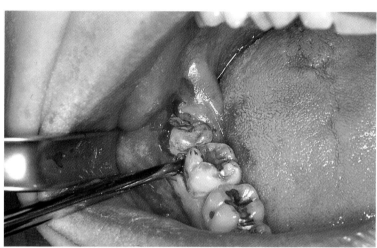

141 Seldin elevator

When using this instrument, care must be taken to avoid damage to the adjacent second molar. If the adjacent tooth is missing, particular care is required to avoid damaging restorations or otherwise compromising adjacent teeth.

Left: Seldin elevators for use on the left and right sides.

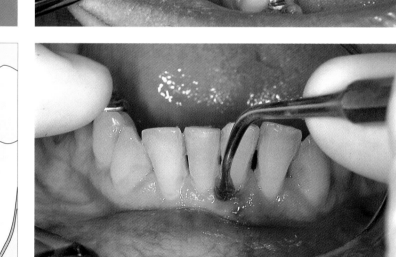

142 Extraction of mandibular anterior teeth

Tooth removal is achieved by buccolingual movement of the tooth.

Left: Using a narrow, straight elevator, removal of the root can be accomplished by applying a gentle rotatory force in the apical direction.

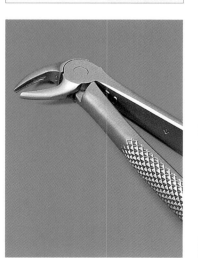

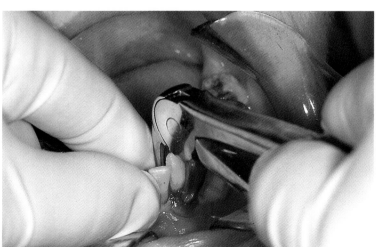

143 Use of the forceps

The tooth is extracted using the forceps, and the alveolar walls are compressed by finger pressure.

Left: This forceps is indicated for extracting mandibular teeth with narrow roots.

Tissue Flap Reflection

Access for ostectomy is achieved by reflecting a muco-periosteal flap created by an incision at the gingival margin and one or two lateral releasing incisions. The incision must take account of local anatomy. When work is being carried out in the premolar region of the mandible, the mental nerve must be uncovered at its point of exit from the mental foramen.

To maintain ridge height and avoid lateral osseous defects, the ostectomy is performed apically, and the root fragment is luxated coronally using the Cryer elevator. Removal of the buccal wall of compact bone to extract a root fragment is a clinical procedure that we do not recommend.

144 Removal of root fragments—soft-tissue flap reflection
The flap is reflected to reveal the buccal bony plate completely to the apical extent of the roots. In this case, the surgical removal of root fragments from teeth 34 and 35 is shown; the mental nerve should be exposed at its exit point from the foramen in order to avoid any unintentional nerve damage. A round burr is used to penetrate the cortical bony plate in the region of the root apex.

Right: Radiograph showing the roots of teeth 34 and 35.

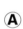 **A**

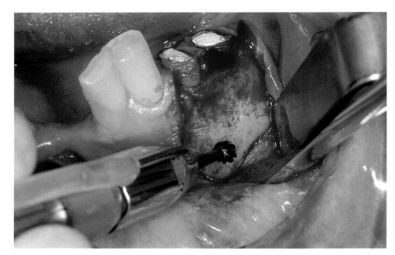

145 Apical osteotomy
The osteotomy provides an opening through which the root fragment can be forced out coronally without sacrificing the remaining buccal alveolar wall.

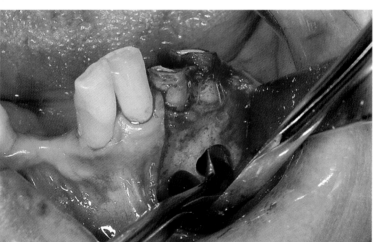

146 Luxation from the apical access
A pointed forceps is applied to remove the root fragments, and the soft-tissue flaps are sutured over the osseous wound. The empty alveoli repair themselves underneath the soft-tissue flaps by secondary osseous regeneration.

Right: Creating a groove in the apical region of the root fragment provides a purchase point for the tip of the elevator.

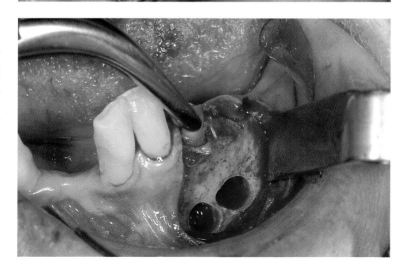

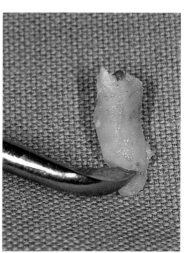

Retained Root Tips

In order to preserve the alveolar crestal bone, old root tip fragments should be surgically removed by means of lateral apical ostectomy. Dual-plane radiography must be used to locate old root fragments or foreign bodies. A wax baseplate with variously shaped and positioned metal bodies (e.g., paper clips) can serve as a radiographic stent for definitive spatial localization within the jaw as depicted on a radiograph. In extreme cases, and if the anatomical risks are high, a computed tomogram (CT) is warranted.

The indication for removal of root fragments must be determined on a case-by-case basis. Basically, root fragments showing signs of inflammation should be removed before any dental reconstructive treatment is performed in the area. Since root fragments represent potential foci of infection, it is imperative to remove them before radiotherapy or immunosuppressive therapy.

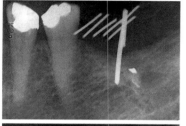
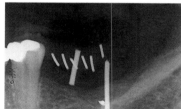
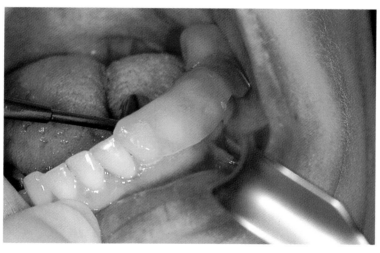

147 Locating a retained root fragment
An old, healed-in root fragment first has to be localized. An important aid for this purpose is a wax stent with metal wires placed buccally and lingually; with the stent in place, two radiographs are taken with different projection angles.

Left: These two radiographs, taken at different projection angles, reveal the lingual position of the foreign body.

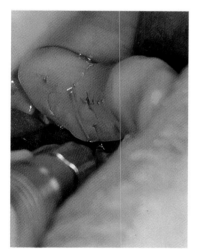
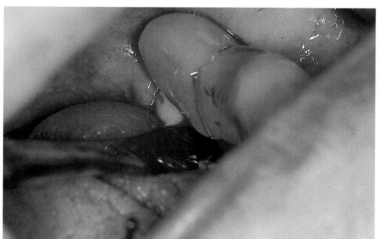

148 Lingual flap reflection
With the wax stent in place, the root fragment is removed from its lingual position. To do this, a soft-tissue flap extending from teeth 37 to 42 was necessary in order to ensure adequate visual access from the lingual aspect.

Left: Ostectomy carried out following the guidance provided by the wax stent.

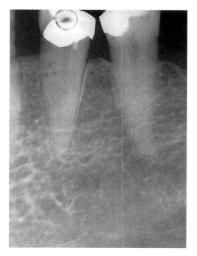
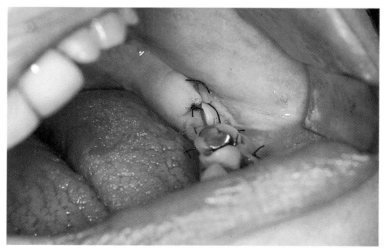

149 Radiographic check
When the surgical procedure is complete and the wound margins have been closed, a radiograph should be taken to ensure that the residual root fragment has been completely eliminated.

Left: Wound margins were closed using interrupted sutures and mattress sutures at the ostectomy site.

Complications

Postextraction Pain

If a clot fails to form within the alveolus, or if the coagulum disintegrates or is later dislodged (due to infection or during mouth rinsing, for example), localized osteitis may ensue (alveolitis sicca dolorosa or dry socket, fibrinolytic alveolitis).

These disturbances of wound healing are accompanied by severe local pain, and usually occur two or three days after tooth extraction.

The clinical examination often reveals erythema of the surrounding gingiva and mucosa, and severe pain when the area is palpated. The alveolus is usually empty, or filled with detritus (Zimmermann et al. 1992). Granulation tissue is not in evidence, and the surface of the bone is clearly visible.

150 Complication—postextraction pain
Treatment consists of carefully cleaning the alveolus to remove any remnants of degenerated coagulum, rinsing with hydrogen peroxide (3%) and placing an analgesic dressing such as iodoform–Vaseline gauze with lidocaine gel.

Right: The therapeutic dressing in the alveolus.

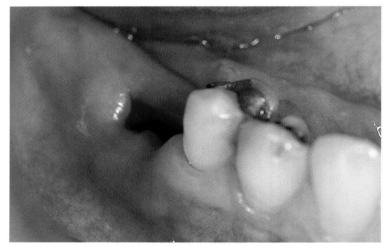
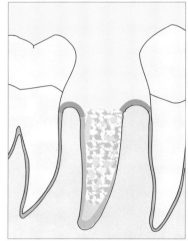

Treatment
The clinician must first make certain that there is no other cause for the infectious condition (e.g., a remaining root fragment). It is advisable to take a new radiograph. After administration of local anesthesia, the wound is carefully cleaned by gentle curettage and rinsing with hydrogen peroxide or saline solution. Then a dressing consisting of iodoform gauze coated with an anesthetic gel is placed. This procedure, including a change of dressing, is repeated every three days until the pain subsides and granulation tissue becomes visible within the alveolus. In cases in which this routine therapy fails to bring relief, it may be necessary to revise the wound under local anesthesia. An antibiotic regimen is indicated if there is evidence that an infection is spreading.

Tooth Fracture and Dislocation of Roots

An important consideration during treatment planning for tooth extraction should include the possibility of root fracture and root tip retention.

Treatment
If a root fragment from an infected tooth is forced into surrounding trabecular bone, it must be carefully removed surgically. Antibiotic coverage to prevent infec-

tion should be instituted whenever appropriate (Freyberger 1971, Paulsen and Reimann 1979).

Osseous Fracture

This usually involves a fracture of the alveolar process, which is generally quite localized and unilateral, either buccal or lingual.

Treatment
In most cases, the bone fragment can be repositioned, and sutures can be used to stabilize the wound margins. Expansive defects can result from the loss of bony fragments, often requiring a wound dressing and subsequent reconstructive procedures.

Damage to Adjacent Teeth or Tooth Buds

Careless use of instruments can lead to damage or even luxation of adjacent teeth.

Treatment
Reposition the tooth and monitor it for at least six months to allow further intervention if required. The patient should be fully informed of the situation, and should be spared any additional fees for necessary treatment; this may help to prevent subsequent legal action.

Postoperative Hemorrhage

This involves recurrence of continuous bleeding from the extraction site, which begins hours or days postoperatively. The causes may include failure by the patient to heed postoperative instructions, poor surgical technique involving injury to soft or hard tissues, and hemorrhagic diathesis (unknown clotting disorders or anticoagulation, abuse of analgesics), high blood pressure, or excessive physical exercise by the patient. Potential infection must be excluded (Becker 1974, Oatis et al. 1986).

Treatment

Temporary hemostasis via tamponade and compression. Assess the patient's systemic condition, and estimate the severity of blood loss. Monitor pulse and blood pressure. If bleeding has persisted over a long period of time, hematocrit should be measured.

Closer scrutiny of the medical history may reveal undetected factors. Contacting the patient's physician will often provide useful information.

The source of the bleeding must be identified, usually under local anesthesia. It is important to avoid infiltrating anesthetic solution into the area immediately adjacent to the hemorrhagic site, as the hemostatic effect of the anesthetic may prevent recognition of the source of the bleeding.

Bleeding from soft tissue can usually be stopped by means of tamponade. An iodoform–Vaseline strip, which may be combined with sutures and thermoplastic material (stent) for compression, serves the purpose very well. Visible bleeding from a vessel is an indication for ligation or coagulation (electrosurgery). Placing compression sutures is often sufficient to bring the bleeding to a halt.

When there is bleeding from bone, percussion of the bleeding site is often effective. If blood is oozing from the trabecular bone, it may be necessary to harvest a piece of compact bone from the immediate vicinity and tap it into place on the spongy bone. Sterile lyophilized bone from a bone bank can be used for this purpose. Such procedures must take account of the local anatomy (mandibular canal). Application of a stent along with forceful tamponade may be effective.

If there is a coagulation disturbance, the use of fibrin adhesives is very effective (Ilgenstein et al. 1987, Fuchsjäger 1984).

The effect of any measures undertaken should be carefully observed for at least 30 minutes before the patient is released. In critical situations, or in patients with circulatory instability, hospitalization may be indicated.

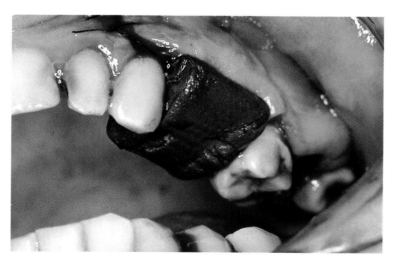

151 Postoperative hemorrhage
Debride the area and identify the source of the bleeding. Local tamponade often arrests the seepage.

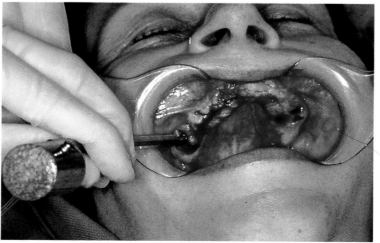

152 Postoperative hemorrhage
Bleeding from the soft tissues can be stopped by placing tight sutures. The success of any measures taken to stop postoperative hemorrhage should be monitored.

Extraction of Deciduous Teeth

The root shape and the presence of permanent tooth buds must be taken into account. Deciduous molars should be sectioned, and the pieces removed individually. Resistant root fragments may be allowed to remain in the bone, in order to protect the subjacent permanent tooth bud. In these exceptional cases, the patient and his or her parent or guardian should be informed. There is an extensive literature concerning the deciduous dentition and extraction of deciduous teeth, to which reference may be made for further details.

153 Extracting deciduous teeth
Forceps for extracting deciduous teeth are generally smaller, due to the size and shape of the teeth themselves and the patients' smaller oral cavities.

Right: Handling of a forceps is improved by spring-loaded handles.

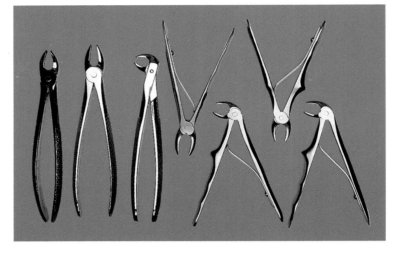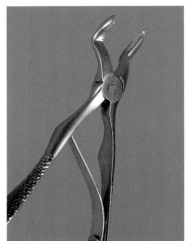

154 Sectioning a deciduous molar
Deciduous molars with roots that have not yet been resorbed are best separated, with subsequent removal of the individual halves. This is necessary because of the extreme divergence of deciduous molar roots.

Right: The radiograph shows the small deciduous molar, with exceptionally divergent mesial and distal roots.

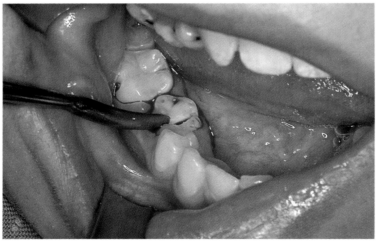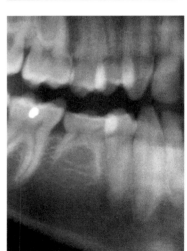

155 Deciduous molar extraction
Removing individual roots using forceps.

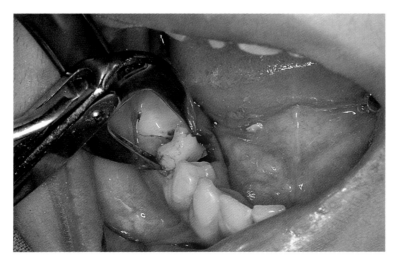

Retained (Non-Erupted) Teeth

Introduction

Definitions

A "retained tooth" is defined as one that does not erupt into the oral cavity at the normal time.

The term "impacted tooth" refers to a retained tooth that is completely surrounded by bone.

"Aberration" or "ectopic tooth" are terms applied to a tooth that develops distant from its normal location.

Multiple retained teeth often accompany the following syndromes: cleidocranial dysostosis, congenital brevi-collis dystrophy, Klippel–Feil syndrome.

Various pathological conditions often accompany retained teeth. These require a particularly careful medical history and precise evaluation of the radiographs. In cases of atypical healing or unexplained manifestations, histopathological analysis should be carried out. Retained teeth require individual and special attention to all clinical and radiographic findings, with due consideration also being given to the preventive aspects of diagnosis and therapy.

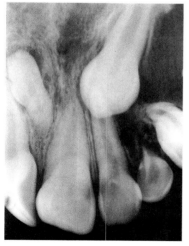

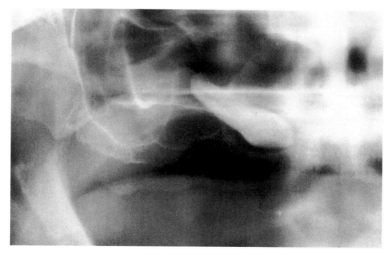

156 Retained teeth—cyst formation
Retained teeth are often associated with the formation of cysts, as in this 68-year-old edentulous patient. This panoramic radiograph reveals the cysts in the region of retained tooth 13.

Left: This occlusal radiograph depicts the mesiodens and retained tooth 23, which appears to be surrounded by a cystic formation around the crown. The root of the persisting deciduous tooth has been partially resorbed by follicular cysts.

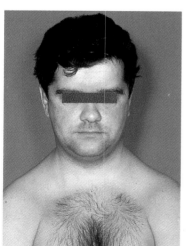

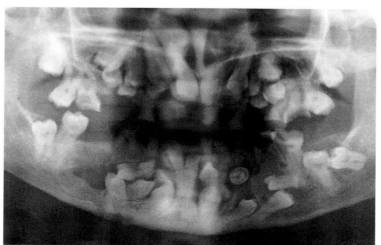

157 Cleidocranial dysostosis
Individual medical syndromes are often associated with multiple cysts, as depicted here in a case of cleidocranial dysostosis.

Left: One particular clinical symptom of this syndrome is the complete absence of the clavicles.

Indications for Removal

The simple fact that a tooth has not erupted at the normal time does not represent an indication for removal. This decision has to be taken individually in each case. In principle, only those retained teeth that harbor a pathological potential should be removed. The indications for removal can be categorized as follows:

—Difficult eruption accompanied by local infection (pericoronitis).
—Retention with cyst formation, e.g., follicular, keratin, and periodontal cysts.
—Partially erupted teeth should be removed even if there are no inflammatory symptoms evident; this can be regarded as a prophylactic measure, since even healthy-appearing conditions may harbor pathogenic microflora (Mombelli et al. 1990).

158   Indications for removal of retained teeth
This graph shows the different indications leading to the removal of retained teeth (Department of Oral Surgery, University of Zurich, 1995). In the case of mandibular third molars, the indication was mainly infection, while extraction of retained teeth elsewhere was primarily for prophylactic reasons.

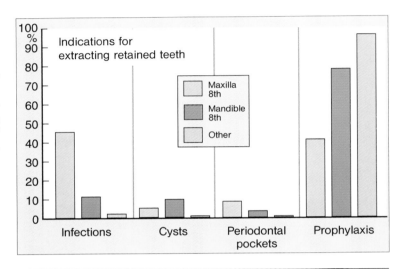

159   Pericoronitis
Infection that occurs around erupting third molars may cause local swelling of the soft tissues, as well as pain, lymph-node enlargement, difficulty in swallowing, and limited ability to open the jaw.

Right: This 24-year-old man shows the classical symptoms of third molar eruption.

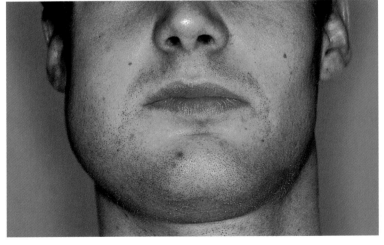
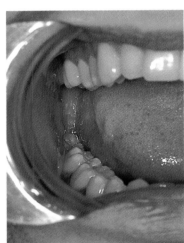

160   Pericoronitis
The mandibular right third molar has partially erupted; it is surrounded by edematous, swollen gingiva.

Right: The radiograph shows an arcuate zone of radiolucency distal to the crown of tooth 48, indicating chronic infection.

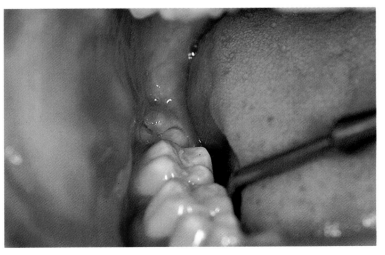
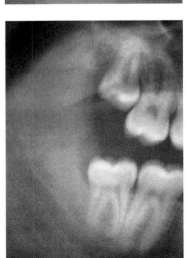

—Caries and impending pulpitis of retained teeth are only possible if there is a connection between the oral cavity and the tooth; this may constitute an indication for tooth removal. Undermining resorption of adjacent teeth is also an indication.

—If the patient complains of indefinite pains in the jaws and facial area, it is necessary to clarify whether retained or impacted teeth may be the cause of such pain. In doubtful cases, tooth extraction may be a reasonable course.

—Periodontal pocket formation toward an adjacent tooth.

—Inhibition of eruption of other teeth.

—Before prosthetic reconstruction, retained teeth may be extracted if there is an expectation that such teeth may be disturbed. An impacted tooth should never be allowed to remain beneath a fixed prosthetic replacement, because subsequent removal can lead to esthetically and functionally undesirable defects.

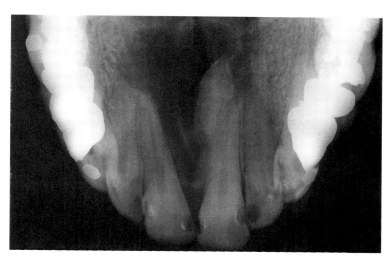

161 Pathological alteration accompanying a retained tooth—follicular cyst
This 42-year-old woman was suffering from pressure-sensitive swelling in the medial subnasal region. The radiographic examination revealed a retained partial tooth in the midline of the maxilla, which was surrounded by a heart-shaped osteolytic zone with sclerosing borders.

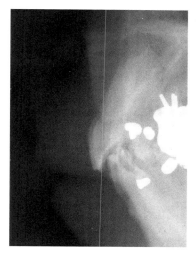
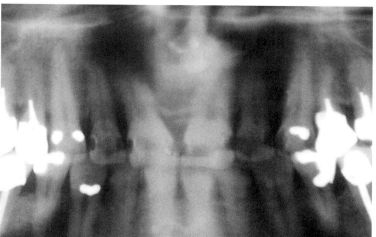

162 Follicular cyst
The panoramic radiograph reveals the expanse of the cystic formation laterally and between the roots of teeth 11 and 21, which have been displaced laterally.

Left: The lateral cephalometric radiograph also reveals the incompletely formed tooth immediately below the floor of the nose.

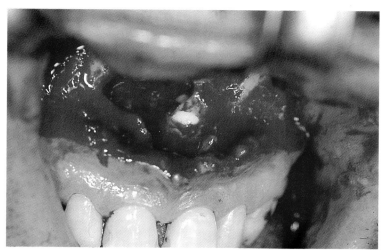

163 Follicular cyst
Removal of the retained tooth and creation of a communication between the follicular cyst and the floor of the nose were carried out in this case by mobilizing the maxilla (Le Fort I osteotomy) with repositioning.

Further Indications for Removal

—Orthodontic reasons.
—Supernumerary teeth.
—On a fracture line: teeth that are present on a fracture line and show signs of inflammation should be removed, since they may inhibit repositioning and fixation of the bones (p. 340).

—Before orthodontic surgical procedures, e.g., prior to performing sagittal sectioning of the ascending ramus of the mandible (Obwegeser 1965).
—In the course of removing a focus of infection to prevent a potential source of infection, particularly prior to radiotherapy, the removal of retained teeth is often indicated (see sections on medical history, surgical principles and tooth extraction).

164 Keratocyst
This type of cyst may be associated with a retained tooth; however, in contrast to follicular cysts, the crown of the tooth does not lie within the lumen of the cyst. In the case of the young patient depicted here, the keratocyst has compressed the bud of tooth 18 and has also prevented normal eruption of tooth 17.

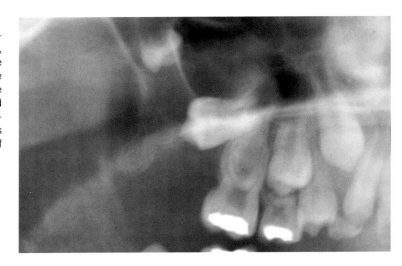

165 Periodontal cysts
These normally reside lateral to the tooth root, as shown in this radiograph of tooth 48.

Right: Note the expansive cyst on the root of tooth 48.

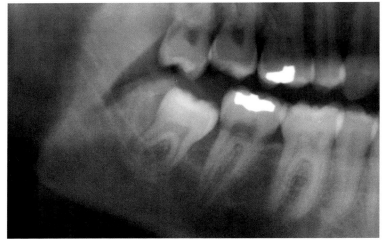
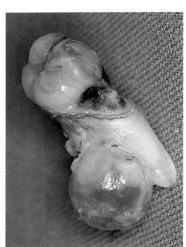

166 Tumors
The formation of a tumor may also represent an indication for removal of retained teeth, as in this case, where a complex odontoma is inhibiting eruption of the third molar.

Right: The incompletely developed dental components forming the odontoma.

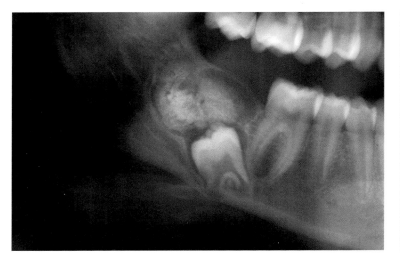
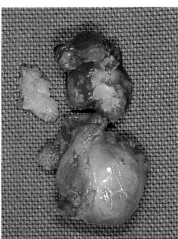

Prognosis for Retained Teeth

Eruption of the mandibular third molars can be expected as early as age 16. No data are available with regard to other retained teeth; however, it is reasonable to assume that when the period of tooth development has elapsed, any teeth still retained are highly unlikely to erupt spontaneously. Since complications are more frequently encountered with increasing age, the indication for removal or forced eruption of retained teeth should be assessed whenever possible before age 20.

In every case, the patient must be informed about the presence of retained teeth and about their potential for causing future difficulties such as cyst formation and the resorption of adjacent teeth.

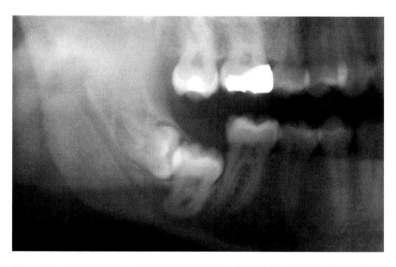

167 Impeding the eruption of adjacent teeth
The panoramic film depicts the intimate relationship between the mandibular second and third molars ("kissing teeth").

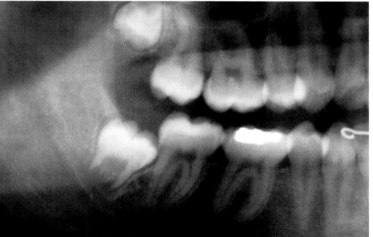

168 Inadequate space at the angle of the mandible
Insufficient space often leads to tooth retention, as shown here at the conclusion of orthodontic treatment.

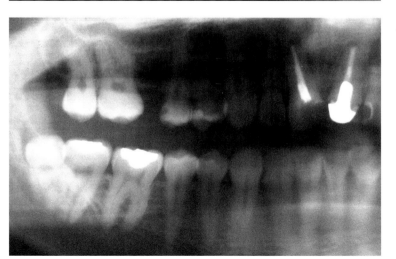

169 Supernumerary teeth
Whenever prudent, supernumerary teeth or tooth buds should be removed, since they may disturb normal tooth development, as in the case of this tooth 49.

Tooth Removal: Degree of Difficulty

Although the removal of retained teeth represents one of the most common oral surgical procedures—a routine task in everyday practice—intraoperative problems occur from time to time, and these relate to an incorrect or inappropriate appraisal of the technical difficulties of the surgical procedure. An estimation of the degree of difficulty of the planned surgical procedure must be made before the operation, and the patient must be fully informed. The surgical team must be prepared for unanticipated surgical difficulties.

Caution
Only surgical procedures in which the complications that arise can be dealt with successfully may be performed.

170 Retained tooth within a fracture line
If there is a retained tooth on the line of an alveolar fracture, and if it is in communication with the oral cavity, it should be removed, provided this will not inhibit proper repositioning of the bone segments.

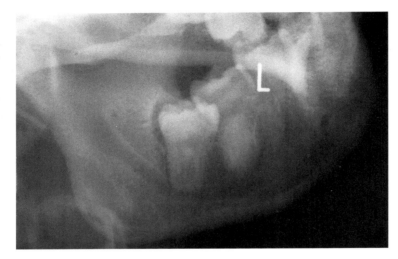

171 Caries, pulpitis, and resorption of adjacent teeth
These conditions present a clear indication for removal of the offending tooth.

Right: In rare instances, actual fusion of teeth may occur if there is intimate contact between the retained tooth and the root of its neighbor.

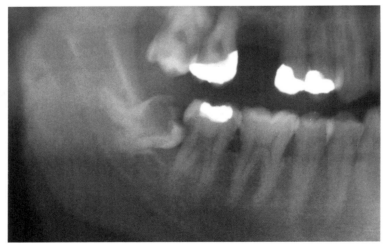
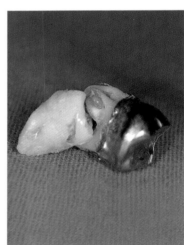

172 Before radiotherapy
In these cases, retained teeth present a potential source of infection. In each individual case, a decision must be taken on whether to extract such retained teeth. In the case depicted in this radiographic view, a 58-year-old man presented before radiotherapy for a laryngeal carcinoma. Intraorally, a communication was noted between this retained tooth and the oral cavity, so that a possible focus of infection was present; this represented an indication for removing the retained tooth.

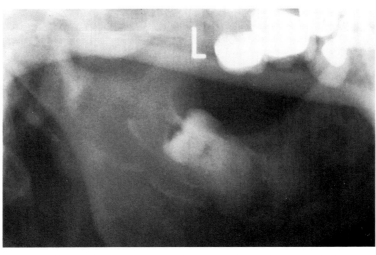

Surgical Procedure

Preparation for the operation:
—For treatment of retained, impacted, or malposition-ed teeth, we recommend the arrangement of the surgical area and the patient described on page 24.
—For removal of tooth fragments that persist after extraction, the procedure described on page 66 can be used. Antibiotic coverage is advisable.
—The patient should be prepared as described on page 26.
—For information on perioperative medication, see page 49.

The following surgical procedures are required:
—Creation of adequate visual access by reflecting mucoperiosteal flaps and possible ostectomy.
—Division of the tooth into segments to allow mechan-ical removal, with preservation and protection of the surrounding tissues.
—Careful wound treatment to ensure complication-free healing by primary intention or guided wound healing, depending on the individual situation.

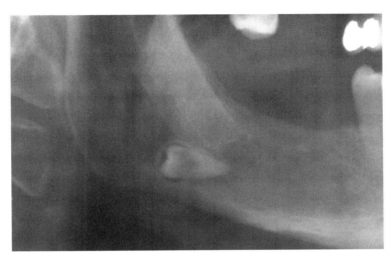

173 Nebulous pain
In this 47-year-old woman, chronic facial pain had persisted for eight years without any demonstrable etiology. This would be a possible indication for removal of the deeply impacted molar, even with-out any clinical or radiographic indications.

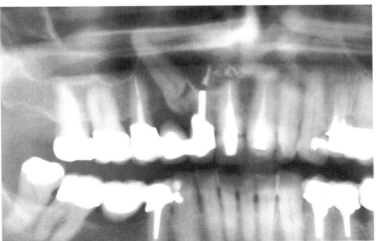

174 Retained tooth below fixed bridgework
Teeth such as this should be removed immediately, unless the patient refuses treatment even after being informed of the risks involved when subsequent compli-cations occur.

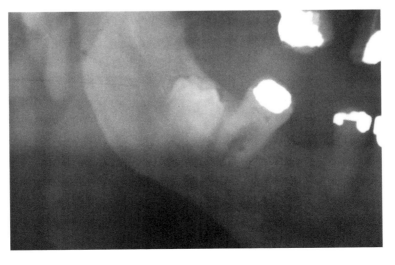

175 Focal infection
In an attempt to remove any possi-ble focus of infection, an otherwise undisturbed retained tooth may be extracted because of the possible source of infection it represents. In the case shown here, the patient was expecting a kidney transplan-tation with subsequent immuno-suppressive therapy, and was referred for elimination of possible foci of infection. Tooth 48 present-ed a possible focus of infection, and its removal was recommend-ed.

Contraindications for Removal

Absolute contraindications are rare. However, it is advisable to avoid surgical removal on an outpatient basis in the situations described below. The degree of difficulty of the operative procedure should also be considered. Usually, any contraindication is temporary, and after appropriate treatment or preventive ancillary measures, normal surgical procedures can be carried out.

Temporary contraindications:
—Existing acute infection in the surgical region, e.g., pericoronitis.
—Hemorrhagic disturbances, e.g., subsequent to aspirin abuse or anticoagulation treatment.

—Undiagnosed pathological changes in the area surrounding a retained tooth. Clarification and a definitive diagnosis is necessary, by means of biopsy if needed.
—Poor general health of the patient.
—Immunosuppression.
—Conditions that require treatment under general anesthesia, including extremely aberrant location of the tooth or lack of cooperation from the patient.
—Hospitalization provides a better infrastructure for dealing with nerve exposure or extremely unusual root forms or aberrations.
—Retained teeth in an area that has been irradiated. Removal of such teeth should only be carried out by an experienced specialist.

176   Contraindication—acute infection
One contraindication for surgical removal of retained teeth is the presence of acute infection. This 24-year-old woman had been suffering increasing swelling on the right side and difficulty in opening the mouth and swallowing for 14 days. It was only when the symptoms became severe that she visited the dentist.

Right: The clinical photograph shows highly inflamed and partly necrotic gingiva surrounding tooth 48.

177   Acute infection
Right: The radiograph shows the retained tooth 48 with distocoronal, sickle-shaped osteolysis. Attempting to remove this tooth in the patient's current condition would involve a risk of spreading the local infection.

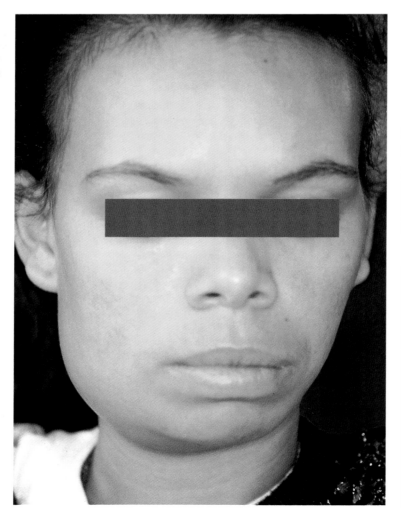
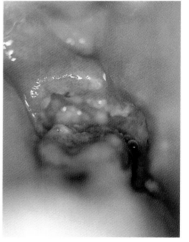
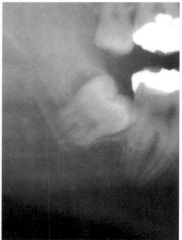

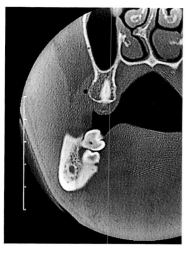

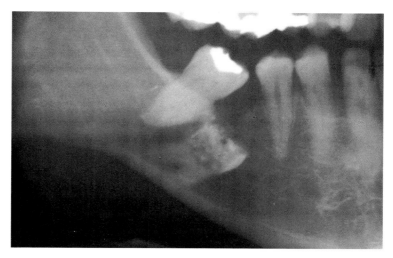

178 Extreme tooth position

This retained and partially ankylosed tooth 46 should not be removed on an outpatient basis, due to the difficulty of its position in the mandible.

Left: The CT shows the position of the mandibular canal and its extremely close relationship to the retained tooth.

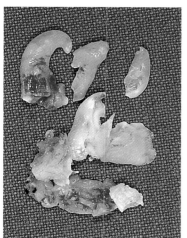

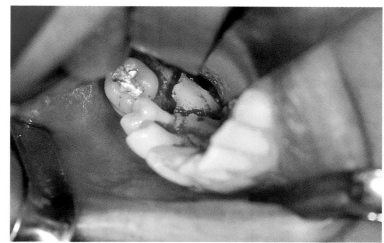

179 Removal

The retained tooth was removed under general anesthesia in a clinic. The lingual cortical plate of bone was removed, and the tooth was carefully sectioned.

Left: The individual pieces of the tooth were checked to ensure complete tooth removal.

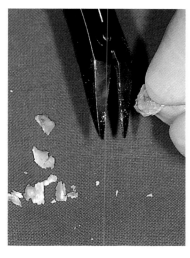

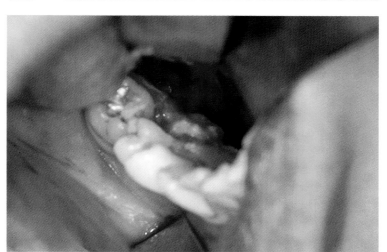

180 Filling the defect

The cortical bone that had been removed was mixed with lyophilized cartilage to fill the defect.

Left: Use of a bone cutter to reduce the cortical bone to small particles.

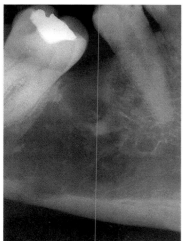

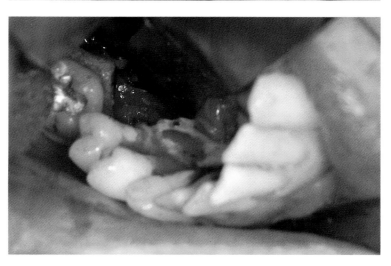

181 Clinical and radiographic view

The clinical photograph reveals the lingual defect before it was filled with the mixed cortical bone and lyophilized cartilage.

Left: This periapical radiograph was taken immediately postsurgically to ensure that the retained tooth had been completely eliminated.

Mandibular Third Molars

Surgical removal of retained mandibular third molars is one of the most frequent outpatient surgical procedures performed in dental and oral surgical practice.

Indications for Removal

In the 20-year-old age group, the incidence of retained mandibular third molars is about 84%. Depending on the position of the tooth, up to 97% will remain in situ (Ventä 1993). The incidence of retained mandibular third molars appears to be increasing, probably because measures to prevent decay have led to less tooth loss in the molar region (Rajasuo et al. 1993). In principle, it is growth relationships in the mandible and insufficient space in the retromolar region that are responsible for retention of mandibular third molars. Even as early as 13 years, radiographic examination can provide an assessment of the likelihood that the third molars will erupt normally (Ganss et al. 1993). However, the indication for surgical removal of retained teeth must always be made on an individual basis (Jaquiéry et al. 1994).

Indications for surgical removal of mandibular third molars include:
—Pericoronitis and *dentitio difficilis*.
—Resorption and caries on adjacent roots.
—Cystic expansion of the follicular space, or tendency for cyst formation.
—Orthodontic indication to eliminate crowding.
—To prevent infection and during removal of foci of infection.
—Facial pain of undetermined etiology.
—Combined surgical procedures during removal of cysts.
—Mandibular fracture in the presence of pathological processes.
—Preparation for oral prosthesis.

182 Indications for removing mandibular retained third molars

I *Dentitio difficilis* and pericoronitis
II Small cysts
III Possible source of infection
IV Inadequate space
V Caries, pulpitis
VI Vague, undiagnosed pain

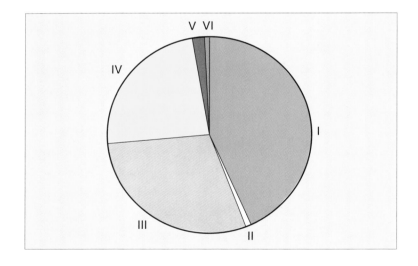

Any difficulties that can be expected depend on the position of the tooth and its relationship to neighboring structures, the surgical procedure itself, and particularly the type of postoperative care (pp. 96, 140). Usually, retained mandibular and maxillary third molars on one side are removed during a single appointment.

Clinical Tip
It is very important to give the patient preoperative information about the potential risks of the surgery, as well as the possible consequences of postponing the procedure.

Timing of the Extraction

The indication for extraction should be assessed when the patient is between the ages of 18 and 25. During this time, the risks of complications from all aspects of the surgical procedure are at the lowest point (Pajarola and Sailer 1994). It is not uncommon that the removal of totally impacted third molars from older patients leads to unanticipated complications—so that one should "let sleeping dogs lie."

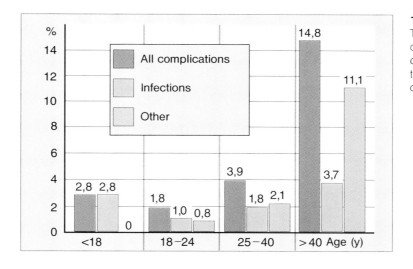

183 Timing of the extraction
This graph depicts the frequency of complications according to age category. It is recommended that third molars should be extracted during young adulthood.

Postoperative Course

The normal postoperative course will include some edematous swelling of the surrounding soft tissues for two or three days, and moderate pain on opening for up to ten days. Patients may find they are unable to open the mouth completely.

Types of Impaction

Since tooth position and root form play important roles in determining the technique for removing retained teeth, these will be discussed in more detail here. Before any attempt at surgical removal, the position of the tooth, its spatial relationship with neighboring structures, and the exact shape of the roots must be determined. Before commencing any procedure, the surgeon must formulate a plan for the technique to be used, based on the clinical situation and the radiographic evidence.

Seven types of *impaction* can be differentiated:

Type 1 Tooth bud with fully formed crown, which sits like a sphere in the follicular space. This type of tooth cannot be removed using an elevator; it simply rotates inside the space.

Type 2 Incomplete root growth; the crown is surrounded by a relatively broad follicular space. Due to the incomplete growth, resistance to extraction forces is usually low.

Type 3 Completely formed tooth with normal axial orientation. The technique for extraction depends on the shape of the root.

184 Impaction type 1
Tooth bud with fully formed crown.

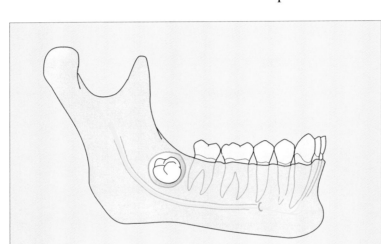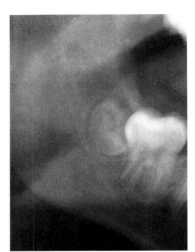

185 Impaction type 2
A "young" tooth, whose root development is approximately two-thirds complete.

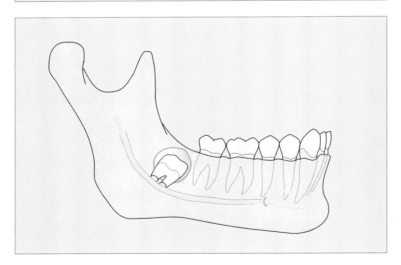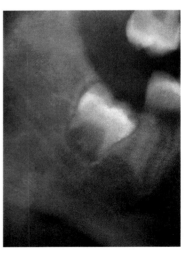

186 Impaction type 3
Retained tooth in a normal position.

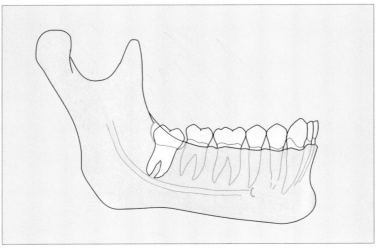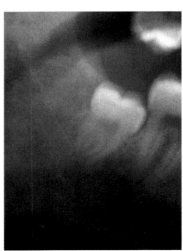

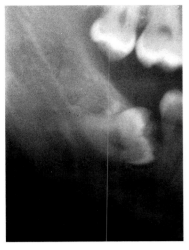
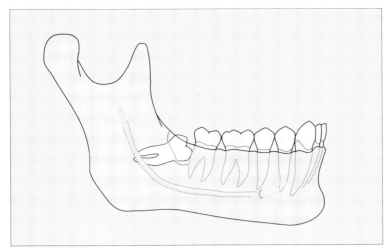

187 Impaction type 4
Mesially tipped tooth.

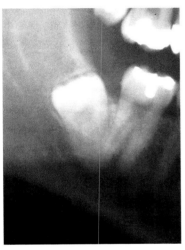
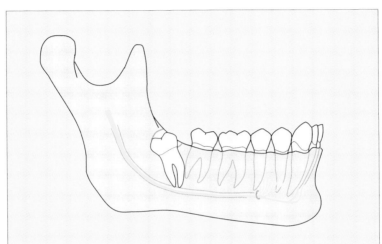

188 Impaction type 5
Distally tipped tooth.

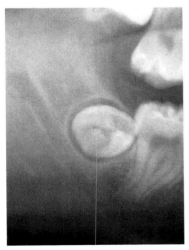
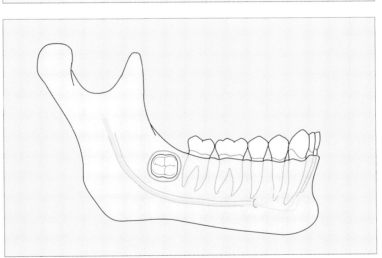

189 Impaction type 6
The tooth is positioned transverse-ly within the alveolar process.

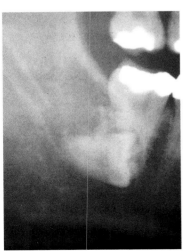
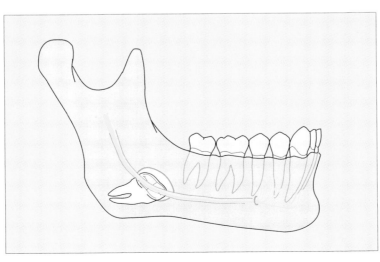

190 Impaction type 7
A widely aberrant third molar.

Type 4 The tooth is positioned with its crown tipped mesially. Contact with the distal root of the second molar may be very tight.

Type 5 The tooth is positioned with its crown tipped distally. The roots of the third and second molars may be in very close proximity to each other.

Type 6 The tooth is positioned transversely within the alveolar process, with the occlusal surface oriented buccally or, less often, lingually.

Type 7 The tooth is displaced considerably from its normal position. The tooth position can be quite bizarre—for example, subjacent to the mandibular canal or within the substance of the ascending ramus.

Careful analysis of the radiographs can prevent surprises. On the other hand, even the most targeted periapical radiograph cannot always provide every detail. In unclear situations, therefore, the surgeon should expect to encounter some problems. If the relationship of the roots to the mandibular canal is uncertain, further clarification using computed tomography should be considered; direct coronal sections (1.5 mm layer thickness) in the axis of the impacted tooth should be requested. Often it is not possible, even with a recalculated image, to achieve the precision required to determine the spatial relationship of the roots to the inferior alveolar nerve.

Root Formation

In tooth extraction, not only the tooth's position but also the configuration of the roots are of importance.

Root types:

Type A Single post-like root. This root form usually presents no technical difficulties.

Type B Divergent, blunt roots. It is usually necessary to section the tooth before extraction.

Type C Hook-like projections at the end of one or more roots. It is necessary to section the tooth and the roots before extraction.

Type D Conglomeration of the roots. Sectioning into several pieces is necessary.

Type E Beak-like roots. These cause particular problems when in close relationship to the mandibular canal; sectioning is necessary.

191 Root types
A radiograph does not always allow precise visualization of root shape and form. Impacted third molars often have grotesque root shapes. This panoramic radiograph shows an impacted tooth 48, type 4, with roots extending into the mandibular canal.

Right: Surprisingly, the tips of the roots closely approximated each other near the apex. The inferior alveolar nerve passed through the opening.

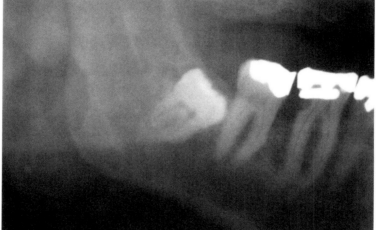
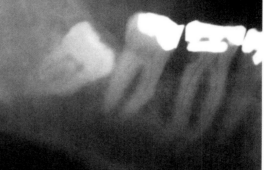
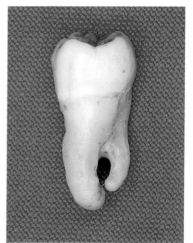

192 Root types
In this radiograph, the deeply impacted type 3 third molar appears to have several roots.

Right: The real arrangement of the roots only became clear after the tooth had been removed.

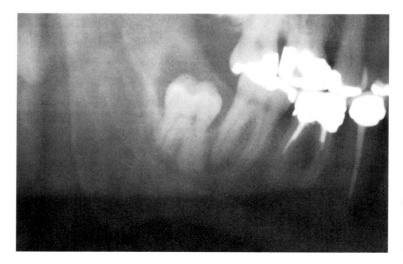
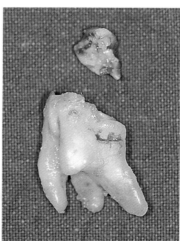

Surgical Procedure

Documentation
Panoramic radiograph or separate lateral views of the mandible. If the tooth appears to be in close proximity to the inferior alveolar nerve, additional radiographs will be necessary: a frontal tomogram or computed tomogram (CT) with radial sections (dental scan) to depict the course of the mandibular canal (Feifel et al. 1991).

Armamentarium
For surgical removal of mandibular third molars, the basic instrument set is augmented by adding:
—Straight elevators, wide and narrow.
—Cryer elevators, right and left.
—Root forceps with diamond-coated beaks.
—Surgical handpiece.
—Round burrs for osseous surgery.
—Carbide steel burrs for sectioning teeth.

A contra-angled handpiece and special luxation instruments may be added if necessary.

Anatomy
The course of the lingual nerve and inferior alveolar nerve within the mandibular canal are important, as well as the shape and number of roots, and the spatial relationship of the crown and roots to the nerves.

Lingual nerve. Its course to the tongue is through the soft tissues of the floor of the mouth, lingual to the mandible. The anatomical relationship of the nerve to the lingual bony margin of the retromolar region varies considerably, and cannot be predicted.

Inferior alveolar nerve. The relationship of this nerve to a third molar tooth must be deduced from the radiograph. If the situation is critical, especially when the narrowing of the mandibular canal is obvious radiographically near a root, the need for additional clarification (e.g., a coronal CT) should be discussed with the patient.

The root form should be classified preoperatively in order to plan the technical procedure properly.

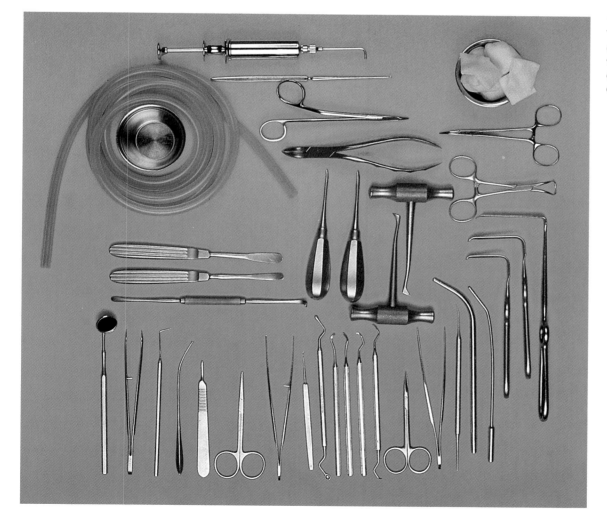

193 Instrumentarium
The basic instrument set is enhanced by addition of the Cryer elevator, wide and narrow straight elevators, and a root forceps with diamond-coated beaks.

Anesthesia
1. Block anesthesia of the inferior alveolar nerve.
2. Infiltration anesthesia of the long buccal nerve.
3. Infiltration anesthesia within the vestibule.

Access
The orientation is over the crown of the second molar onto the external oblique line of the ascending ramus. The thumb is used to stretch the mucosa laterally against the ascending ramus, to keep the incision line on bone and to prevent slipping off in the lingual direction.

Primary Incision
The shape of the mucoperiosteal flap will depend primarily on the postoperative care that is anticipated. The incisions depicted in this chapter are designed with open postoperative treatment in mind.

The primary incision is approximately 20 mm long, extending from the distolingual bony margin of the second molar in a distobuccal direction toward the ascending ramus, at an angle of approximately 45° buccal to the dental arch segment. Contact of scalpel blade with bone must be continuous, and avoid slipping off in the lingual direction.

194 Minnesota retractor
This wound retractor is used to deflect the soft tissues that are displaced buccally.

Right: The V-shaped indentation is placed directly on the bony surface of the ascending ramus.

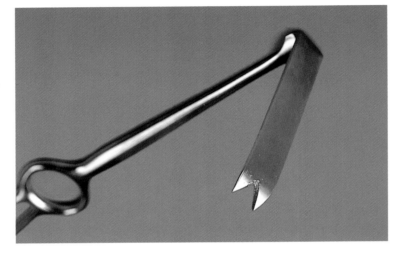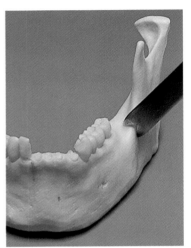

195 Flexible spatula
The flexible, wide metal spatula, which can be bent into any shape desired, is used to protect the soft tissue that is reflected toward the lingual.

Right: Positioning of the spatula on the internal oblique line.

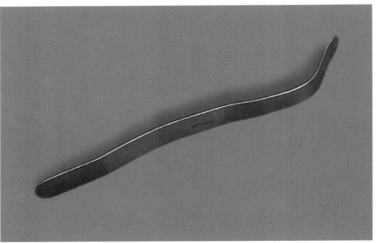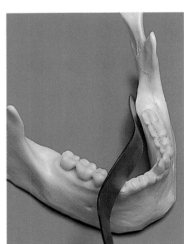

196 Straight and contra-angled handpieces
Buccal ostectomy is carried out using surgical burrs in a handpiece with continuous water cooling. The contra-angled handpiece can be used in difficult situations to achieve the desired direction for the ostectomy, or for sectioning the teeth.

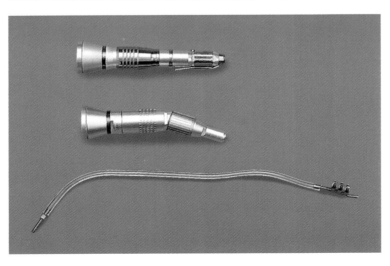

The second incision is placed distal to the second molar, and perpendicular to the vestibular incision. The mesially diverging incision line leaves a section of bone denuded for open postoperative treatment, which also may delay wound healing and increase postoperative pain.

The third incision is at the margin, lingually and within the gingival sulcus of the second molar, with the scalpel moving distally. Any deviation can lead to injury to the lingual nerve (Pajarola et al. 1994).

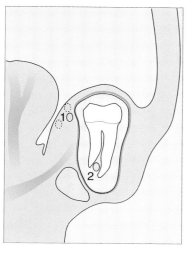 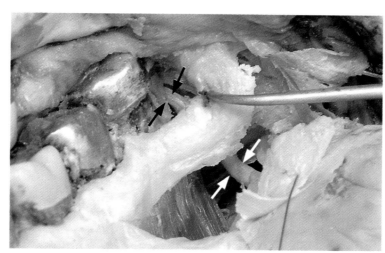

197 Anatomy of the lingual nerve
This cadaver preparation shows the internal surface of the mandible and the relationship of the lingual nerve to the gingiva near a mandibular third molar.

Left: The most common variations in the location of this important nerve.

1 Lingual nerve
2 Inferior alveolar nerve

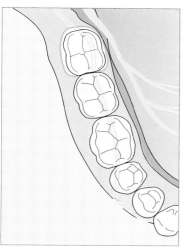 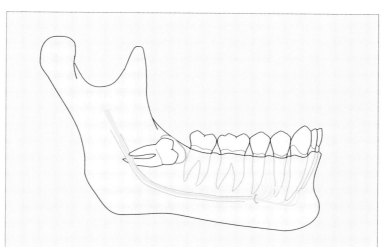

198 Anatomy of the inferior alveolar nerve
The potentially close spatial relationship between the roots of tooth 48 and the mandibular canal.

Left: Course of the two important nerves in the area of the mandibular third molar.

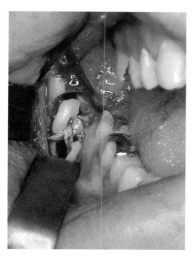 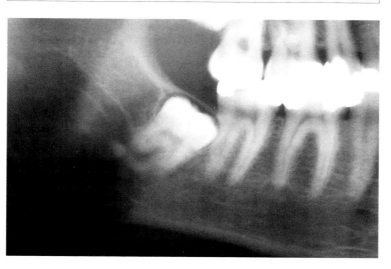

199 Critical course of the inferior alveolar nerve
This section from a panoramic radiograph clearly shows the curving course of the mandibular canal around the distal root of tooth 48.

Left: During the surgical procedure, the inferior alveolar nerve is clearly seen coursing between the roots of tooth 48. Injury to the nerve can only be avoided by separating the roots.

200 Documentation—radiograph

In addition to the clinical examination, radiographic documentation is especially important. In the case of retained or impacted teeth, it is important to have comprehensive imaging of the tissues surrounding the tooth, as well as the dimensions of the mandible.

Right: This periapical radiograph is not adequate for presurgical evaluation.

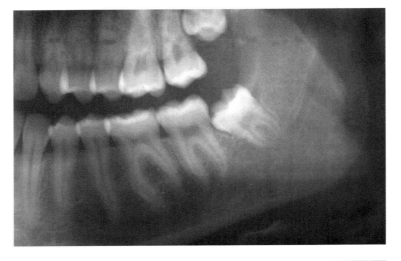 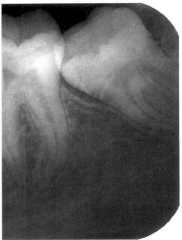

201 Documentation—CT

In particularly critical cases, a CT can provide important information about the relationship between the root and the mandibular canal, in virtually any direction desired (radial sections are used in this example).

Right: This lateral radiograph of the angle of the mandible can provide additional information.

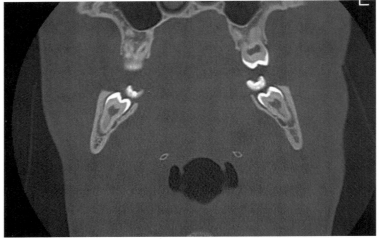 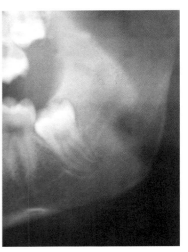

202 Anesthesia

For extraction of mandibular third molars, block anesthesia of the inferior alveolar nerve is used, as well as local anesthesia of the long buccal nerve and infiltration buccal to the second molar.

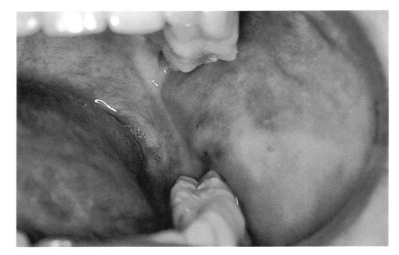

203 Access

Access for removal of a mandibular third molar with ostectomy is achieved from the buccal aspect by creating a vestibular mucoperiosteal flap.

Right: The three incisions.

1 Perpendicular within the vestibulum
2 Along the ascending ramus
3 Within the sulcus, lingual to the second molar

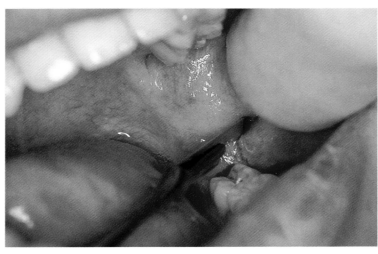 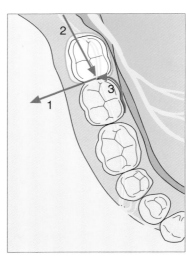

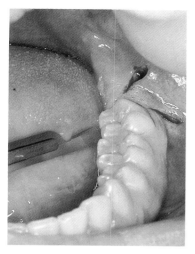
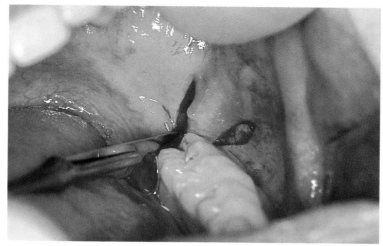

204 Flap reflection
After severing the mucoperiosteum, a tissue flap is created, which can be reflected distally toward the ascending ramus.

Left: Careful incision within the lingual gingival sulcus of the second molar.

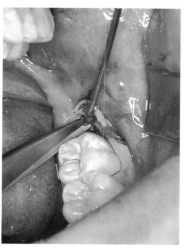
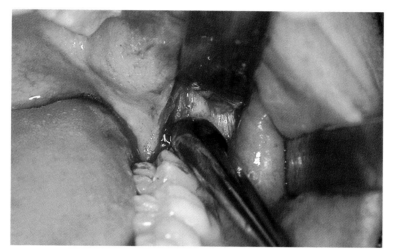

205 Protecting the soft tissues: Minnesota retractor
The Minnesota retractor is useful for holding the soft tissues in a cranial position, simultaneously improving visual access to the field.

Left: Indurated adhesions can be separated under direct vision using scissors or scalpel.

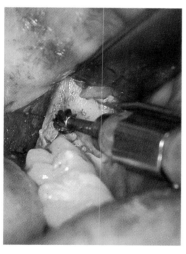
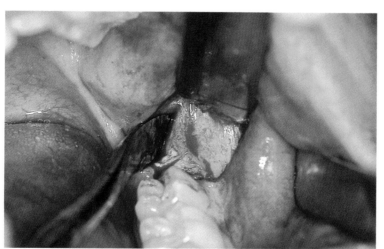

206 Flexible spatula
For protection of the lingual soft tissues, a wide elevator or an individually adapted metal spatula is inserted between the bony surface and the soft tissues.

Left: Note the metal spatula that is deflecting and thus protecting the lingual soft tissues during the ostectomy procedure.

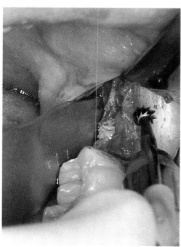
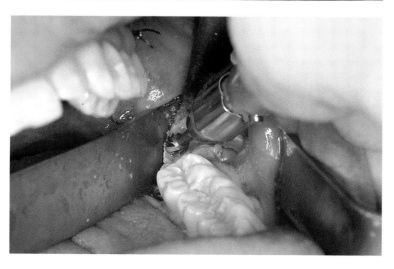

207 Ostectomy
Surgical drills are used with constant saline cooling solution to carry out the necessary ostectomy. The flexible metal spatula protects the soft tissues.

Left: The flexible metal spatula can be bent as needed to provide protection for the lingual soft tissues.

208 Anatomy—tooth position and root geometry

This cadaver preparation shows the relationships to the important nerves: the lingual nerve may course very near to the gingival margin under the mucosa.

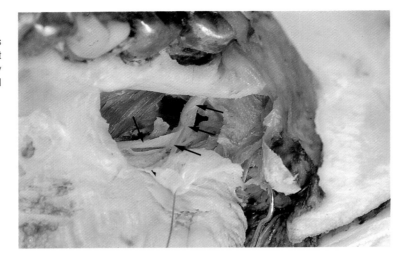

209 Tooth extraction, type 1

Note that the tooth primordium shows no root formation and lies in an apparently hollow space, surrounded by the membrane. This section from a panoramic radiograph shows the situation in a 14-year-old boy who was undergoing orthodontic treatment. It was planned to extract the mandibular third molars to avoid any subsequent negative spatial relationships.

Right: The impacted tooth crown.

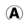

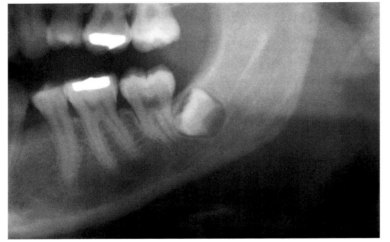 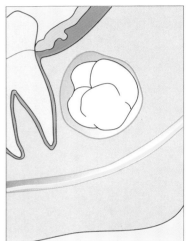

210 Sectioning the crown

After ostectomy from the buccal aspect, the crown can be sectioned under direct vision. The sectioning is necessary because the crown simply rolls within its space if an elevator is applied.

Right: Sectioning of the crown after the ostectomy.

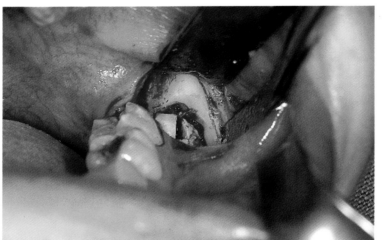 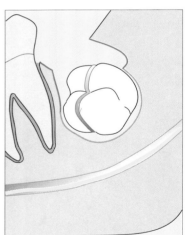

211 Removal of the sectioned parts of the crown

A Cryer elevator is used to remove the two parts.

Right: Luxation of the crown fragments using the Cryer elevator.

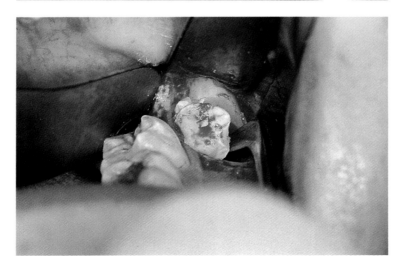 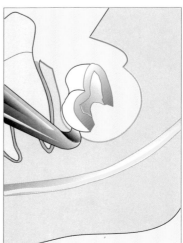

Tooth Extraction

Type 1 Buccal ostectomy, sectioning crown using carbide fissure burs, removal in two pieces.

Type 2 The crown is exposed from buccal or from occlusal. A groove is milled on the buccal aspect, and the Cryer elevator is used to luxate the tooth occlusally. If space is limited, the crown can be sectioned.

Type 3 A groove is milled at the level of the cemento-enamel junction. The Cryer elevator uses the groove as a purchase point to luxate the tooth coronodistally. It may be necessary to separate the crown from the root and remove the two pieces individually.

Type 4 Sectioning of the crown and use of an elevator or a root forceps to remove the fragments. Further sectioning of the crown and root is sometimes necessary.

Type 5 Ostectomy, sectioning of the crown and luxation of the roots individually. Additional sectioning or ostectomy may be necessary.

Type 6 Ostectomy, sectioning the crown with a contra-angled handpiece, and removal of the roots, sometimes with additional sectioning.

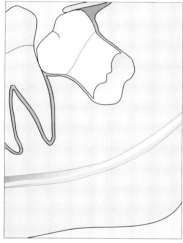

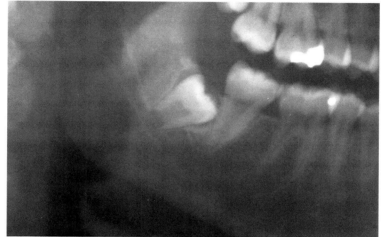

212 Tooth extraction, type 2
Tooth 48 shows incomplete root growth and is scheduled for extraction after orthodontic treatment in an 18-year-old man; the goal is to prevent recurrence of crowding in the lower arch.

Left: The tooth bud, with incomplete root formation.

Ⓢ

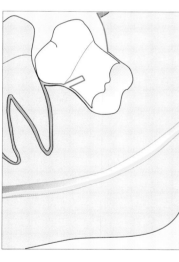

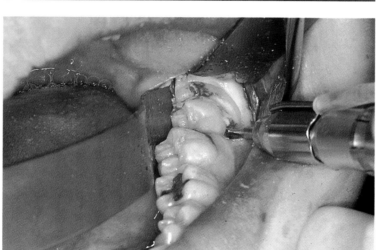

213 Milling a groove
After buccal and distal ostectomy, a groove is milled into the tooth from the mesial aspect at the junction of crown and root.

Left: The groove, which serves as a purchase point for the Cryer elevator.

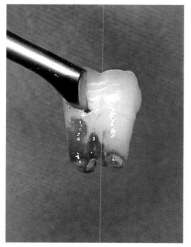

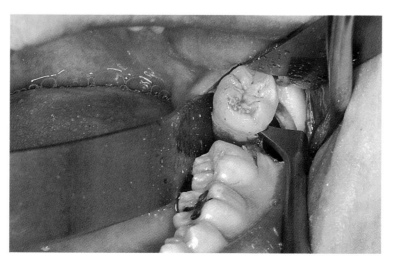

214 Cryer elevator
Using the mesial groove in the tooth as a purchase point, the Cryer elevator is used to luxate the tooth distally.

Left: The mandibular third molar, showing incomplete root formation, was extracted using the Cryer elevator.

215 Tooth extraction, type 3
The panoramic radiograph reveals tooth 38 retained in a vertical position. The roots extend to the level of the mandibular canal. If there is direct contact of the root with the nerve, the postoperative course will inevitably include some disturbance of sensitivity in the region served by that nerve. The same is true for the lingual nerve.

Right: Note the proper positioning of the metal spatula after flap reflection and ostectomy.

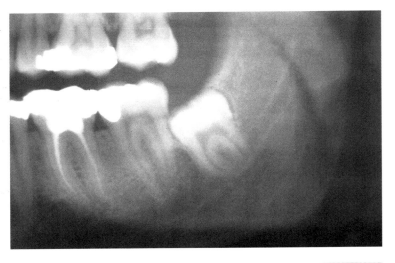
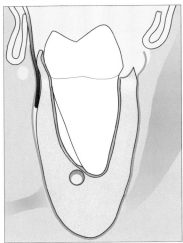

216 Spatula
After buccal flap reflection and placement of a Minnesota retractor, the mucoperiosteum is also deflected lingually to allow placement of the metal spatula in direct contact with the bone. This prevents trauma to the lingual nerve. The crown is exposed, sectioned into three pieces using a fissure burr, and broken off using a straight elevator or Cryer elevator.

Right: The tooth immediately before removal of the crown segment.

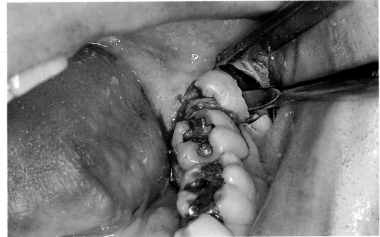
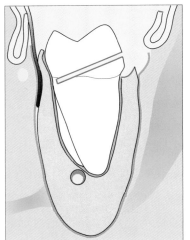

217 Sectioning the root
After removal of the crown, a groove is cut vertically into the root, and the straight elevator is used to separate the two roots.

Right: Removal of the crown using the Cryer elevator.

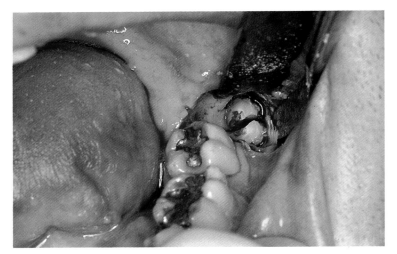
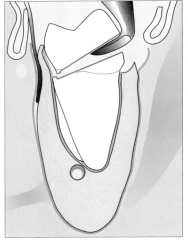

218 Removal of the individual roots
The roots are now carefully luxated. Depending on the curvature of the root, an additional groove at the root margin may allow appropriate movement. During the entire procedure, the metal spatula should remain motionless in place.

Right: Partial sectioning of the roots before separation using a straight elevator.

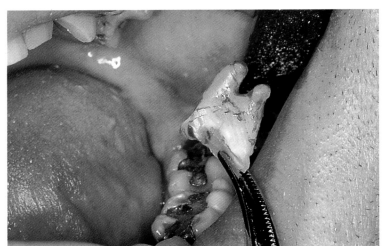
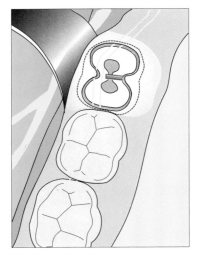

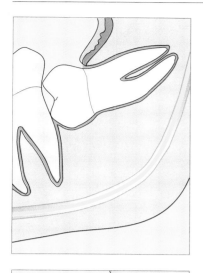

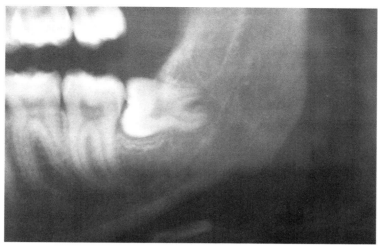

219 Tooth extraction, type 4
The panoramic radiograph shows a mesially tipped third molar lying immediately distal to the second molar. Note the sclerotic zone immediately subjacent to the third molar crown; this is a sign of chronic inflammation. In the mouth, the tooth is partially visible, and acute infection can develop at any time in this situation.

Left: Overview.

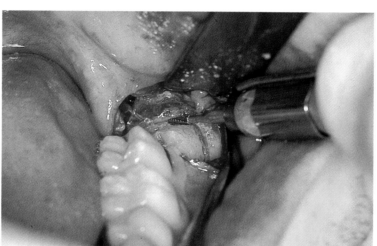

220 Sectioning the crown
The crown of the mesially tipped tooth is exposed from the buccal approach, and then sectioned perpendicular to its long axis. The depth of the groove should not include the lingual enamel wall. If it becomes necessary to expose the crown from the lingual approach, the metal spatula should be appropriately placed to prevent injury to the lingual soft tissues.

Left: The depth of the groove separating the crown from the roots.

221 Sectioning the roots
After the crown has been removed, a fissure burr is used to separate the two roots.

Left: Grooves for separating the roots.

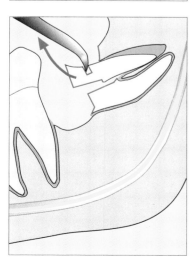

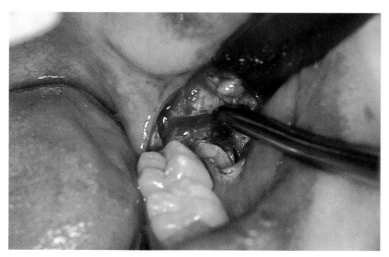

222 Removing the individual roots
If necessary, a small groove can be milled into the root to provide a purchase point for an elevator. Depending on the root curvature, the roots are removed one at a time using the Cryer elevator. In particularly difficult cases, it may be advisable to cut the roots into smaller pieces to reduce trauma during removal.

Left: Cutting a small groove in the root provides a purchase point for the elevator.

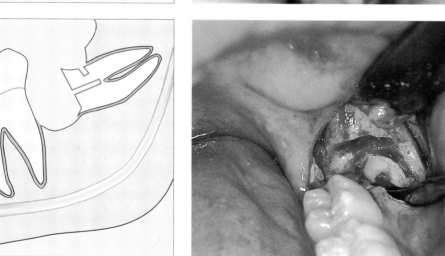

223 Tooth extraction, type 5
The panoramic radiograph shows a distally tipped third molar; note the very close proximity to the distal root of the second molar. A deep carious lesion in the crown of the third molar is visible as a distinct radiolucency.

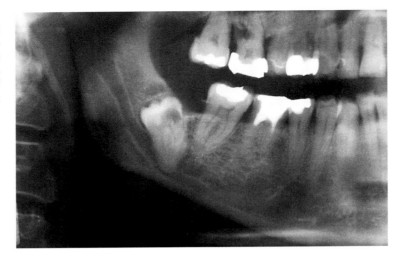

224 Segmenting the root
Access through soft and hard tissues is obtained as described above in extraction types 3 and 4. After the crown has been removed, the roots can be extracted into the space formerly occupied by the crown.

Right: Extraction of the roots. The direction of luxation will be determined by the root curvature.

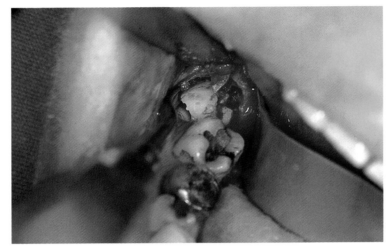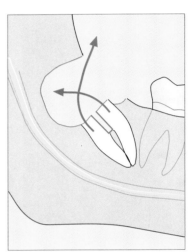

225 Tooth extraction, type 6
The CT shows that the impacted third molar is positioned horizontally in the alveolar process. The indication for tooth extraction is elimination of a potential infectious focus.

Right: A cross-section of the mandible through the long axis of the tooth. Note the deep groove that has been cut perpendicular to the long axis to facilitate removal of the crown. If the situation requires, the crown itself can be segmented before removal.

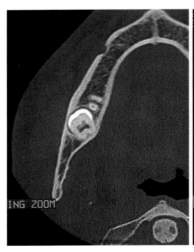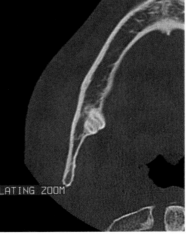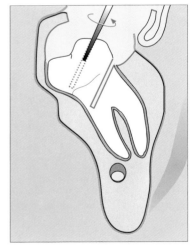

226 Segmenting the roots
Access is gained by reflection of a buccal flap and appropriate ostectomy. Once the crown has been removed, sufficient space is available for removal of the roots, either together or as separate fragments.

Right: Removal of the two roots.

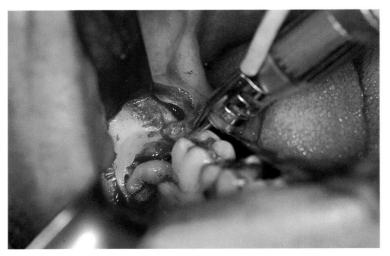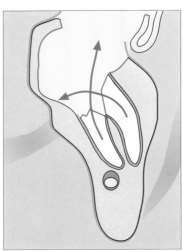

Unusual Location and Accompanying Pathology

Severely impacted third molars demand particularly careful clinical and radiographic examination. Treatment of these cases requires considerable experience on the part of the surgeon. The procedures required are complex, and usually involve a synthesis of several different surgical techniques. This type of operation is at the limits of what is possible in an outpatient oral surgery practice.

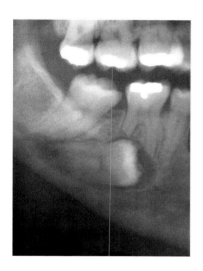
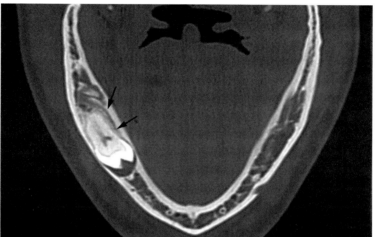

227 Tooth extraction, type 7
This severely impacted third molar is surrounded by a cystic cavity. There is extremely close proximity to the mandibular canal, but the precise spatial relationship cannot be detected from the radiograph. A CT provided clarity concerning the expanse of the cyst and the position of the mandibular canal (arrows).

Left: The radiograph reveals the impacted tooth within a cystic cavity, and severe resorption of the distal root of the second molar.

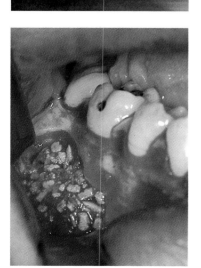
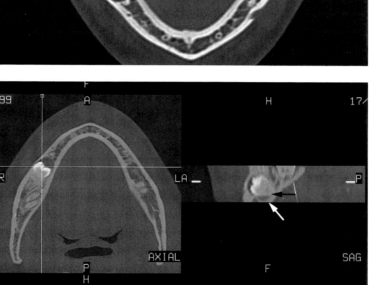

228 Tooth extraction, type 7— dental scan
Reformatting the axial CT into sagittal sections shows the relationship of the impacted tooth (arrows) to the mandibular canal.

Left: This radiograph was taken seven months after removal of the impacted molar.

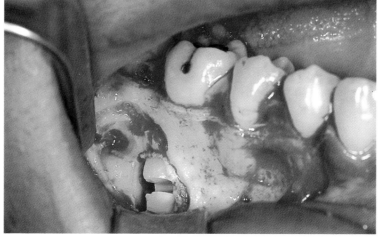
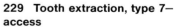

229 Tooth extraction, type 7— access
Access is obtained from the buccal aspect. An extensive mucoperiosteal flap is reflected, which can be repositioned postsurgically and firmly affixed with sutures to close the considerable osseous defect. The crown has been segmented and separated from the roots. After removal of the tooth, the inferior alveolar nerve is seen in the expected position, lingually and caudally.

Left: The large osseous defect is filled with lyophilized cartilage chips before primary closure.

Wound Treatment

After ensuring that all fragments of the third molar have been completely removed, any remaining follicular tissue is removed. Any remnants of the periodontal ligament tissue on the distal surface of the second molar root are allowed to remain in situ.

Using a large, round burr, sharp bony margins are smoothed; this applies also to any areas that were crushed by the elevator. The water spray is used buccally and lingually to completely rinse away all osseous fragments and chips.

The condition of the osseous defect distal to the second molar is carefully checked using a mirror and a probe. Any denuded root segments are measured using the periodontal probe and noted on the chart.

The buccally reflected mucoperiosteal flap is then repositioned in such a way that all bone segments are completely covered. The flap is covered with a loose iodoform–Vaseline strip, which helps to maintain the flap during healing. A coagulum forms in the depth of the alveolus, and is maintained there by the secure flap closure. One week postoperatively, the wound dressing is changed.

The area is rinsed after removal of the dressing, and if the rinse remains clear, a new strip is applied.

230 Wound treatment—debridement
Granulation tissue and any remnants of the follicular sac are removed using a sharp spoon excavator or the Black excavator, with care being taken not to infringe on the marginal periodontal tissues of the second molar.

Right: A hemostat is used to remove the cyst-like follicular sac.

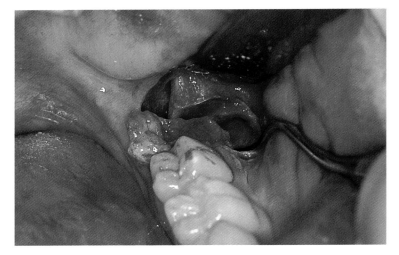 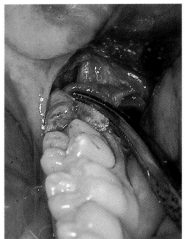

231 Smoothing the bone
Localized osseous necrosis can be avoided by carefully smoothing any sharp bony edges or any osseous tissue that has been crushed by the use of elevators.

Right: Buccal and lingual soft tissues must be protected during the bone-smoothing procedure.

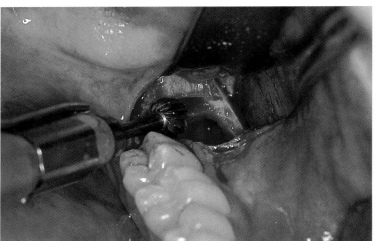 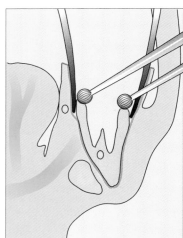

232 Rinsing the wound
The surgical field is thoroughly rinsed using physiological saline solution. This should wash away all bony fragments from between the cortical bone and the periosteum. The clean wound can then be examined. The condition of the tissues distal to the second molar is carefully inspected, as well as the position of the inferior alveolar nerve if it has been exposed during the surgical procedure. All clinical observations are recorded in the patient's chart.

Right: Rinsing of the surgical area.

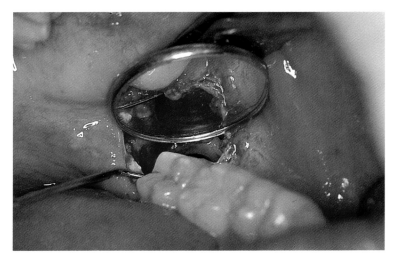 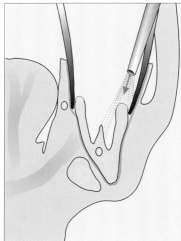

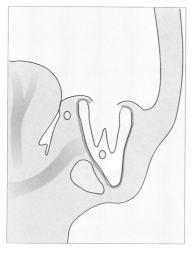
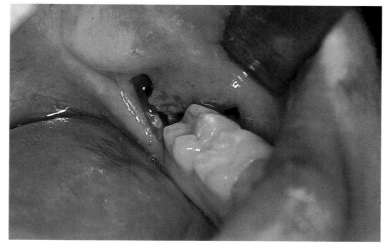

233 Wound dressing
The buccal mucoperiosteal flap is reflected back into the osseous defect. The wound is left open for healing by secondary intention.

Left: After repositioning of the buccal and lingual soft tissues.

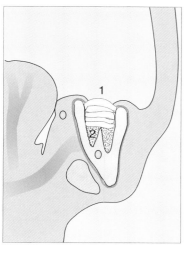
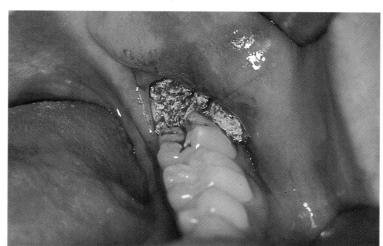

234 Iodoform–Vaseline drain
The wound is covered using a loose iodoform–Vaseline drain (IVD). A blood coagulum should be left at the base of the wound.

Left:
1 Iodoform–Vaseline drain
2 Coagulum

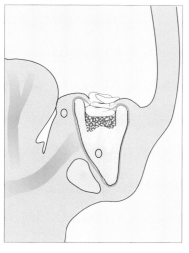
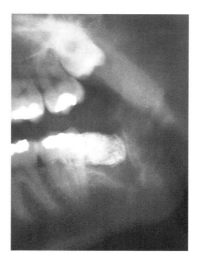
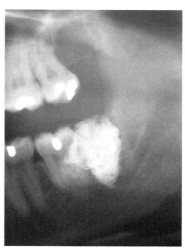

235 Wound healing, first week
Left: Correct positioning of the wound dressing immediately after the first dressing change.

Center: Correct positioning of the IVD.

Right: In this case, the IVD was forced too deeply into the defect, effectively preventing the formation of a coagulum.

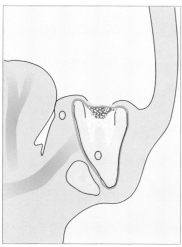
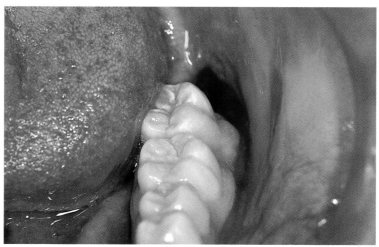

236 Healing period, week two
The dressing is changed seven to ten days postoperatively. The area is thoroughly rinsed, and a fresh IVD dressing is placed. This procedure is repeated once or twice at ten-day intervals. With time, the surgical defect becomes flatter, and reepithelialization proceeds inward from the wound margins.

Left: The condition immediately after removal of the drain.

Potential Complications

Immediate or delayed infection (osteomyelitis). Open wound treatment after extraction of mandibular third molars rarely leads to postoperative infection. Other types of complications depend on the surgical technique and the anatomical situation surrounding the third molar. Instances of chronic osteomyelitis with radiographic manifestations have been reported.

Fractures. When ostectomy has been extensive in the course of removing mandibular third molars, fracture of the jaw is not uncommon, occurring usually within three weeks of the operation, especially if the mandible is atrophic. If there is a danger of mandibular fracture, patients should be advised to take only soft nutrition, and prophylactic splinting may be indicated. If a fracture occurs nevertheless, appropriate treatment must be instituted immediately (p. 333).

Other potential complications include nerve damage, postoperative hemorrhage, sensitivity of adjacent teeth, ostectomy defects, as well as root fractures and dislocations.

237 Complication—fracture
Chronic infection was the indication for extracting tooth 38 in this 65-year-old man. The postsurgical healing appeared to be normal until the 18th postoperative day, when the patient experienced swelling and pain at the angle of the mandible after experiencing a noticeable snap.

Right: This detail of a mandibular radiograph clearly depicts the dislocated fracture near the site from which the impacted wisdom tooth had been extracted.

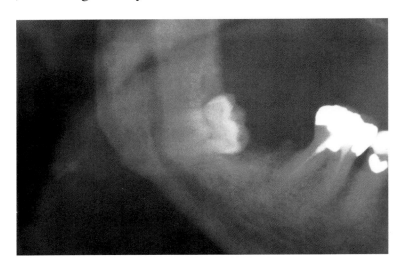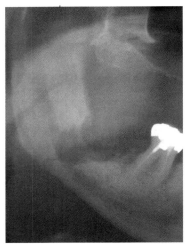

238 Splinting
Complication-free healing and consolidation of the fracture was observed four weeks after intermaxillary fixation of the jaws in centric occlusion and prophylactic administration of antibiotics.

Right: Radiographic view four months postoperatively.

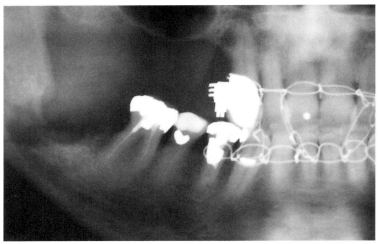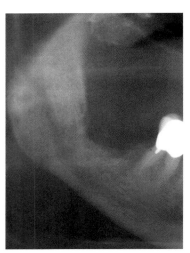

239 Remaining fragments
Inadequate visualization and inadequate checking during the surgical procedure can result in fragments of the tooth remaining in situ after the procedure. These may subsequently cause infection, requiring an additional surgical procedure, and possible legal consequences.

Right: This radiograph clearly reveals that fragments of the third molar were not removed during the extraction procedure.

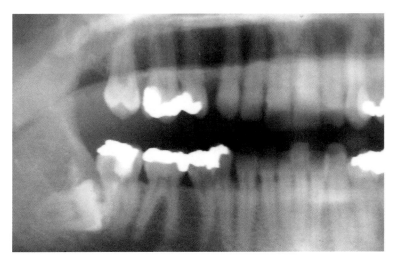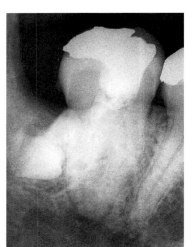

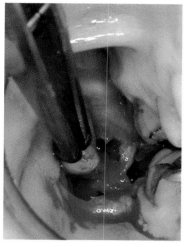
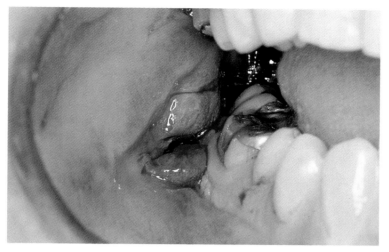

240 Sequestration
In this case, wound healing was delayed, and there were local signs of inflammation accompanied by pain in the surgical area. Follow-up radiographic examination revealed a sclerosed fragment, which was removed after reopening of the wound. Open healing followed, as after the primary intervention.

Left: The sequestrated fragment is removed using a forceps.

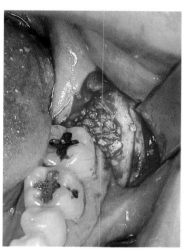
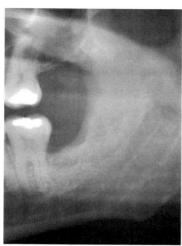
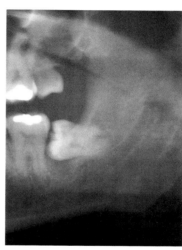

241 Pocket formation on the adjacent tooth
Left: After extraction (type 4) of the third molar, the distal surface of the root of the second molar was exposed. The defect was filled with lyophilized cartilage and the wound was closed. The patient received antibiotics.

Center: Osseous regeneration after one year.

Right: This preoperative radiograph shows the initial situation.

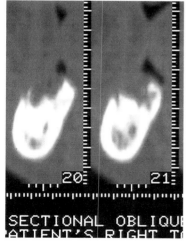
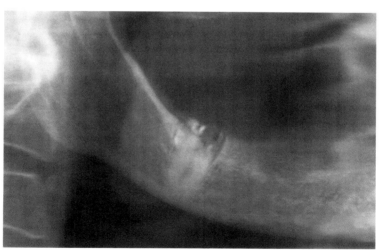

242 Severing the inferior alveolar nerve
Immediate reconstructive procedures have to be undertaken if the inferior alveolar nerve is severed. This radiograph depicts an impacted tooth 48.

Left: The coronal CT images indicate that the course of the mandibular canal runs between or through the roots of tooth 48.

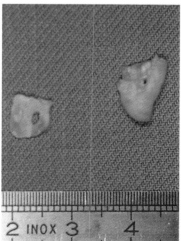
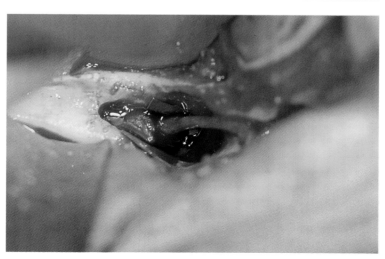

243 Nerve approximation
While the tooth was being extracted, the nerve was severed. On the same day, nerve reapproximation was attempted in a hospital setting. Three months postsurgically, sensitivity in the area was partially restored.

Left: The nerve had actually passed directly through the roots of tooth 48.

Mandibular Premolars and Canines

Indications for Extraction

Retention or impaction of premolars and canines occurs less frequently in the mandible than in the maxilla. It is usually the persistence of a deciduous tooth that reveals retention of its subjacent permanent counterpart. The reason for persistence of the deciduous tooth must be identified radiographically. The indication for removal must be established on a case-by-case basis. In an otherwise healthy young adult dentition, a retained tooth should be extracted if it becomes clear that there is no hope of bringing it into normal occlusion or if this is not indicated.

The position of the roots of the adjacent teeth should be taken into account, as well as any pathological alterations adjacent to or surrounding the retained tooth (e.g., sclerosis, cyst formation, or tumors). Often, the indication for extracting a retained tooth coincides with treatment for a pathological process in the jaw. It is usually advisable to consult an orthodontist regarding whether or not tooth extraction is necessary or recommended.

244 Anatomy of the mental nerve
There is a close relationship between the impacted premolar and the mandibular canal and the foramen, where the mental nerve exits from the alveolar process.

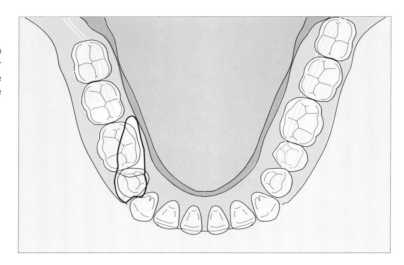

245 Floor of the mouth
This cadaver preparation shows the structures in the anterior portion of the floor of the mouth.

1 Anterior lingual artery
2 Duct of the submandibular gland
3 Mylohyoid muscle
4 Lingual nerve

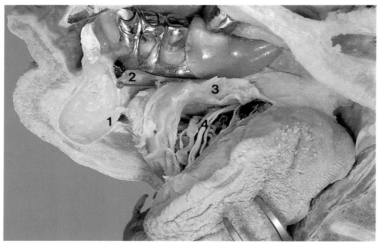

Surgical Procedure

Presurgical Documentation
The clinical examination should include examination of the teeth, vitality testing, periodontal pocket measurements, and soft-tissue palpation. The function and sensitivity of the mental nerve should be ascertained.

A panoramic radiograph is necessary to provide an overview for planning the surgical procedure. The precise location of the impacted tooth within the jawbone, and its positional relationship to adjacent teeth, are assessed using individual periapical radiographs taken in two directions (i.e., from mesial and distal).

Occlusal radiographs can provide additional information. Computed tomography may be necessary if radiographs fail to provide sufficient information.

The reason for extracting the tooth, and the details of the surgical procedure, including any attendant risks, must be discussed with the patient or his or her parents. If the case involves retained deciduous teeth, the longer-term consequences and possible treatment modalities should also be discussed.

Anatomy

The course of the inferior alveolar nerve and its site of exit through the mental foramen are important, and also the relationship of the crown and root of the impacted root to the adjacent teeth. If the impacted tooth is to be removed using a lingual approach, precise knowledge of the anatomical relationships of the musculature of the floor of the mouth and the contents of the lingual soft tissues is necessary.

Anesthesia

1. Block anesthesia of the mandibular nerve.
2. Infiltration anesthesia near the mental foramen.
3. Infiltration anesthesia in the buccal vestibule and into the floor of the mouth if the surgical approach is from the lingual.

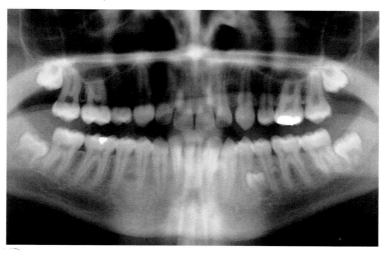

246 Documentation—panoramic radiograph
The panoramic radiograph provides an excellent overview, and is indispensable for assessing the indication for surgery, as well as in planning the procedure.

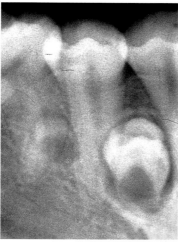 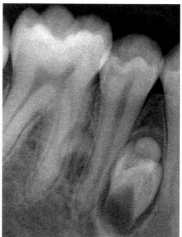

247 Positional determination
Radiographs taken using different central ray projections are necessary to determine the exact position of the impacted tooth, and for planning the surgical procedure.

Radiographs taken from distal and mesial angles show that the supernumerary tooth is positioned toward the lingual aspect of the adjacent tooth roots.

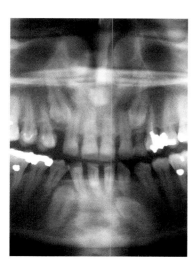 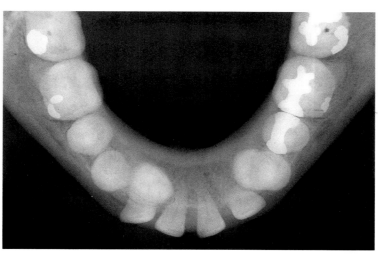

248 Occlusal film
A mandibular occlusal radiograph does not always show the precise position of the impacted tooth. In this film, the impacted mandibular canines are scarcely visible.

Left: This section from a panoramic radiograph clearly reveals the impacted canine.

Buccal Approach

If the impacted tooth is positioned buccally, access for the extraction procedure is achieved by reflecting a vestibular tissue flap, as described earlier (p. 66) for the removal of root tips. The releasing incisions in the vestibule must be kept distant from the mental foramen. Depending on the individual situation, the width of the tissue flap should extend from the canine region to the region of the first molar or beyond. The mental nerve should be carefully exposed as it exits the foramen. The nerve must be constantly protected using a periosteal elevator during the operation.

Lingual Approach

If the tooth is positioned lingually, access is achieved by means of an incision along the lingual gingival margin, extending from the anterior segment back to the molar region. Releasing incisions are normally not required. If additional mobilization of the flap toward the lingual is necessary, the marginal incision can be extended toward the opposite side of the arch.

Lingual position of the crown. The lingual soft tissues are reflected using an elevator held in direct contact with the bone, until visual access is adequate. A broad retractor is used to reflect the soft tissues toward the

249 Anesthesia
A unilateral block of the inferior alveolar nerve is carried out, as well as infiltration bilaterally near the mental foramina.

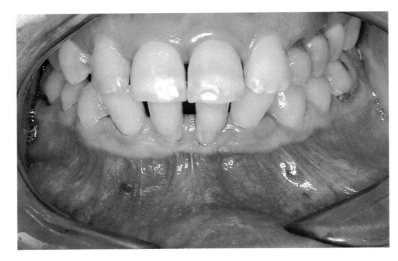

250 Buccal approach
Possible incision lines *(red)*. Care must be taken to avoid injuring the nerve where it exits from the mental foramen. Releasing incisions must be located in such a way as to avoid trauma to the mental nerve.

Right: View from the occlusal aspect.

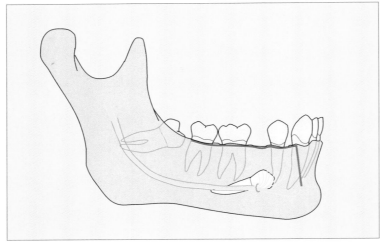
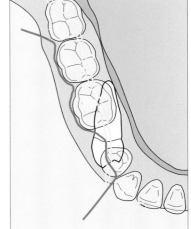

251 Flap design
For removal of a retained mandibular canine 43, a mucoperiosteal flap is created using an intrasulcal incision and a vertical releasing incision near the midline. The flap is carefully reflected in order to expose the mental nerve as it exits from the mental foramen; this ensures that it can be protected during the subsequent procedures.

Right: Radiograph showing the position of tooth 43. Note the close proximity of the crown to the root of tooth 42.

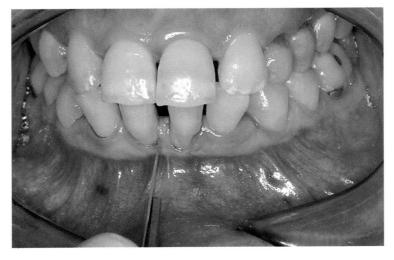
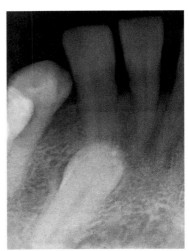

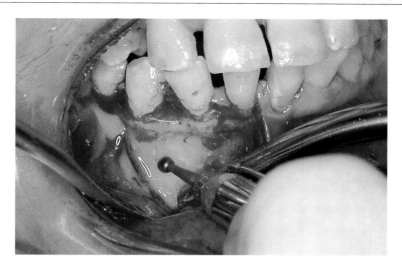

252 Tooth removal
A round bone cutter is used for ostectomy over the region of the impacted crown, exposing it. The mental nerve and surrounding soft tissues are protected using an elevator.

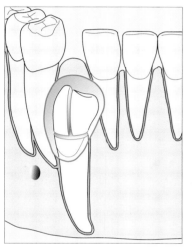
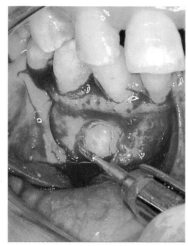
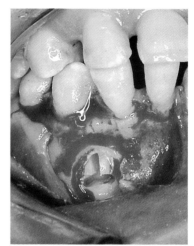

253 Sectioning the crown
Using a Lindemann bone cutter, the crown is sectioned *(right)* and separated from its root *(center)*.

Left: Sectioning the crown keep the ostectomy to a minimum.

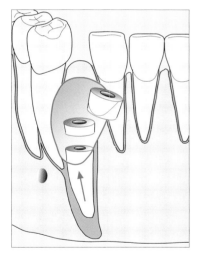
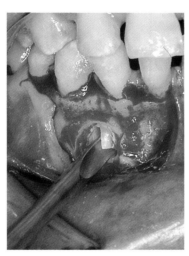
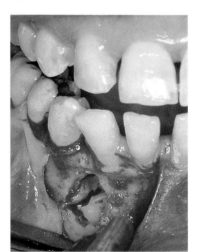

254 Root removal
The root is mobilized. The space that is created by removal of the crown is insufficient for removal of the remaining root in toto. However, in order to maintain the marginal alveolar bone and prevent any damage to adjacent teeth, no additional ostectomy should be performed. Instead, the root is simply lifted very carefully in its alveolus and removed in small slices.

Left: Slice-by-slice removal.

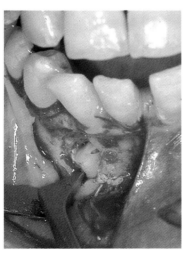
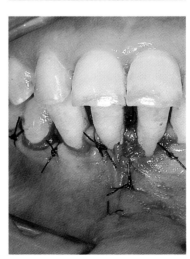

255 Wound closure
A small groove is made in the apical root segment to receive the beak of a Cryer elevator *(left)*. The root tip is removed, the surgical area is cleaned and rinsed, and the soft-tissue flap is then repositioned and secured using interrupted sutures.

tongue. A round bone cutter is used to open the intra-osseous space surrounding the crown. Depending on the position of the tooth, removal can be accomplished using either a straight elevator or the Cryer elevator.

In most cases, it is advantageous to separate the crown from the root.

Buccolingual position. The initial approach should provide access to the crown from the buccal or lingual approach, depending on the position of the tooth. With root types B and C, it may be necessary to open from both the buccal and lingual aspects. This results in a "tunnel-like" defect, which requires special treatment (described in the section on osseous defects).

Position subjacent to the apices of adjacent teeth. The buccal approach should be used, as it provides better visual access (caution: mental foramen).

Sharp bony margins should be smoothed, and any remnants of the follicle should be removed. Check whether adjacent roots have been exposed or injured.

Secure with interdental sutures.

Postoperative Care

Sutures are removed one week later. Sensation in the areas supplied by the mental nerve, as well as the vitality of the adjacent teeth, should be ascertained.

256 Lingual approach
The primary incision *(red line)*. With a lingual approach, vertical releasing incisions are usually not necessary, but the sulcal primary incision is carried further anteriorly to provide more extensive flap mobilization. Anesthesia is achieved as described in Fig. 94.

Right: This occlusal radiograph depicts the lingual location of the impacted tooth 44.

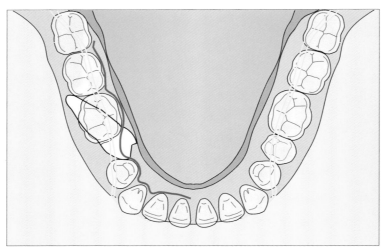
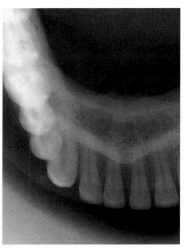

257 Flap mobilization
The sulcal primary incision extends from tooth 46 to tooth 32, allowing lingual flap reflection.

Right: Flap reflection, ostectomy, and sectioning of the crown.

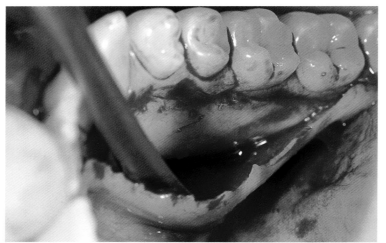
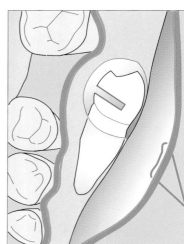

258 Tooth removal
The crown is exposed using a round burr, and sectioned using the straight elevator. After removal of the fragments, the wound is thoroughly cleaned, and the flap is replaced and secured with interrupted sutures.

Right: Severing the crown with a straight elevator.

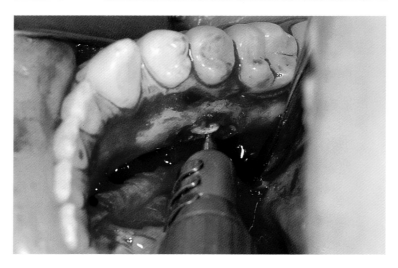
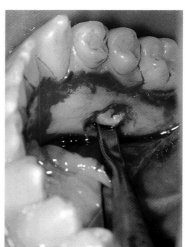

Potential Complications

If there is postoperative infection, some of the sutures are removed, and the wound is rinsed and drained. This procedure must be carried out daily until the signs of acute infection subside. The vitality of adjacent teeth should be checked to ensure that they are not affected by the infectiously involved.

Any disturbance of sensation in the region of V/3 must be carefully followed up during the healing phase. If the surgical procedure has been performed carefully, any hyposensitivity will be reversible.

Hemorrhage from the soft tissues of the floor of the mouth: Apply temporary compresses or ligate individual vessels if necessary. Caution: submandibular duct.

Hemorrhage from the mandibular canal: Gentle, temporary application of pressure. Check for possible nerve damage and document the course of healing.

Damage to adjacent tooth roots: If devitalization occurs, endodontics and root tip resection are performed.

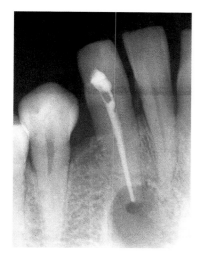 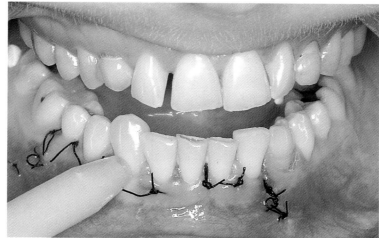

259 Complications—devitalization of adjacent teeth
During removal of the follicular sac around the impacted tooth, the apex of the root of tooth 43 was exposed. Subsequent examination, including a vitality test, showed that the tooth had been devitalized. A root canal treatment can be performed at the time of oral surgery if conditions allow it and the situation is stable.

Left: The radiograph shows adequate filling of the root canal of tooth 43.

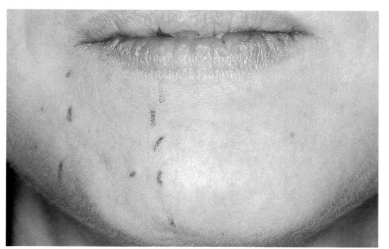

260 Disturbance of sensation
Occasionally, when the patient returns for suture removal, hypoesthesia may be found in the area of the chin innervated by the mental nerve. The affected region is outlined on the skin surface for documentation.

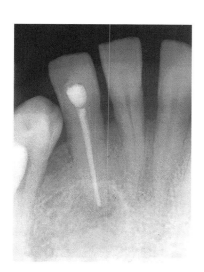 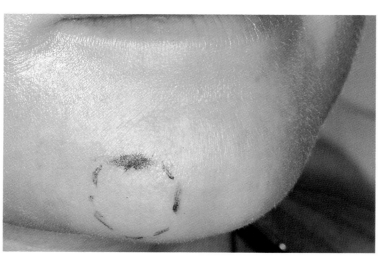

261 Subsequent appointment
An examination two weeks later showed that the area of desensitization had become significantly smaller, suggesting a favorable prognosis.

Left: A radiograph taken six months postoperatively shows normal healing at the apex of tooth 43.

Maxillary Third Molars

Indications for Extraction

Impaction of maxillary third molars is seen slightly less often than mandibular third molar impaction. This is probably mainly due to the more favorable spatial relationships in the maxilla. Maxillary third molars can deviate buccally. They are often found in this position, directly beneath the mucosa, or covered only by a paper-thin layer of bone over the crown. Because of this more favorable topography, the clinical symptoms of pericoronitis are observed less frequently in the maxilla. Depending on how severely the third molar is tipped, there may be close contact with the root of the second molar. Actual fusion of the roots of second and third molars is sometimes seen. The position and location of impacted maxillary third molars can also be given a general classification (types 1–6). There is particularly wide variation in the shape of the root, and it is often difficult to depict the root shape radiographically. A primary anatomical concern is the immediately adjacent maxillary sinus.

In general, the indications for removing mandibular third molars also apply in the maxilla.

Surgical Procedure

Documentation

In addition to clinical inspection, there should be radiographic examination including panoramic films and, if indicated, axial maxillary projections. With severe impactions, a lateral cephalometric radiograph or an anteroposterior skull film can provide additional topographical information. A computed tomogram can provide particularly useful information about the position of impacted teeth and their relationship to the adjacent structures. Standard periapical radiographs often provide precise details about root shape, location, and anatomical relationships.

> **Caution**
> In radiographs, the muscular process of the mandible is often superimposed over the maxillary tuberosity.

Anatomy
Adipose tissue will be encountered in the soft tissues of the buccal aspect, and further cranially lies the posterior superior alveolar artery. The palatine artery exits from the palatal foramen. Maxillary and nasal sinuse may be in close proximity.

262 Types of impaction
Left: **Type 1**—tooth bud.

Center: **Type 2**—incomplete root formation.

Right: **Type 3**—impaction with normal position and axis orientation.

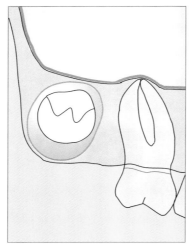
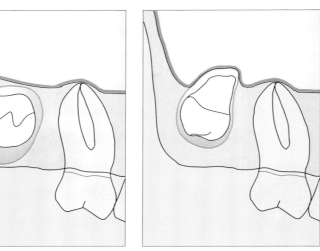
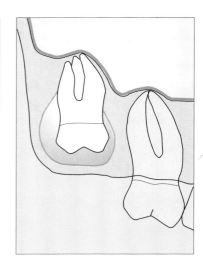

263 Types of impaction
Left: **Type 4**—mesially tipped tooth.

Center: **Type 5**—distally tipped tooth.

Right: **Type 6**—buccopalatal third molar impaction.

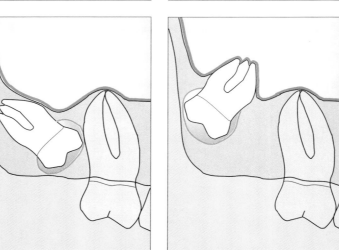
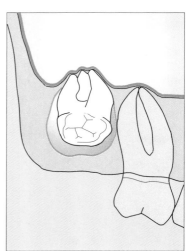

Anesthesia

1. Infiltration near the tuberosity.
2. Infiltration near the palatal foramen.
3. Vestibular infiltration anesthesia near the first molar, from the buccal approach.

Access

The primary incision should be made in such a way that tight wound closure of the osteotomy wound can be achieved. As the mucoperiosteal flap is reflected buccally, the buccal fat pad should be protected, since if the periosteum is severed, adipose tissue may extrude and make subsequent procedures more difficult. Further cranially, the posterior superior alveolar artery must be protected. Care must be taken while the third molar is being removed, since the second molar is probably in close proximity. The roots of these two teeth are often in quite intimate contact, and root fusions are possible.

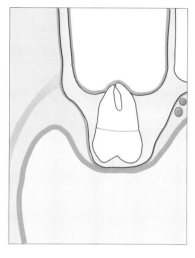

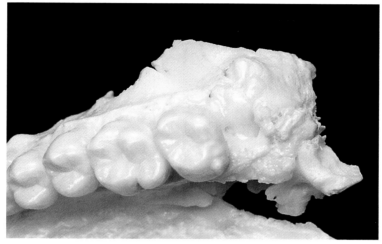

264 Anatomy
The osseous structure of the maxilla is characterized by thin cortical bone and coarse spongy (trabecular) bone. Impacted maxillary third molars are most often positioned with the crown toward the buccal aspect.

Left: Buccal positioning of the crown, covered by a thin layer of cortical bone on the buccal aspect.

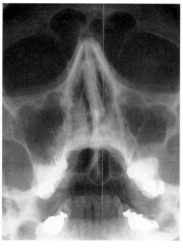

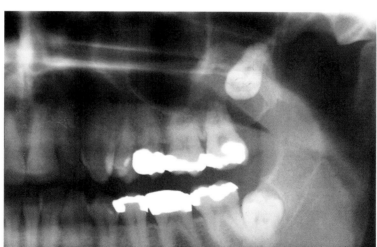

265 Documentation—radiography
A panoramic film is generally sufficient. A standard periapical radiograph often does not depict the relationship of the impacted tooth to the maxillary sinus.

Left: In special circumstances, an axial projection of the maxilla will provide additional information about the condition of the maxillary sinuses. In this film, note the spherical soft-tissue indurations at the base of the left maxillary sinus, representing signs of a follicular cyst at tooth 18.

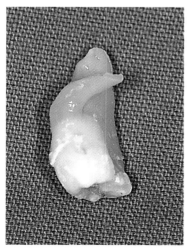

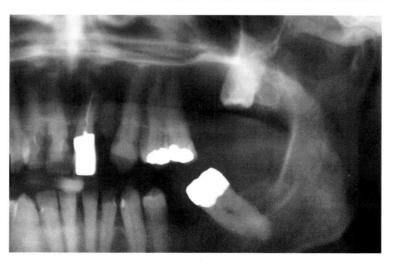

266 Root dilaceration
Radiographs do not always identify every detail of root form.

Left: The unusual root dilaceration in this maxillary third molar was not detected in the panoramic radiograph.

Tooth Extraction

Types 1 and 2:—The crown is approached from the buccal aspect. The Cryer elevator is engaged from the palatal direction, and the tooth is luxated toward the occlusal. The elevator must engage the crown completely on the palatal aspect, otherwise there is a danger of luxation into the maxillary sinus or into the vestibular soft tissues.

Type 3:—The impacted crown, exposed from the buccal approach, is engaged palatally with the Cryer elevator, and luxated distobuccally. The force applied to the elevator must *not* be directed only distally, since this is associated with a risk of fracturing the tuberosity.

If the roots of the impacted third molar are widely divergent, it is often advisable to section the tooth and remove the roots separately. This avoids the danger of small root fragments; such fragments might be forced into the maxillary sinus during further attempts to remove them.

267 Anesthesia
For removal of an impacted tooth 28, infiltration anesthesia is applied near the palatal foramen and in the vestibule near the tuberosity. In addition, anesthetic solution is injected high in the vestibule, apical to the first molar.

Right: This section from a panoramic radiograph clearly reveals the impacted third molar.

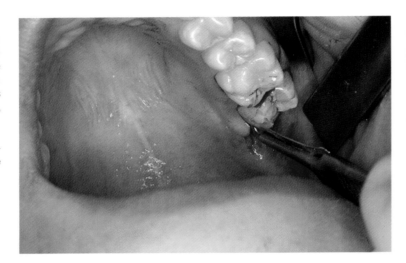
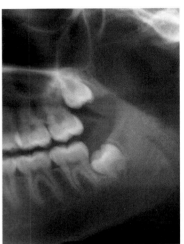

268 Access
The maxillary third molars are most often positioned with the crown facing in the buccal direction. Access is therefore usually achieved after reflecting a buccal flap.

Right: The primary incision *(arrowed red line)*.

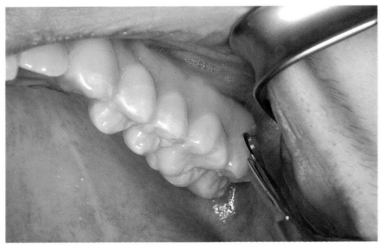
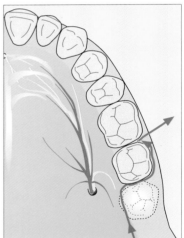

269 Creating the flap
The primary incision is made vertically, mesial to the second molar; the second incision is made intrasulcally around this tooth; and the third incision is over the maxillary tuberosity from the palatal direction *(see diagram above)*. This type of flap allows uncomplicated closure if the maxillary sinus is inadvertently opened.

Right: Reflecting the mucoperiosteal flap, originating at the line of the releasing incision.

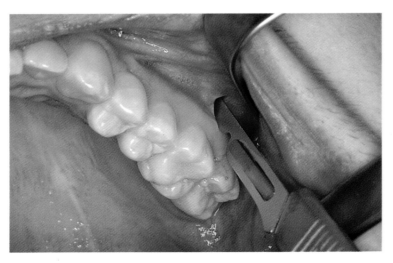
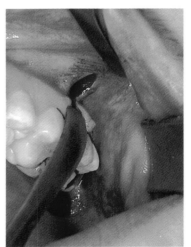

Types 4 and 5:—There is usually intimate contact with the second molar. It is strongly recommended to separate the crown from the root. The anatomical situation will determine whether the crown is removed first, or whether the root can be luxated to begin with. The force vector of the elevator is always directed from the apical toward the occlusal. If the tooth is severely impacted in a cranial position, opening the maxillary sinus and using the Cryer elevator from above may be the only solution.

Type 6:—It is always advisable to section the third molar if there is intimate contact with the second molar. If there is no contact, the Cryer elevator is used to luxate the third molar from the palatal direction.

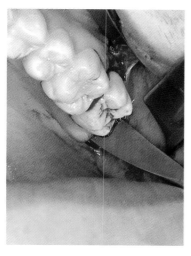 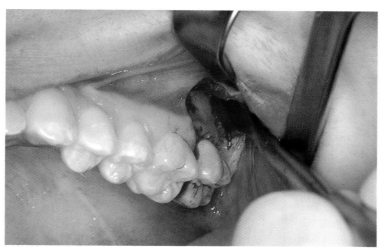

270 Ostectomy
A mucoperiosteal flap is reflected using an elevator, and kept free of the surgical site using a Langenbeck retractor. During the ostectomy procedure, the soft tissues are protected by placement of a periosteal elevator or metal tissue retractor.

Left: Using the flat periosteal elevator to release the mucoperiosteal tissues in the tuberosity region.

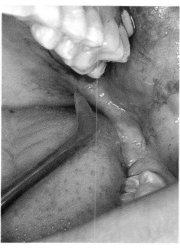 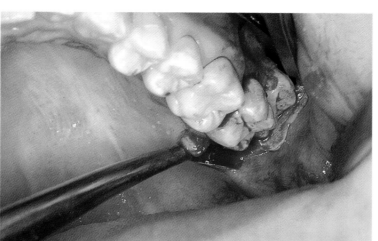

271 Tooth removal
Once an extraction pathway has been created toward the buccal direction, the tooth can be engaged from the palatal approach using the Cryer elevator, and dislodged distobuccally.

Left: Correct positioning of the Cryer elevator to engage the impacted third molar on its palatal surface.

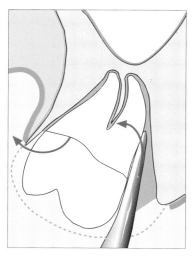 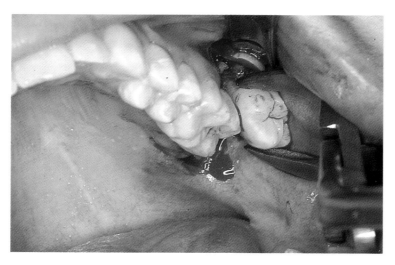

272 Protecting the soft tissues
The tooth is extracted using an appropriate forceps. During the extraction procedure, the retractor remains in place to prevent the tooth from becoming embedded in the soft tissues.

Left: The direction of tooth removal *(red arrows),* with palatal engagement of the elevator.

Eccentric Positions

Maxillary third molars are usually quite easy to locate via a vestibular approach. The problems associated with maxillary third molar extraction generally relate to the tooth roots, which are often very thin and severely dilacerated, and have a tendency to fracture. Additional difficulties may result from the lack of visual access due to the tightly restricted surgical field.

Third molars that are impacted in an extreme cranial position may be impossible to remove using the buccal approach. The removal of these teeth can be achieved by creating a vestibular window in the canine fossa toward the maxillary sinus.

Perforation of the nasal sinus is possible, and resulting hemorrhage is difficult to control. In cases in which the third molars are impacted beyond the boundaries of the alveolar process, surgical specialists must be called in. Cases of this type present too many risks to be treated on an outpatient basis.

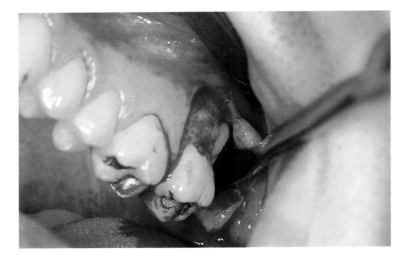 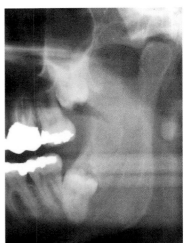

273 Divergent roots
If the maxillary third molar that is to be extracted has multiple, divergent roots, it is best to remove the crown first from a buccal approach, after ostectomy.

Right: A maxillary third molar with widely diverging roots.

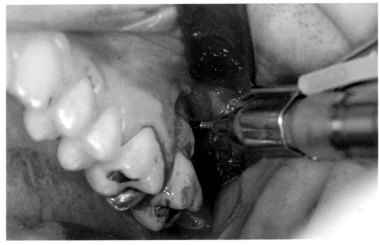

274 Sectioning the tooth
From a buccal approach, a groove is milled through the crown, which can then be separated using a straight elevator.

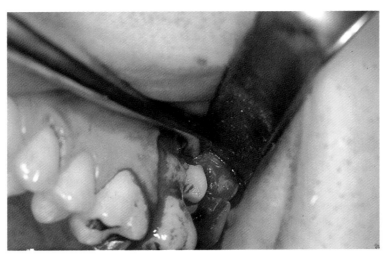

275 Separating the roots
If necessary, the roots can be multiply segmented and removed piece by piece using the Cryer elevator or a straight elevator. (Caution: do not force the roots into the maxillary sinus).

Wound Treatment

Opening of the sinus can be ruled out by carefully checking the extraction site with a large, blunt probe, and by having the patient hold the nose and blow.

Sharp bony margins are smoothed, and any remnants of the follicular sac are excised without damaging the periodontium of the second molar. Tissue flaps are repositioned and affixed using interrupted sutures vestibularly and across the maxillary tuberosity. If the sinus has been opened, wound closure should be especially tight. The patient should be advised to leave the mouth open when sneezing.

Antibiotic coverage is indicated if there is any potential for developing emphysema.

In contrast to the mandible, the bone of the maxilla is primarily trabecular, very well vascularized, and covered by a thin cortical plate.

Postoperative Care

It is not necessary to treat the wound daily. The patient should be recalled one week after the operation for removal of the sutures.

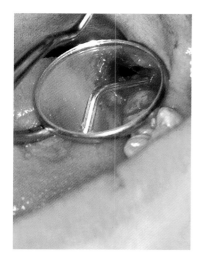
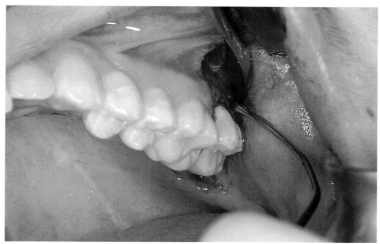

276 Wound debridement
The alveolus is cleaned, and any sharp bony margins are smoothed. A blunt probe is used to determine whether the maxillary sinus has been perforated.

Left: A mirror and a probe are used to inspect the extraction site and determine whether the adjacent tooth has been compromised.

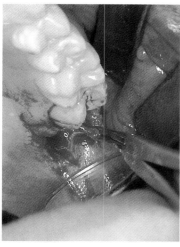
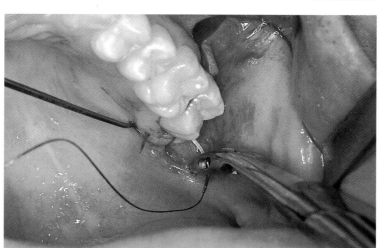

277 Dental sac
The soft-tissue flaps are repositioned and sutured palatally, distal to the second molar.

Left: A hemostat is used to remove remnants of the follicular sac.

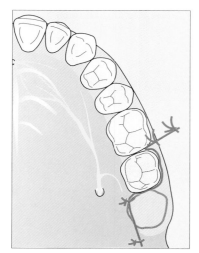
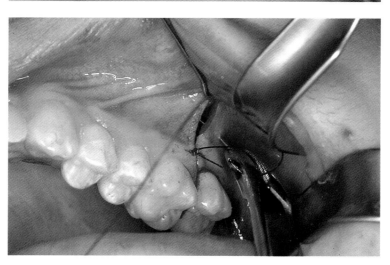

278 Suture closure
Additional sutures are used to close the vertical releasing incision. If the maxillary sinus has been opened, additional sutures should be placed to ensure tight closure of the wound.

Left: This diagram depicts suture placement for secure wound closure.

Potential Complications

Complications during the Operation

During the surgical procedure, hemorrhage from the soft tissues may occur in the region of the tuberosity. Since visual access in this area is severely limited, the primary treatment consists of applying compresses to the vestibular soft tissues to achieve hemostasis. If a vessel has been injured, ligation using resorbable suture material may be necessary.

If the maxillary sinus has been opened, extra care must be taken to ensure proper flap repositioning and tight suture closure. If the flap has to be extended by severing the periosteum, the buccal adipose tissue may extrude, and it has to be repositioned. During this procedure, the suction device should not be used, as it tends to encourage mobilization of the adipose tissue.

The distal root surface of the second molar can be exposed during extraction of the third molar. If simultaneous opening of the maxillary sinus does not occur, the osseous defect can be compensated by application of lyophilized cartilage (see p. 307, osseous defects).

279 Complications—extrusion of buccal adipose tissue
Care must be taken when using the suction device, since it may pull out the adipose tissue lying loosely in the surrounding connective tissue. If this occurs, the fatty tissue is carefully repositioned, and the wound is closed in the usual way.

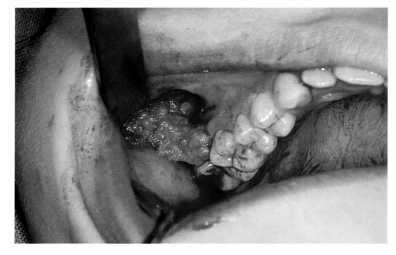

280 Tuberosity fracture
If the distal portion of the tuberosity is fractured away during tooth removal, it is likely that the maxillary sinus has been perforated. If the bony fragment remains attached to its periosteum, it can be repositioned and securely attached beneath the tissue flap. Bony fragments that are completely detached are removed, and the soft tissues are used to cover the defect.

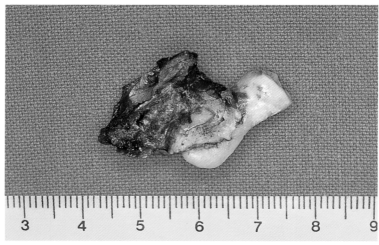

281 Root fusion
In these cases, third molar extraction cannot be carried out without damaging the adjacent second molar, and both teeth usually have to be extracted. This risk should be explained to the patient before surgery, so as to avoid any legal problems.

Right: The radiograph shows virtual confluence of teeth 28 and 27.

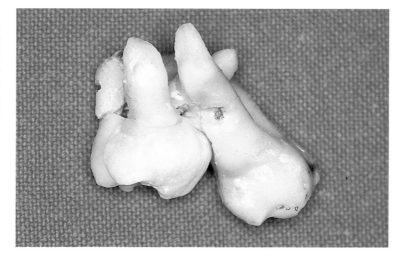

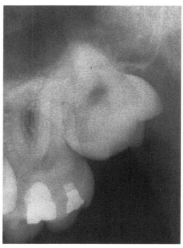

If fracture of the tuberosity occurs, the bony fragments can be repositioned and stabilized using the sutured tissue flaps. Small bony fragments are removed.

If the tooth is forced into the sinus cavity, it must be immediately removed, or the patient must be referred to a specialist. Antibiotic coverage is indicated.

If the tooth is dislocated in the vestibular direction, additional radiographs must be taken to precisely locate it, and it should be removed immediately; it may be necessary to refer the patient to a specialist. If it is not possible to remove the tooth on the same day, antibiotic administration is imperative.

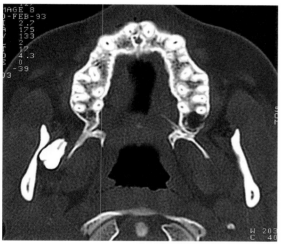
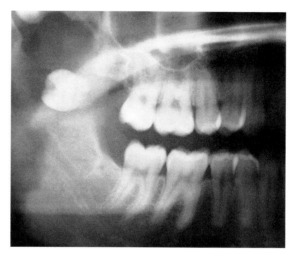

282 Dislocations
It is advisable to refer the patient to a specialist if a displaced tooth cannot be immediately located and mobilized.

Left: The CT clearly reveals the third molar between the ascending ramus of the mandible and the lateral pterygoid process.

Right: The radiograph shows the dislocated tooth 28 positioned within the infratemporal fossa, in a 22-year-old woman.

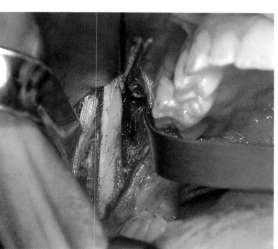
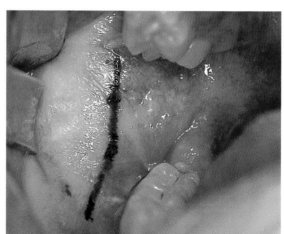

283 Removal from the infra-temporal fossa
Left: In an exploratory procedure, the soft tissues are reflected. The tooth is located by touch using a blunt probe.

Right: With the patient under general anesthesia, an incision is made parallel to the ascending ramus of the mandible.

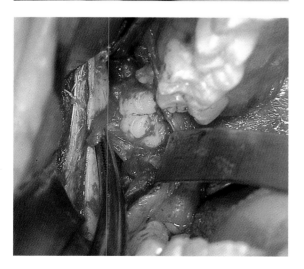
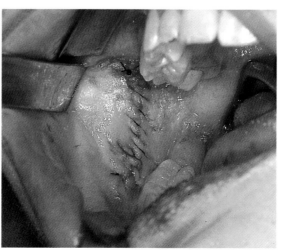

284 Extraction and wound closure
Left: The tooth is removed using a diamond-coated forceps or clamp.

Right: Very careful closure of the soft-tissue wound.

Postoperative Complications

Infection may occur following the surgical procedure. Infections should be treated as described on page 155.

If a hematoma develops, a suture should be removed to allow rinsing and drainage.

> **Caution**
> Do not use a high-velocity suction tip, as the buccal adipose tissue might be aspirated. Antibiotic coverage is indicated.

If there is emphysema—for example, after the maxillary sinus has been opened due to excessive pressure in the nasopharyngeal area (sneezing, nose blowing)—the patient must be informed about this situation in order to allay any fears. Again, an antibiotic regimen is indicated.

285 Infections
Formation of abscesses can be expected after lengthy surgical procedures involving traumatization of the soft tissues or hematoma formation. Abscesses can spread into the retromaxillary infratemporal fossa and even into the orbit (p. 145). Situations of this type require immediate surgical intervention.

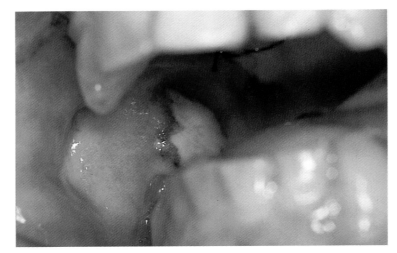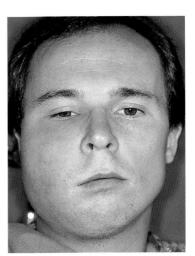

286 Development of emphysema
If the sinus cavities are opened, and especially if the periosteum is severed, air can escape into the soft tissues. The patient will experience a sensation of pressure, rapidly developing swelling, and a typical crackling sound (crepitus) on palpation. This CT shows extensive areas of air in the soft tissue in the midfacial region on the left side.

Right: This patient blew his nose a few hours after the extraction of tooth 28, and experienced sudden swelling of the soft tissues on the left side of the face.

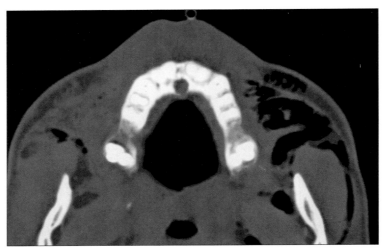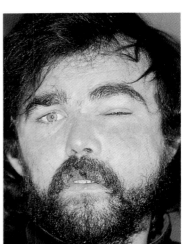

Maxillary Premolars and Canines

Indications for Extraction

Impaction or retention of maxillary canines is the most frequent form of impaction after third molars. Less frequently, the maxillary premolars may be impacted within the maxilla. The indication for removing these impacted teeth may vary from one case to another. Extraction may be indicated because of a retained deciduous tooth. Any attendant pathology must be clarified. In some cases, it may be possible to bring the impacted tooth into functional occlusion by ortho-dontic means. With young patients, consultation with an orthodontist is advisable.

In all cases, preoperative measures will include precise determination of the location and position of the impacted tooth, definitive diagnosis of any accompanying pathological conditions, and providing the patient—or, in the case of children, the patient's parents—with full clarification and information.

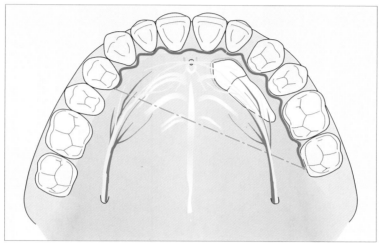

287 Impacted maxillary canine—anatomy
The primary incision *(red line)* in the gingival sulcus on the palatal aspect, for creation of the mucoperiosteal flap. Note the anatomical position of the major palatine artery and the accompanying nerves.

The incisal artery and nerve will be severed as the flap is reflected; coagulation may be necessary to stop any hemorrhage.

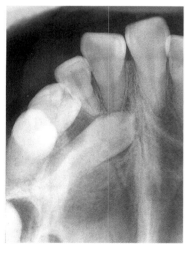
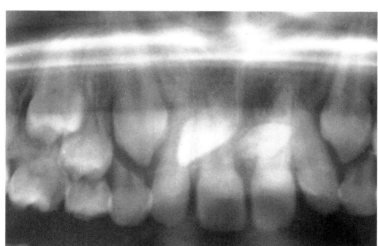

288 Documentation—panoramic radiograph
Diagnosis and planning for the surgical procedure must be accomplished using radiographs, including a panoramic film as well as periapical films.

Left: This maxillary occlusal projection shows the impacted canine clearly.

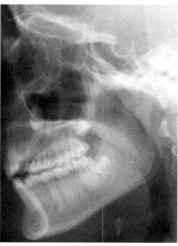
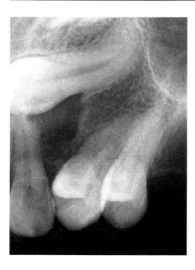
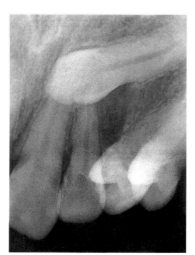

289 Location
Left: In extreme cases, a lateral cephalometric radiograph may provide additional information; for example, the impacted tooth 21 in this case is lying immediately subjacent to the floor of the nose.

Center: Periapical radiograph taken from a distal angle.

Right: Periapical radiograph taken from a mesial angle. By comparing the two radiographs, it can be seen that the impacted tooth is located palatal to the roots of teeth 22 and 24.

Surgical Procedure

Documentation

The relationship between the impacted tooth and the roots of the adjacent teeth must be clarified radiographically. A panoramic radiograph provides a broad overview, which can be enhanced by lateral cephalometric films and axial projections of the maxilla. Periapical radiographs taken with the central ray projected from the mesial or distal aspect will provide information about the exact position of the impacted tooth in the vestibulopalatal dimension. An occlusal radiograph of the maxilla can provide additional information.

Anatomy

The spatial relationships among the impacted tooth and the floor of the nose and the maxillary sinuses, as well as the incisal canal, the palatal foramen, the course of the palatine artery, and the position of the infraorbital foramen, must be taken into account.

Anesthesia

1. Infiltration near the infraorbital nerve, bilaterally.
2. Infiltration near the palatal foramen.
3. Infiltration at the incisal foramen.

The impacted tooth may be vital.

290 Access from the palatal aspect
This 23-year-old man presented with palatal impactions of teeth 13 and 23.

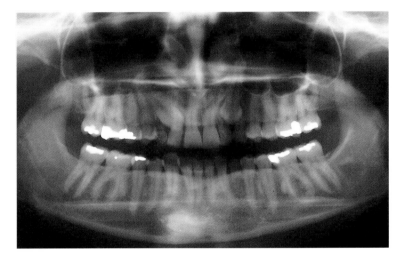

291 Determining the position
The periapical radiograph and the occlusal film *(right)* provide sufficient information to determine that the impacted tooth is positioned palatally.

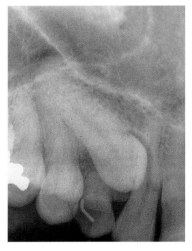
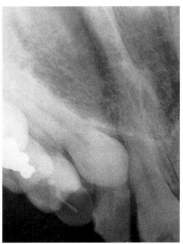
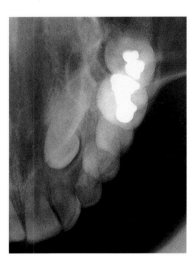

292 Anesthesia and access
Anesthetic solution is infiltrated bilaterally at the palatal foramen, with additional infiltration at the incisal foramen, and block anesthesia of the infraorbital nerve on the right side. The mucoperiosteal flap is outlined by an intrasulcal primary incision extending from the first molar to the canine on the palatal aspect of the maxilla.

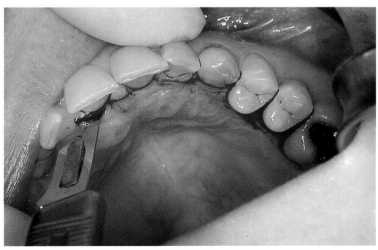

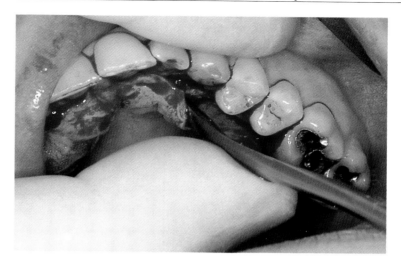

293 Flap reflection
As the palatal flap is being reflected, the tip of the elevator should be kept in direct contact with bone at all times. The palatine artery courses within the mobilized flap.

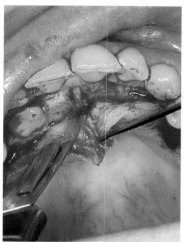
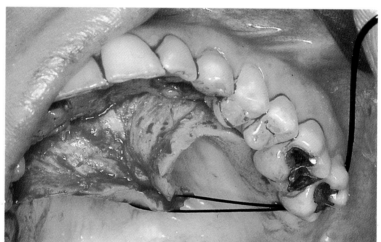

294 Incisal nerve
A 2–0 silk suture (Vicryl) is used to keep the palatal flap clear of the surgical site.

The tiny neurovascular bundle emanating from the incisal foramen is severed *(left)*; any resulting hemorrhage is staunched by applying pressure, or electrosurgically.

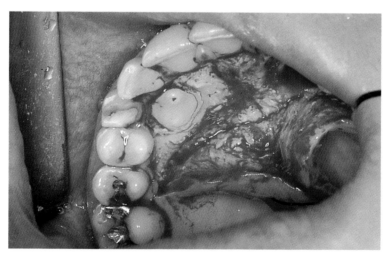

295 Ostectomy
A round burr is used to remove bone overlying the impacted crown.

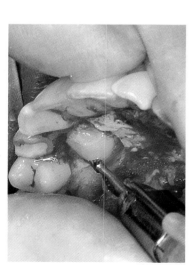
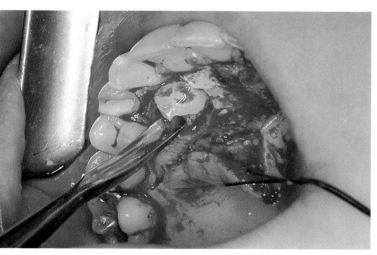

296 Tooth extraction
The crown is first notched deeply using a fissure burr *(left)*, and it is then snapped off by forceful application of the straight elevator. The proximity of the roots of adjacent teeth must be taken into account.

Access for Palatal Impactions

The primary intrasulcal incision extends from the palatal aspect of the canine on the opposite side to the first molar on the working side. Flap reflection must include the periosteum, in order to avoid injury to branches of the palatine artery. Special care is needed when working near the palatal foramen. The small neurovascular bundle emanating from the incisal foramen is severed.

A round bone cutter is used to expose the crown of the impacted tooth, and the crown is then sectioned using a carbide fissure burr. If the impacted crown is located near the crestal margin, it may be necessary to divide the crown into several smaller pieces, to avoid destroying the narrow bony margin.

The root is exposed and extracted using the Cryer elevator.

A hemostat is used with great care to remove any remnants of the follicle, but without damaging adjacent tooth roots.

The surgical site is cleaned and carefully inspected for the presence of any bony pockets or root exposures.

297 Ostectomy
It is usually necessary to carry out additional ostectomy around the root before it can be engaged by the elevator.

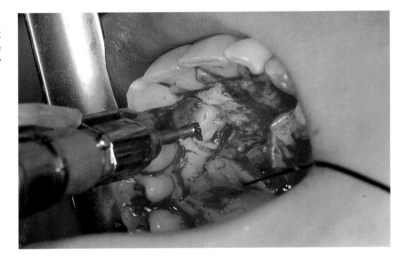

298 Root extraction
The luxated root is removed using a hemostat or a small root forceps.

Right: The root must be inspected to make sure that the apex is intact.

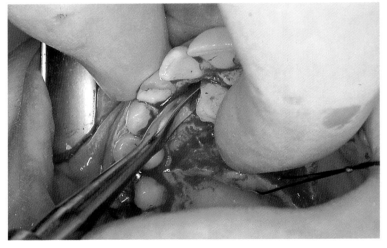
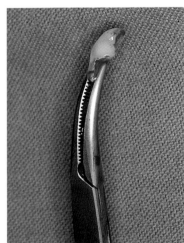

299 Wound treatment
After removal of any remnants of the follicular sac, the surgical site is inspected for any encroachment into the nasal or maxillary sinuses, exposed root surfaces, or a bony pocket communicating with the surgical defect.

Right: A hemostat is used carefully to remove the follicular sac, without destroying the marginal osseous bridge.

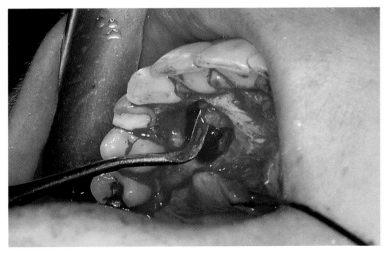
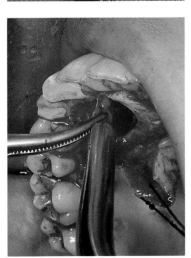

Palatal Wound Closure and Dressing

The soft-tissue flap is repositioned and secured with interrupted interdental sutures. Hematoma formation and the attendant risk of infection can be avoided by applying pressure to the site. Young patients can be instructed to use the thumb to apply pressure to the roof of the mouth during the first hour after surgery to prevent hematoma formation. A custom-made palatal plate is an excellent aid in the prevention of palatal hematoma, and can also assist with compression if postoperative hemorrhage occurs. A palatal plate is indicated for adults and for less cooperative children. If a palatal plate has not been fabricated, gauze squares can be pressed onto the palate and secured tightly with sutures. This type of compress should be inspected 24 hours later and removed for reasons of hygiene.

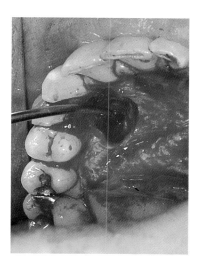
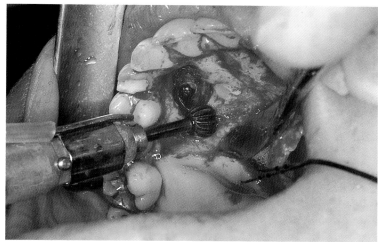

300 Wound cleaning
After the surgical site has been rinsed and inspected, any sharp bony margins are removed, with copious rinsing. The palatal flap is then repositioned.

Left: Inspecting and rinsing the surgical site.

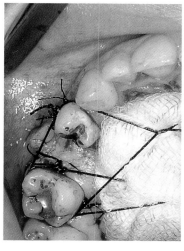
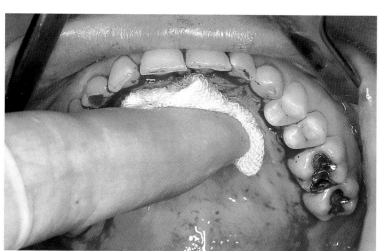

301 Compression
To prevent hematoma formation, the flap is compressed against the bone.

Left: A thick piece of gauze can be attached with sutures, as shown here.

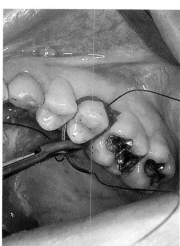
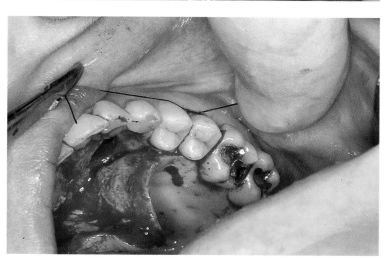

302 Suture closure
The flap is secured using sling sutures or mattress suturing around the teeth *(left)*.

Right: The sutures should be knotted on the buccal aspect.

303 Palatal plate
A palatal plate with retentive clasps can be used postsurgically to apply pressure on the palate, to prevent hematoma formation and reduce the risk of infection. The transparent plate allows visual inspection of the wound. The patient must remove the plate in the evening, clean it thoroughly and perform routine oral hygiene before reinserting the plate. The plate should also be cleaned after each meal.

Right: Clinical view after suture placement.

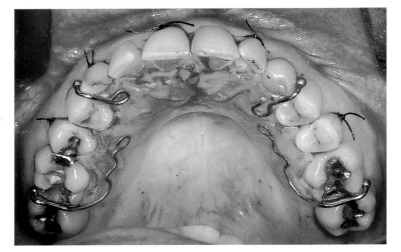 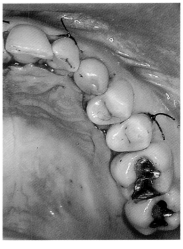

304 Follow-up
At an early check-up on the third day after surgery, the palatal plate is removed and the wound is cleaned. During the healing phase, patients may be more comfortable if they continue to wear the palatal plate, but it must be removed and cleaned, along with brushing the teeth, after every meal.

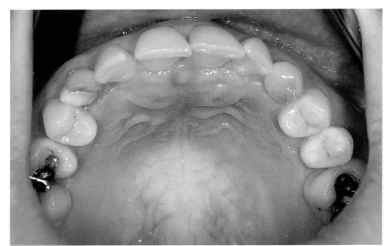

305 Suture removal
One week after surgery, the sutures are removed and the teeth are tested for vitality. In special cases, radiographic evaluation of bone regeneration in the defect is indicated.

Right: Radiographic view six months postsurgically.

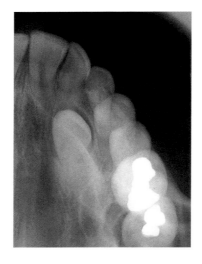 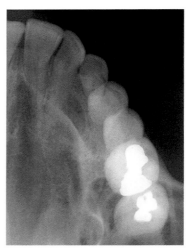

Making a Palatal Plate

The acrylic palatal plate to prevent hematoma formation under a palatal mucoperiosteal flap should be constructed before the operation. Simple alginate impressions of the maxilla and mandible are needed. The plate is made using prefabricated components (ball-end clasps) and transparent, autopolymerizing resin.

With the plate in situ after the operation, it should be possible to visualize the surgical area through the plate. The plate is not removed during the first two postoperative days. Oral hygiene during this period should be enhanced with a disinfecting (antimicrobial) mouthwash. After two days, the plate can be removed and then reinserted as necessary, e.g., when eating.

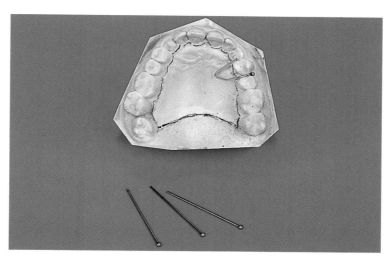

306 Materials used in making a palatal plate
A stone model, autopolymerizing resin, and clasp wires are required. The ball-end wires are bent into the configurations necessary for adequate retention, and attached to the plaster model with sticky wax. For stability, four clasps are usually incorporated two between the premolars bilaterally, and two between the molars bilaterally.

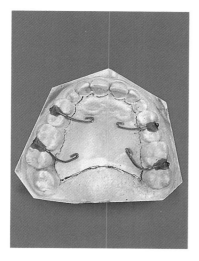

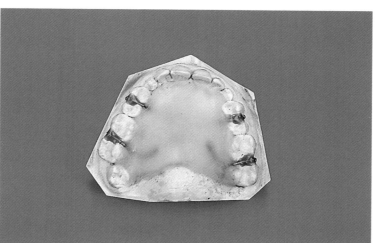

307 Application of resin
Transparent, autopolymerizing resin is applied to the palatal surface to create a plate about 2 mm thick.

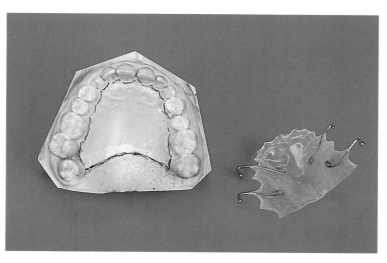

308 Finishing
The plate is finished using conventional laboratory methods, and then polished to a high gloss.

Access from a Vestibular Approach

The surgical approach here is the same as that described for removing retained root tips: a primary intrasulcal incision and two lateral releasing incisions. The flap should be wide enough to provide adequate visual access during the procedure and to ensure that suture closure will occur on an osseous base.

If the tooth is impacted horizontally, i.e., with the long axis lying in a faciopalatal orientation, the initial surgical approach should access the crown first. If the roots are severely dilacerated, it may be necessary to open from the palatal aspect as well.

This results in a tunnel-like defect, which is treated by implantation of lyophilized cartilage (see under osseous defects, p. 307).

Postoperative Care

The patient should be seen three days postoperatively to check for the possibility of palatal hematoma formation; the wound is rinsed and drained as necessary. Sutures can be removed after one week. The vitality of all the teeth in the vicinity of the surgical procedure must be ascertained.

309 Vestibular approach—documentation
The panoramic radiograph shows that tooth 11 is impacted near the anterior nasal spine. Precise location of these teeth can be achieved using a maxillary occlusal film and a lateral cephalometric radiograph. The case presented here resulted from trauma when the patient was nine years old. An orthodontist was able to close the space by moving tooth 12. The impacted tooth 11 could be palpated high in the vestibulum.

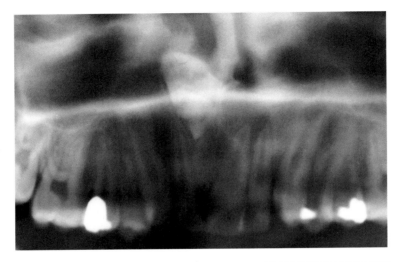

310 Anesthesia and access
Infiltration anesthesia of the right infraorbital nerve, infiltration in the vestibulum near tooth 11 and on the opposite side, as well as infiltration at the incisal foramen. The floor of the nose is also treated with a topical anesthetic.

Right: The flap is defined by an intrasulcal incision and bilateral vertical releasing incisions distal to teeth 12 and 21. Note that the thumb is used to prevent slipping as the flap is reflected using an elevator.

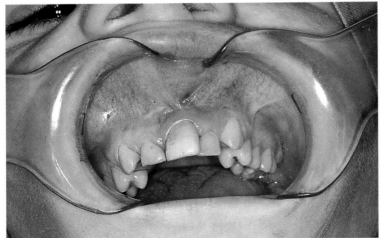
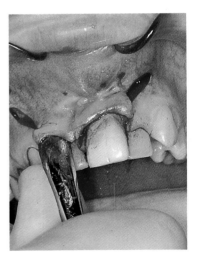

311 Flap reflection
When the flap is fully reflected, the protuberance of the cortical bone near tooth 11 can be visualized.

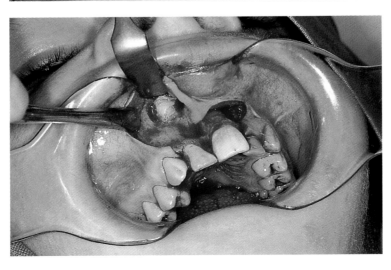

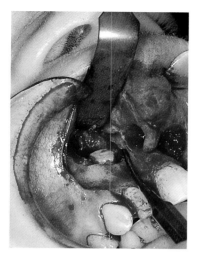

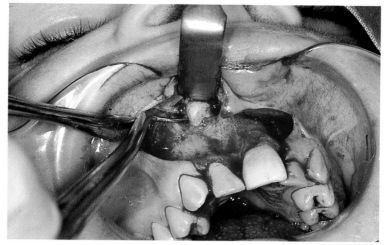

312 Tooth luxation
The crown is uncovered by ostectomy, and the tooth is then luxated using a Cryer elevator.

Left: Here, a Black excavator is used carefully for initial luxation.

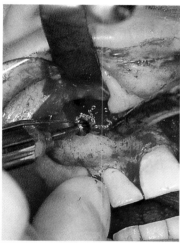

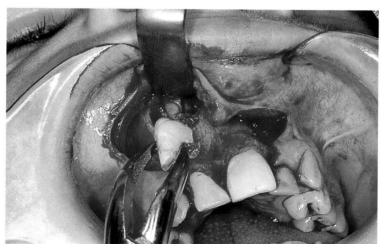

313 Tooth removal
A forceps with diamond-coated beaks is used to remove the partially developed tooth.

Left: The bony margins are smoothed.

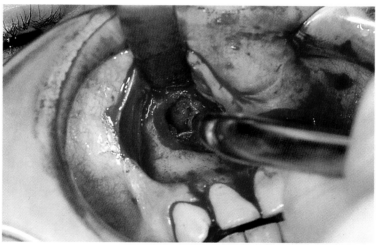

314 Inspection
After removing all the remnants of the follicular sac, the wound is inspected for possible perforation into the nasal cavity.

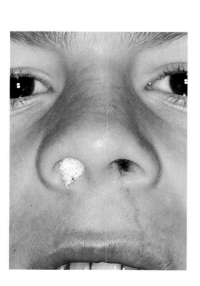

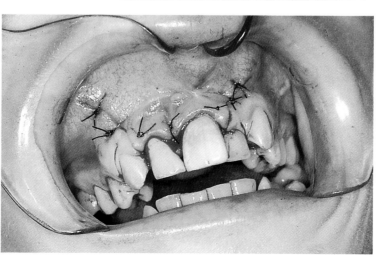

315 Wound closure
The flap is repositioned, and interrupted sutures are placed to close the releasing incisions; sling sutures are then used to approximate the gingival margins around the teeth.

Left: Because of the possibility of hemorrhage, a piece of Vaseline-coated gauze is placed at the front of the nostril.

Complications

Complications during the Surgical Procedure

If hemorrhage occurs from the palatal soft tissues due to injury of branches of the palatine artery, the vessel should either be coagulated or ligated using resorbable sutures.

If hemorrhage occurs from the palatal foramen, the bone is crushed using the closed end of a hemostat.

Compression may also be used to staunch hemorrhage directly from the surgical site. Caution should be exercised when adjacent roots are in close proximity.

No special procedures are indicated if the maxillary sinus is inadvertently opened. The patient should be informed that some slight bleeding from the nose is possible. A fistula via the surgical defect must be ruled out during postoperative appointments.

Similarly, no special treatment procedures are required for inadvertent opening through the floor of the nose. If bleeding from the nose is a problem, a Vaseline-coated gauze strip may be placed for two or three days. The patient should be fully informed about the situation.

Damage to adjacent teeth: if devitalization is confirmed, endodontic therapy should be instituted immediately. If there is any doubt about possible devitalization, a wait-and-see approach can be adopted.

With expansive osseous defects in the cervical region and completely exposed roots, extra care must be taken to ensure that the mucoperiosteal flap is securely repositioned. In some cases, it will be possible to fill the bony defect with lyophilized cartilage. In any case, the prognosis for the tooth is questionable. The situation must be reappraised six months postsurgically, and appropriate further measures undertaken.

Complications after the Operation

If a hematoma develops in spite of careful procedures, a few sutures are removed and the site is rinsed. Applying pressure to the palate using gauze or a palatal plate should inhibit any new hematoma formation.

Postoperative infections are managed by rinsing and drainage. This is repeated daily until all clinical symptoms subside.

Following an infection, a fistula to the maxillary or nasal sinus may remain. If the fistulous tract is long, it is usually adequate to freshen up (de-epithelialize) the wound and place a simple suture. In other cases, it may be necessary to initiate a reconstructive procedure to close the fistula.

A fortunately rare complication is necrosis of the palatal flap. It is possible that this complication results from disturbance of the blood supply. The necrotic tissues are carefully removed, and the wound is allowed to heal by secondary intention under an iodoform–Vaseline gauze drain. If there is also an open connection to the maxillary or nasal sinuses, surgical closure of the defect using a slide tissue flap may be attempted.

Recovery of Impacted Teeth

Definition

The term "recovery" is used here to refer to surgical exposure of the crown of an impacted tooth and attachment of a traction sling to it, in an attempt to move the impacted tooth along its normal path of eruption. This has also been termed "forced eruption."

Indications

Treatment planning is normally carried out in collaboration with an orthodontist (Hotz 1970). The more important issue for the surgeon is therefore possible contraindications. In most cases, the aim will be to bring into alignment a permanent tooth that is positioned in an inappropriate direction of eruption. In some cases, this will involve ruling out possible ankylosis. Often, this can only be ascertained once the crown of the impacted tooth has been surgically exposed. In cases of partial ankylosis, it is sometimes helpful to luxate the tooth slightly before attaching the retraction device to force proper eruption. Impacted teeth are often malpositioned. This requires surgical exposure, attachment of a button to transfer the orthodontic forces, and an open eruption path.

Surgical Procedure

The surgical approach is identical to that used for the extraction of impacted teeth (Bull et al. 1976, Lentrodt and Zentner 1976). The recommended procedure today is to attach the wire ligature to a button that is attached to the tooth using light-cured acrylic; effective hemostasis in the surgical field is therefore necessary. Applying pressure, tamponade, infiltration of local anesthetic solution, hydrogen peroxide rinses, and electrocoagulation may be attempted. Effective hemostasis directly around the crown can be achieved using retraction cord that has been impregnated with epinephrine.

The entire surface of the crown must be exposed. The periodontal fibers must be protected. Bone in the area of the alveolar process at the anticipated eruption site should be removed by ostectomy.

The "eruption canal" that has been created is kept patent by placing iodoform–Vaseline strips. It is very important to note the positions of the adjacent roots and to protect them.

Caution
Epinephrine treatment may cause cardiovascular collapse.

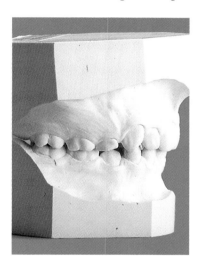

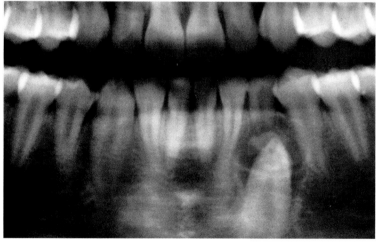

316 Planning
Indications for the procedure are assessed and comprehensive planning is carried out in collaboration between the dentist, orthodontist, and oral surgeon. Panoramic radiographs are absolutely necessary to locate the tooth precisely. This panoramic film shows an impacted tooth 33 with cystic, pericoronal osteolysis.

Left: Study models are used for planning both the surgical and the orthodontic procedures.

Documentation
The patient's chart should include a clear statement of the therapeutic goals. A thorough evaluation will require a panoramic radiograph and periapical films of the impacted tooth; these will provide the dentist with information about the stage of root development of the tooth concerned, as well as its precise location.

Anatomy
During surgery, due caution must be exercised with regard to the individual anatomy when creating the access and exposing the crown of the impacted tooth. In the mandible, beware of the mental foramen.

Anesthesia
Local injection anesthesia is applied as appropriate for the surgical site. Soft-tissue anesthesia is often sufficient.

Access in the Maxilla

Traction for Recovery from the Buccal Aspect

Whenever possible, the buccal approach should be selected, since it provides better visual access and it is considerably easier to isolate against moisture.

The crown is exposed after reflection of a buccal mucoperiosteal flap, and a dry surgical field is established. Careful ostectomy is performed to expose the impacted crown without damaging the tooth itself.

Following the directions of the orthodontist, the anchoring button for the wire sling is affixed to the coronal surface. The wire itself passes beneath the repositioned soft-tissue flap, where it is fastened to an adjacent tooth or to an orthodontic bracket so as not to traumatize the mucosa.

317 Forced eruption in the maxilla—buccal approach
The patient is a 16-year-old boy with an impacted tooth 13, which is located buccally. A panoramic radiograph provides a good overview of the entire masticatory apparatus.

Right: This periapical radiograph reveals the impacted tooth 13, which will be exposed for forced eruption.

Ⓢ

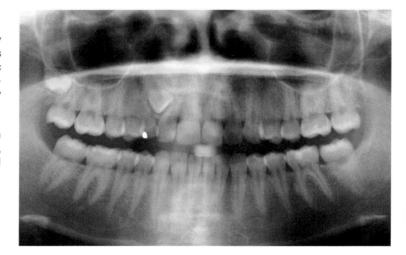
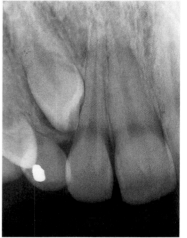

318 Anesthesia and access
An interarch space for tooth 13 is created orthodontically. In most cases, simple infiltration anesthesia on the buccal and palatal aspects is sufficient. Access to the crown of tooth 13 is achieved in this case using an arcuate incision in the buccal soft tissues.

Right: The periapical radiograph shows that adequate space has been created orthodontically.

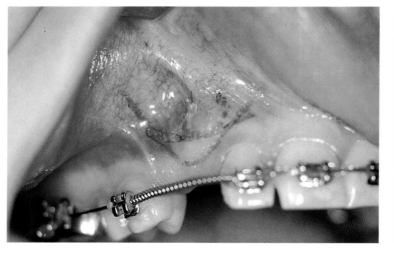
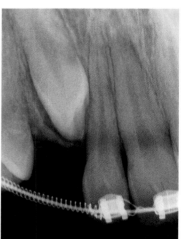

319 Exposing the crown
A round burr has been used on the buccal aspect to expose the crown of the impacted tooth. Caution must be exercised to avoid damaging the enamel surface.

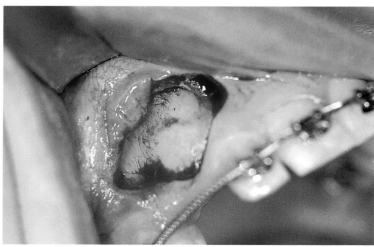

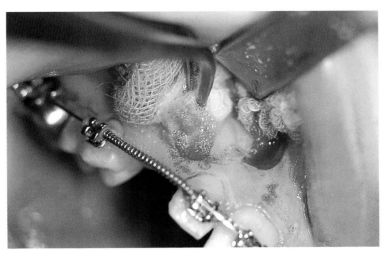

320 Hemostasis
The surgical site is dried by application of the electrotome, followed by swabbing with hydrogen peroxide.

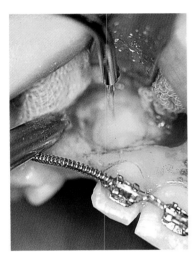

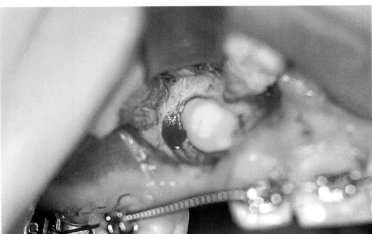

321 Cauterizing the enamel
The dried surface of the tooth crown is cauterized.

Left: After thorough rinsing with water, and subsequent drying, the chalky-colored enamel surface becomes visible.

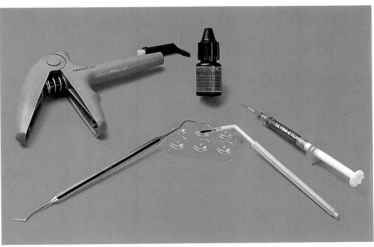

322 Adhesive material
An autopolymerizing, two-component composite system provides a suitable adhesive.

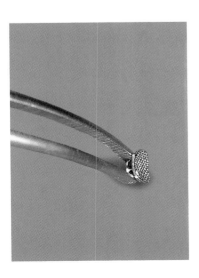

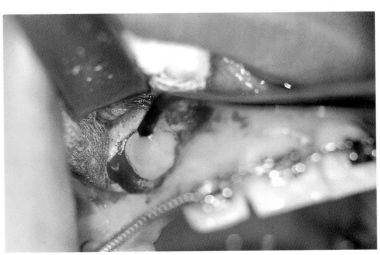

323 Application of the retentive button
The surface of the enamel is painted with the composite adhesive. During this procedure, the area must be kept absolutely dry.

Left: Note that the undersurface of the button has retentive grooves.

324 Application and fixation
The retentive button is applied to the enamel surface and held motionless until the setting reaction of the composite is complete. A precision self-locking forceps or clamp is indicated to hold the button firmly.

Right: Before application, the undersurface of the button is painted with a fluid composite material.

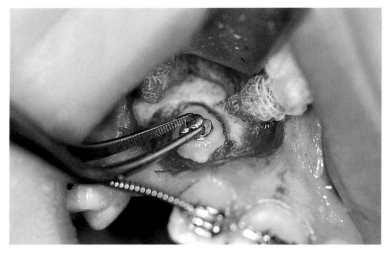
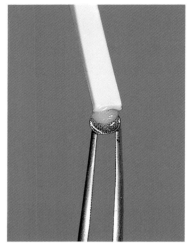

325 Applying the wire ligature
When the autopolymerizing resin has fully hardened, a wire ligature (0.4 mm, soft) is applied, and the ends are twisted securely together.

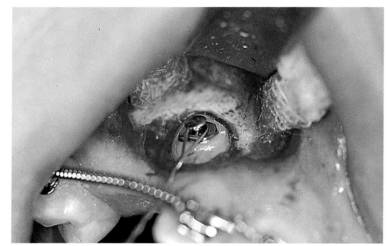

326 Wound closure
The tissue flap is replaced and sutured securely, with the twisted ends of the wire protruding. After suture removal, the orthodontist can initiate active forced eruption of the tooth.

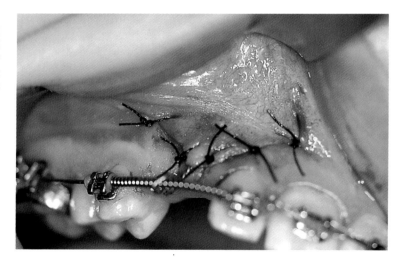

327 Interim clinical view
The eruption status eight months postsurgically.

Right: The radiograph shows an appropriate eruption pathway.

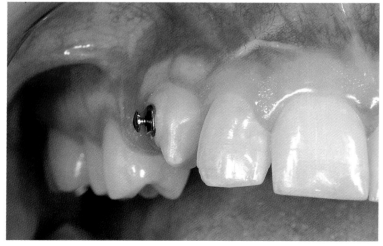
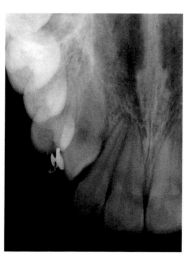

Forced Eruption from a Palatal Approach

The surgical procedure is similar to that for extraction of an impacted tooth. However, care must be taken during the ostectomy procedure to protect the tooth itself from damage.

The ligature wire is attached to the crown as previously described, and the wires course beneath the tissue flap to enter the oral cavity, where they are attached to an adjacent tooth. The ends of the wire must be bent in such a way that tissue trauma does not occur. If a removable orthodontic appliance is in use, it can be used as a surgical stent.

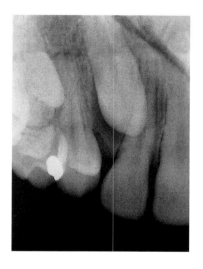
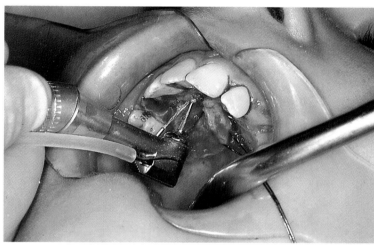

328 Palatal approach for tooth eruption
Anesthesia is identical to the procedure for tooth extraction, but the tissue flap and access are somewhat smaller. The entire surface of the crown has to be exposed.

Left: This periapical radiograph depicts the initial situation.

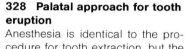

329 Drying the enamel surface
If seepage of blood presents a problem, a retraction cord can be placed to keep the crown dry.

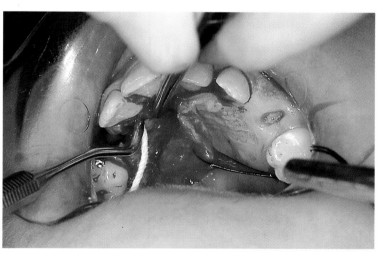

330 Fixation and retention
After etching the enamel, the retentive button is applied using autopolymerizing composite resin.

Left: The cauterized enamel surface of the palatally exposed tooth crown.

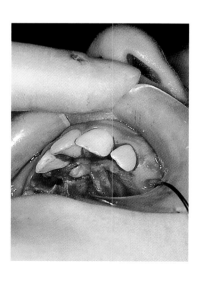
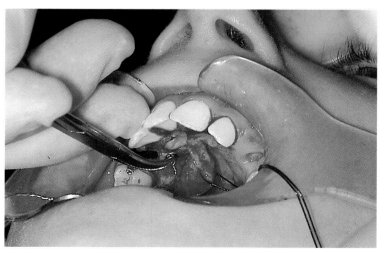

331   Wound closure
The soft-tissue flap is repositioned and secured with sutures. Note the wire ligature leaving the wound area on the palatal aspect of tooth 12.

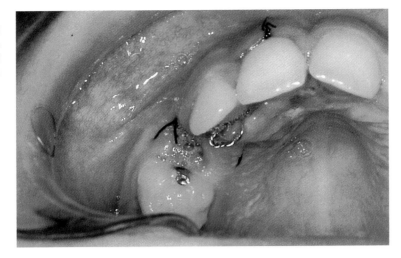

332   Forced eruption
In this case, a removable orthodontic appliance was used with elastic bands to bring the tooth into position. Active orthodontic movement can be initiated as soon as the sutures have been removed.

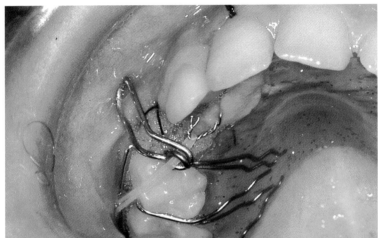

333   Interim view
As the tooth erupted, the retentive button was removed and reattached on the buccal surface, optimizing the force applied to ensure eruption in the proper alignment.

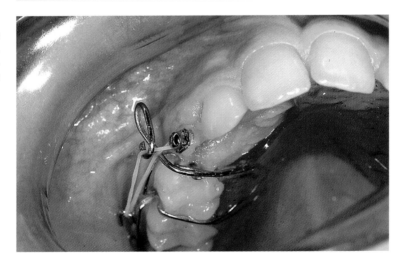

334   Treatment complete
Clinical view eighteen months after surgery. Tooth 13 is in its proper location in the arch.

Right: This periapical radiograph, taken on completion of orthodontic treatment, shows the intact root of tooth 13 and a normal-appearing periodontal ligament.

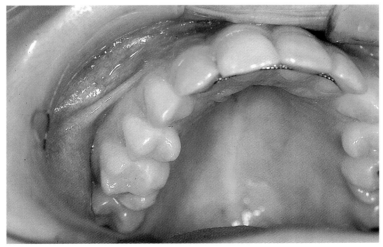
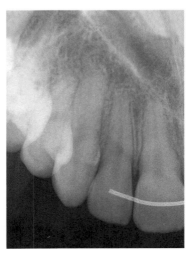

Access in the Mandible

The forced eruption procedure for mandibular impacted teeth is usually carried out using a lingual approach, after reflecting the lingual soft tissues in the same way as in procedures for tooth extraction. Vertical releasing incisions are not used. Extending the primary incision at the gingival margin beyond the midline provides better visual access, and makes it easier to dry the area for attachment of the retentive button.

Access from the buccal approach is the same as in the procedure for tooth extraction (p. 102).

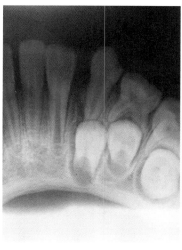
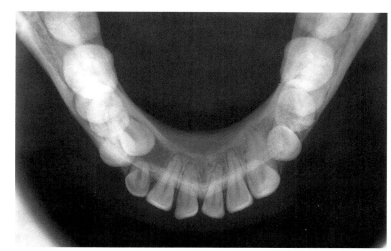

335 Forced eruption in the mandible—lingual approach
This mandibular occlusal radiograph shows a bicuspid impacted in a lingual position, in a 14-year-old girl.

Left: The periapical radiograph shows the spatial relationships. The retained deciduous molar is keeping sufficient space free.

Ⓢ

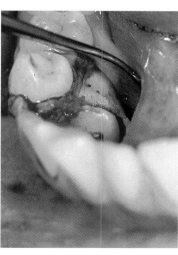
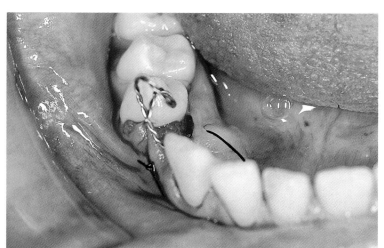

336 Clinical view after wound closure
The surgical procedure is identical to that for tooth extraction. Ostectomy is used to expose the surface of the crown for attachment of the retentive element. Seen here is the clinical view after suture closure; note the extrusion of the twisted wire ligature from the surgical site.

Left: The exposed crown after cauterization of the enamel.

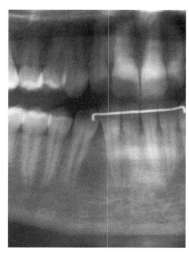
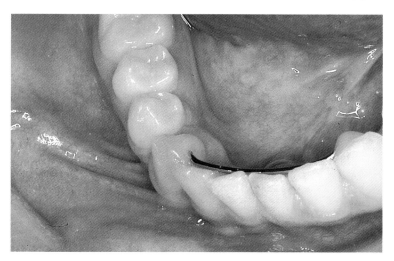

337 Clinical course
Clinical status 14 months postsurgically, showing tooth 44 in its proper position in the mandibular arch at the end of the orthodontic treatment.

Left: Radiograph at the end of treatment, with the fixed retainer wire visible.

Tooth Transplantation

Definition

Tooth transplantation involves implanting a simultaneously extracted autologous tooth into a newly prepared alveolus; the procedure is also termed "autotransplantation." We elect not to perform homologous tooth transplantation.

Indications for Transplantation

It is the orthodontist who usually does the planning and establishes the indication for transplantation. This procedure offers a reasonable alternative when, for example, one arch has a congenitally missing tooth while the opposing arch shows clinical tooth crowding requiring the removal of permanent teeth, or when premature tooth loss makes tooth transplantation, usually of a third molar, attractive for replacement purposes. Additional indications include traumatic tooth loss, tumors, or iatrogenic grounds. In all cases, the developmental condition (root growth) of the tooth intended for transplantation is a critical consideration.

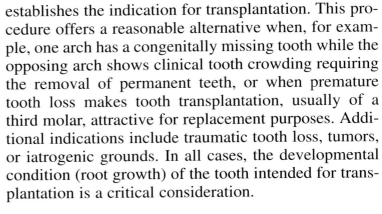

338 Transplantation—documentation
The panoramic radiograph shows that teeth 35 and 45 are congenitally absent, although there is extreme crowding in the maxilla.

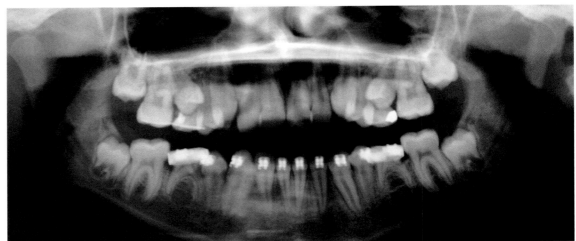

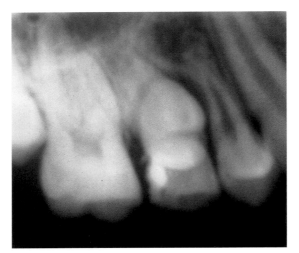
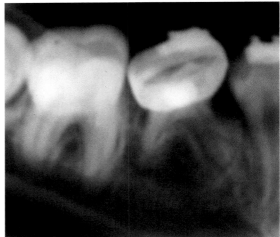

339 Indication and planning
Normally, the dentist, orthodontist, and oral surgeon meet to discuss the indication for tooth transplantation. The crowded maxilla requires extraction of the premolars; these teeth could be used to replace the retained deciduous molar in the mandible. The periapical radiograph provides further information: root development of the maxillary right first premolar is approximately two-thirds complete *(left)*.

Right: The roots of the retained deciduous molar (85) show signs of resorption, and adequate space is available.

The optimum time for transplanting a tooth is when its root development has achieved one-half to three-quarters of the expected root length, and the apical foramen is still wide open (Schultze-Mosgau et al. 1994).

In this type of case, the patients may also be suitable candidates for a dental implant.

Caution
The patient or the patient's parents must be provided with full information, in order to avoid subsequent legal consequences.

Clinical Tip
Maxillary third molars are usually good candidates to replace retained deciduous mandibular molars. The anatomy of the third molar crown often means that it has to be transplanted with a 180° rotation (palatal transposed toward buccal) to enhance proper occlusion and optimum articulation.

If maxillary premolars are transplanted into the mandible, it is also often necessary to rotate the transplanted tooth in such a way that its palatal cusp is oriented buccally.

Surgical Procedure

Documentation
Details clearly stating the goal of the procedure should be entered in the patient's chart. The minimum radiographic documentation will include a panoramic radiograph and periapical films of the tooth intended for transplantation, as well as the recipient site; these radiographs will also show the stage of root development, the precise location, and the osseous structure (residual osteitis, root fragments, etc.).

Anatomy
Due consideration must be given to the anatomical relationships determining the surgical approach used to remove the tooth intended for transplantation.

Anesthesia
The type and location of local anesthesia are determined by the anatomical relationships of the donor and recipient sites.

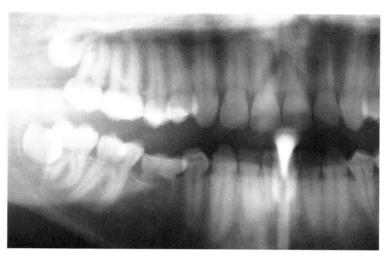

340   Transplantation of tooth 18 into the region of tooth 45
The panoramic radiograph shows congenital absence of the permanent tooth subjacent to the retained deciduous molar (85), and the maxillary third molar (18) is seen with root development about two-thirds complete. The timing for transplantation is favorable.

Ⓐ

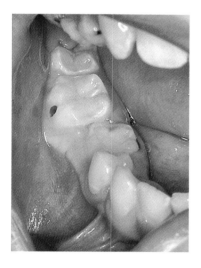
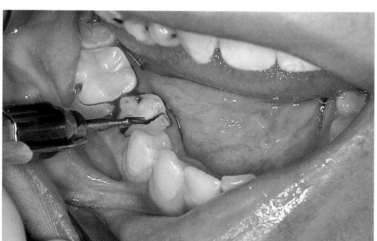

341   Removal of the deciduous tooth
The deciduous molar (85) is first sectioned, and then removed.

Right: Clinical view of the retained deciduous molar.

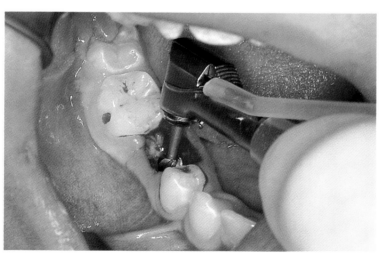

342   Creation of an alveolus
A large round bur is used to create an artificial alveolus (recipient bed) for tooth 18.

343 Removal of tooth 18
The maxillary third molar (18) is carefully removed before being measured and temporarily replaced in its alveolus.

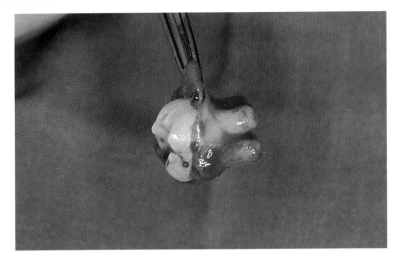

344 Transplantation
Once the artificial alveolus in the mandible has been appropriately adapted, tooth 18 can be seated in its new position. Scissors are used to carefully remove any remnants of the follicular sac.

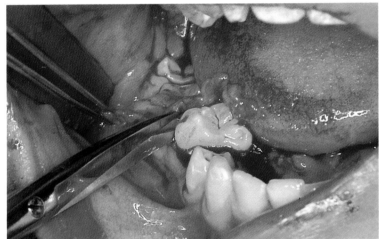

345 Immobilization of the transplanted tooth
Tooth 18 is fixed into the new alveolus using a wire sling suture extending from the two adjacent teeth. Slight mobility within the physiological range is acceptable. Rigid immobilization of a transplanted tooth leads to ankylosis and root resorption.

Right: The transplanted tooth is carefully documented with periapical radiographs.

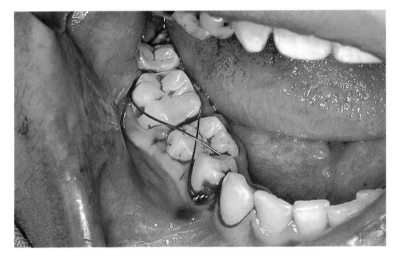
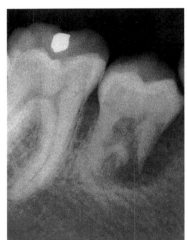

346 Clinical course
The clinical view six months postsurgically. The transplanted tooth is solid, periodontally intact, and shows no symptoms of pulpal necrosis, although it continues to react negatively to the application of cold (CO_2, ice) for vitality testing.

Right: The periapical radiograph shows that root growth has continued, and there are signs of narrowing of the root canals a sign of a vital reaction. Regeneration of the surrounding bone remains incomplete.

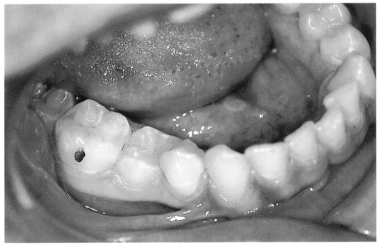
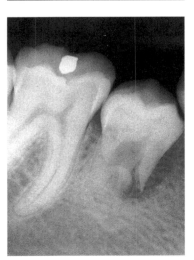

Surgical Procedure

This operation is quite similar to surgery for removing impacted teeth. A major difference, however, is that the tooth intended for transplantation must not be damaged during surgical manipulations. The follicular sac should be left in place as a collar; if the tooth does not fit into the newly created alveolus, it is replaced in its original alveolus.

Retained deciduous teeth are not uncommon. After removal of these deciduous teeth and healing of the residual alveolus (about one month later), a selected tooth can be transplanted. The transplanted tooth should initially lie slightly below the occlusal plane, in order to provide space for the expected continued root growth and development.

Postoperative Visit

The postoperative course is followed up radiographically to document and observe the further development of the transplanted tooth. At the three-month point, the transplanted tooth is examined for vitality, and pocket depth and mobility are tested. Subsequent appointments should be made every six months until the transplanted tooth has reached its final position in the arch. Any orthodontic movement required can be initiated after three months.

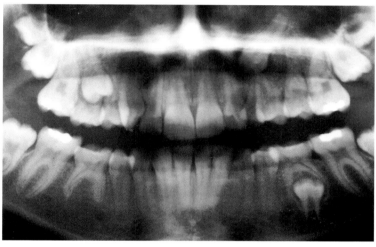

347 Transplantation of tooth 14 into the region of tooth 45— planning and documentation
This panoramic radiograph shows congenital absence of tooth 45. The comprehensive treatment plan includes bilateral premolar extraction in the maxilla. The timing is, however, unfavorable for transplantation, because root development of the premolars has already progressed to three-quarters of the root length.

Ⓐ

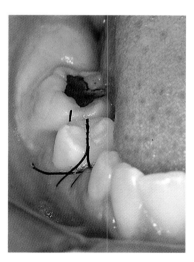
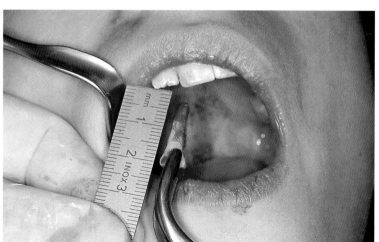

348 Transplantation
After carefully extracting deciduous tooth 5 from the mandible, tooth 14 is removed and measured.

Left: After deepening the new alveolus, tooth 14 was transplanted and secured with a ligature.

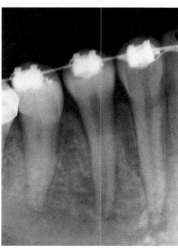
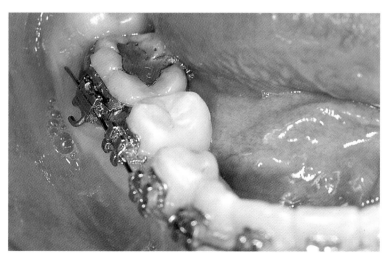

349 Clinical course
After a healing phase of three months, the transplanted tooth 14 is moved orthodontically into the desired position.

Left: This periapical radiograph shows conditions 12 months after transplantation. Root development has stopped, and the root canal is somewhat narrowed; these signs indicate vital processes.

Tooth Transplantation from the Maxilla into the Mandible

The size and shape of maxillary third molars usually make them good candidates for replacing a retained deciduous molar if the succedaneous permanent tooth is congenitally absent. Maxillary premolars that are transplanted to the mandible must be reversed in such a way that the palatal cusp is at the buccal aspect, in order to optimize occlusion. The variable size of these teeth usually means that the space in the mandible has to be closed orthodontically. If tooth transplantation is carried out at the same time as removal of the deci-duous molar, the new alveolus should be prepared to receive either the distal or the mesial root. During the planning stage, the rationale for transplantation should be considered from the point of view of spatial relationships and occlusion.

Clinical Tip
When transplanting a maxillary premolar into the mandible, it must be rotated 180°—i.e., the palatal cusp is positioned at the buccal aspect.

350 Transplantation of tooth 18 into the region of tooth 26—documentation and planning
This panoramic radiograph shows that tooth 26 is severely damaged, and needs to be extracted. The root development of tooth 18 is approximately two-thirds complete. The transplantation will be carried out at the same appointment at which tooth 26 is extracted. (The metal sutures visible here are due to a previous maxillary sliding osteotomy procedure).

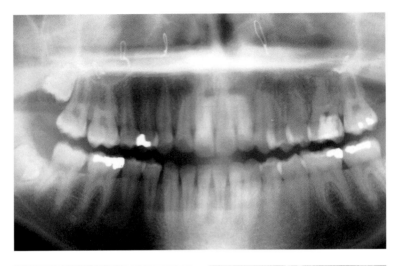

Ⓐ

351 Radiographic course
This series of periapical films shows the course of healing in tooth 18 after transplantation into the tooth 26 region. Comparison of the left and center films shows that root development has progressed.

Right: This film was taken 18 months postsurgically. The root apices are constricted, and there is an intact periodontal ligament space.

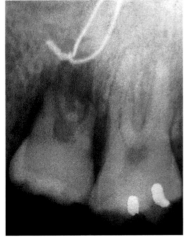
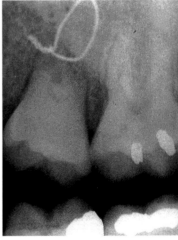
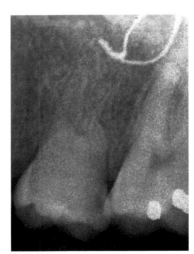

352 Conclusion of treatment
Eighteen months after the transplantation of tooth 18 into the region of tooth 26, physiological, symptom-free conditions are seen. Tooth mobility is within normal limits, and the periodontium is intact.

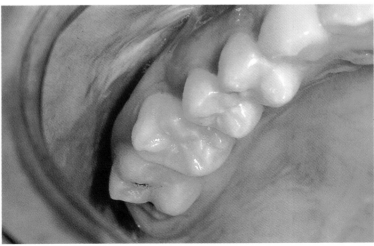

Transplantation within the Maxilla

During the planning stage, it is important to note the available bone at the implantation site. The floor of the maxillary sinus must not be perforated. It is possible to carry out deciduous tooth extraction and tooth transplantation during the same procedure. When replacing a maxillary molar (the usual indication is the impossibility of restoring the tooth adequately for long-term success), a two-stage procedure is more appropriate, because of the chronic apical inflammation that usually accompanies the tooth that is extracted. After the molar has been extracted, the alveolus is allowed to heal for a period of four weeks. This is usually sufficient time for the inflammatory process to subside.

The criteria for transplantation of a premolar are the same as those for molar teeth, and the surgical procedure is also similar. In the premolar region, the danger of sinus perforation is usually slightly lower. Each individual case must be discussed with the orthodontist to establish securely the indication for removal of a premolar on one side in order to replace a congenitally absent tooth on the opposite side. The procedures must be coordinated to prevent any arch discrepancies.

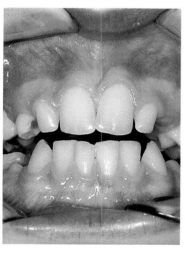
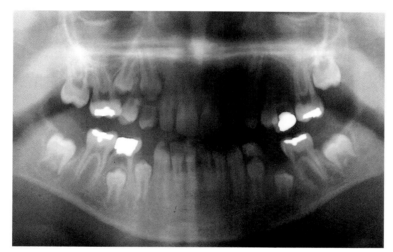

353 Transplantation of tooth 15 into the region of tooth 25— documentation and planning
This panoramic radiograph of a 12-year-old girl shows crowding on the right side of the maxilla, as well as congenital absence of tooth 25. The orthodontist's treatment plan involves removal of tooth 15 and its transplantation into the region of tooth 25, since space closure on the left side is not possible.

Left: Clinical view before transplantation.

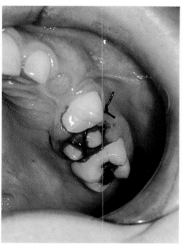
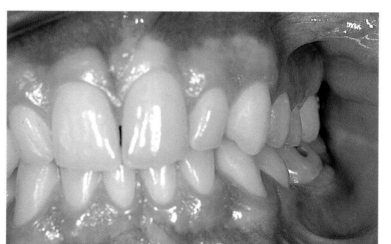

354 Clinical course
Findings six months after surgery; the transplanted tooth has established itself in the occlusal scheme.

Left: Immediate postsurgical view: due to bone availability, tooth 15 is positioned somewhat palatally.

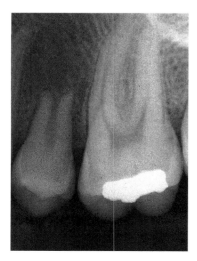
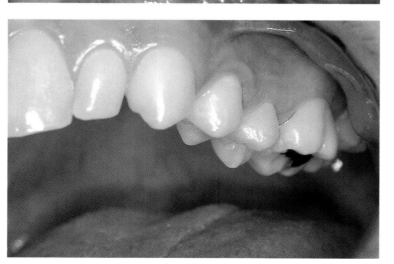

355 Completion of treatment
Clinical view 16 months after surgery; the interarch and intermaxillary relationship are stable.

Left: The periapical radiograph shows incomplete root development, with an open apex and a normal periodontal ligament space. There is no evidence of resorption.

Transposition of a Tooth

The term "transposition" refers to altering the position of a tooth in its usual arch position by means of osteotomy and temporary removal of the tooth.

Planning for the procedure is carried out in collaboration with the orthodontist. Transposition is a risky procedure in relation to achieving the intended goals. For this reason, the planning phase must also take into account alternative therapy in case the procedure fails. It is critically important to inform the patient about the attendant risks.

The surgical procedure will vary individually. It is essential that the tooth being transplanted should be extracted without trauma, and that the osseous defect created should allow reimplantation at the desired location.

Minor corrections using orthodontics can be instituted four to eight weeks postsurgically, with due consideration being given to the clinical condition of the transplanted tooth. Movement of the tooth within an existing osseous defect should only be attempted after bony regeneration.

356 Transposition of tooth 45—planning and indication
It does not seem to be possible to move the impacted tooth 45 into its proper position by means of forced eruption, and extraction of the tooth seems to be indicated. A decision was taken to attempt to bring the permanent teeth into proper position by transposition. The first step was removal of deciduous tooth 75, and space maintenance.

Left: The panoramic radiograph shows the preoperative view.

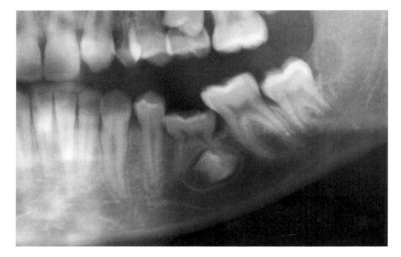
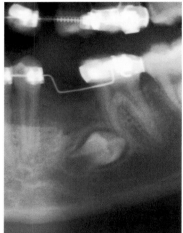

357 Course of therapy
The situation one month postsurgically. The tooth has not yet achieved its proper position in the mandibular arch. Orthodontic movement of the tooth can begin one month later.

Right: Immediate postsurgical view, showing the buccal position of the tooth.

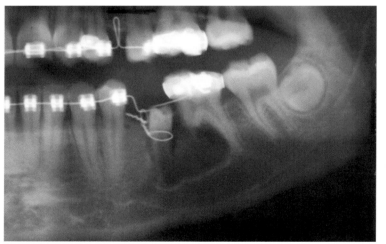
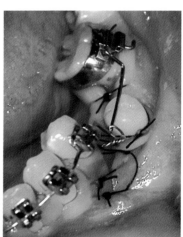

358 Treatment complete
This clinical photograph, taken one year postoperatively, shows the tooth in its definitive position.

Right: These radiographs are unremarkable in their depiction of the transposition of tooth 35 *(above)* and the intermediate stage six months later, when orthodontic movement of the tooth would normally begin.

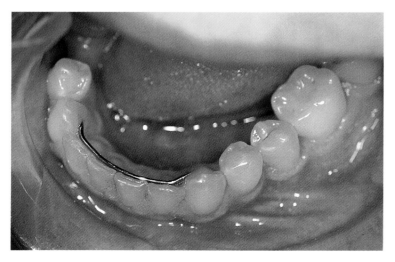
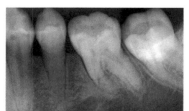
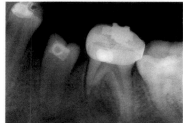

Special Considerations

Timing of the transplantation. If root development is complete at the time of transplantation, pulpal necrosis with possible infection and subsequent root resorption are likely to ensue.

Choice of the tooth for transplantation. The tooth must be easy to access, and it must be possible to extract it atraumatically. The size must correspond to the available arch space. Grinding the tooth to make it fit a smaller space should not be attempted.

Site of transplantation. The transplant bed should consist of well vascularized trabecular bone that allows an alveolus to be created. Teeth should not be transplanted near the mandibular nerve or the maxillary sinuses.

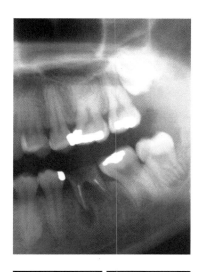
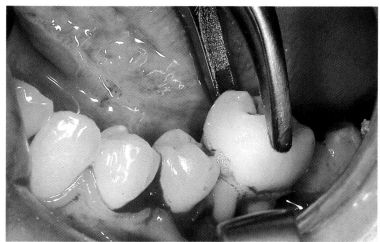

359 Complication—inadequate space
The mesiodistal space is inadequate; tooth 38 is too large for the space created by extraction of tooth 36. Maxillary third molars usually fit into the space of a mandibular deciduous molar.

Left: Preoperative radiograph showing tooth 36, which cannot be saved.

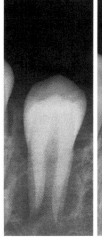
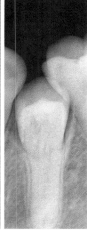
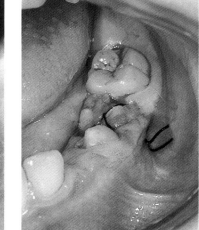
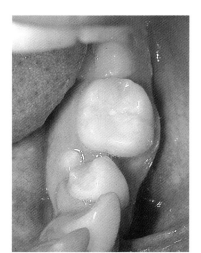

360 Inadequate cooperation
Left: Tooth 24 was successfully transplanted into the region of tooth 35, but subsequent orthodontic treatment was stopped because of inadequate cooperation by the patient.

Center: Immediate posttransplantation clinical view. The mesiodistal space is sufficient.

Right: Clinical view two years after transplantation. Tooth 35 remains incompletely erupted.

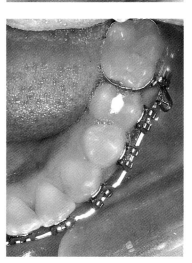
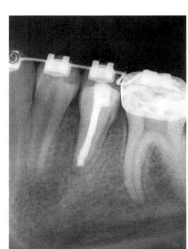

361 Pulpal necrosis
Left: Tooth 24 was transplanted into the region of tooth 35, but subsequently became necrotic, and had to be treated endodontically. The radiograph shows apical inflammatory osteolysis six months after transplantation.

Center: Thanks to careful endodontic therapy, it was possible to achieve clinically and radiographically healthy conditions.

Right: The radiograph taken at the same time shows an intact periodontal ligament space, with no signs of inflammation.

Open Versus Partially Closed Postoperative Care after Mandibular Third Molar Extraction

Up to this point, we have only described open wound treatment after extracting mandibular third molars. We are aware that this method is not widely used; however, in routine everyday practice, it offers significant advantages over other methods of postoperative care.

Complication Rate

There are clear differences between the various treatment methods with regard to complication rates. Two particularly important criteria—healing disturbances and postoperative infection—are known to be directly dependent on the method of postoperative care. When the open method of wound treatment is used, a total of 3% complications can be expected (1% infection, 0.6% healing disturbance, 1.4% other complications); when the partially closed method of wound treatment is used, the complication rate rises to 26% (6% infection and 19.3% healing disturbances, among which 7.3% involve postoperative pain and 12% relate to wound dehiscence). The high percentage of wound dehiscence clearly demonstrates the problems associated with wound closure of mandibular third molar extraction sites involving ostectomy and flap design to protect the lingual nerve. This leads to a clinical situation in which the margin of the soft-tissue flap is only partially supported on the subjacent bone. There can be no doubt that primary healing of the mucoperiosteal flap immediately above to the osseous defect is exceptionally difficult to achieve.

Effect of Oral Hygiene

Healing of an open wound is not delayed if oral hygiene is insufficient. By contrast, with partial closure of the third molar extraction site, a patient with poor oral hygiene can expect to have a higher risk of infection and delayed wound healing.

Costs

The economics of wound healing can be calculated by measuring the duration of therapy and the time required for postoperative appointments. Logically, fewer appointments mean lower costs (in both time and money) for the dentist and for the patient.

Treatment of an open postsurgical site requires, on average, three postoperative appointments for changing or removing dressings. The total treatment time averages 17 days.

With the partially closed method, two postoperative appointments are required, with a total treatment time of 12 days on average. However, 50% of cases treated using the partially closed wound method require extended treatment times. The higher rate of complications with this technique is associated with significantly increased treatment time. Any advantage of a shorter total treatment time is lost in comparison to the 50% complication-free statistic for the open postoperative course.

Conclusions

The results presented here derive from experience in our own clinic. This experience is probably relevant to the general practitioner, since in our clinic we do not pursue absolutely aseptic conditions during the surgical removal of impacted third molars. For example, the coolant water for our handpieces is taken directly from the public water supply, which is known to be less than completely sterile. Our research was aimed at evaluating open postoperative treatment using loosely placed gauze drains, and the clinical results of this technique, in comparison with other postoperative treatment modalities.

In conclusion, open postoperative wound treatment using gauze drains can be regarded as very safe and practical on several criteria. The extent of the postoperative care required is acceptable and, due to the lower complication rate, fully justified for use in a modern dental practice.

Clinical Tip

Open wound treatment after surgical removal of mandibular third molars is the method associated with the fewest complications. The infection rate is extremely low (1%). Systemic antibiotic coverage is not required. Extraction of third molars is mainly indicated in the 18–24 age group. Within this age range, the total treatment time is shortest and the complication rate is smallest.

In view of the risk of complications using the partially closed method, open postoperative care after surgical removal of mandibular third molars appears to be the more cost-saving method. The partially closed method of wound treatment after surgical extraction of mandibular third molars can only be justified for use in patients with perfect oral hygiene, and when the surgical procedure is carried out under aseptic conditions.

Abscess Treatment

Pathology and Diagnosis

Assessment Criteria

Assessment of an infection involves examining the local extent of the process, the patient's general condition, and the virulence of the causative agent.

The clinical examination must determine whether there is a localized infection or whether the symptoms suggest regional spread of the infection, and whether the entire systemic complex is involved.

Local Findings
Dental infections normally produce the classic signs of infection in the immediate proximity of the etiological agent. The microorganisms most commonly involved are streptococci and staphylococci, deriving from necrosis of a nonvital tooth. The most common microorganism is *Streptococcus viridans*. *S. aureus* is very often detected in aspirates, either alone or as one component in a mixed infection.

With periodontal pocket formation, periodontal abscesses are not uncommon, and these have a different bacteriological cause—primarily Gram-negative organisms, accompanied by anaerobes and also actinomycetes (Obwegeser et al. 1989, Schmelzle et al. 1978).

A distinction is made between subperiosteal abscesses and submucosal abscesses.

Cutaneous Fistula
Chronic granulomatous infections, which usually originate from apical infection of the mandibular anterior teeth and molars, may perforate the bone and periosteum and exit externally from the skin surface.

The primary therapy is purely causal—eliminating the causative agent. The primary fistula normally heals spontaneously. Excision or surgical correction is usually only necessary if the fistulous tract has become epithelialized.

Widespread Infections
Widely disseminated abscesses usually originate from a local abscess, and spread along the anatomically demarcated tissue spaces.

If such infections are not controlled, a life-threatening disease process can develop. Sepsis usually ensues, and the abscess may also extend into functionally critical centers. Brain abscesses of dental origin have often been described. Abscesses in the maxilla can spread into the cavernous sinus via the facial vein (where valves are absent) or the angular vein. Symptoms such as periorbital edema or flattened nasolabial grooves are typical.

Diffuse pus formation without demarcation is termed "phlegmon." Typically, it originates in the floor of the mouth, with possible caudal dissemination into the mediastinum. Situations such as this are life-threatening.

Host Resistance Factors
Poor general health or systemic disease can substantially affect host resistance to infection. Poorly controlled diabetes is associated with compromised resistance against bacterial infection. In patients who are immunosuppressed, those undergoing chemotherapy, or patients suffering from leukemia or aplastic anemia, resistance to infection is severely reduced or completely absent. Patients such as these must receive aggressive treatment for their infection, usually on an in-patient basis.

Cardinal Symptoms of Abscess

An abscess represents the acute stage of an infection, and shows the classic signs of inflammation:

—Tumor: caused by edema and pus accumulation.
—Dolor: caused by pressure within tissues and on nerve endings.
—Calor: caused by accelerated local metabolism.
—Rubor: caused by elevated blood flow.
—Functio laesa: caused by a pain reflex.
—Fluctuation: typical sign of fluid accumulation (pus).

Patients do not always present with this full range of symptoms. The diagnosis is based on the course, the possible causes, and the observed pathological alterations. It is important to identify the precise location and the extent of the abscess. This is then followed by surgical therapy, which consists of opening and draining the abscess cavity and, whenever possible, eliminating the etiological factors at the same time (Andrä and Naumann 1991, Becker 1968).

Broadly disseminated abscesses, or those showing an atypical course, should be treated by a specialist (Grätz 1989, Schotland et al. 1979).

362 Cardinal symptoms— tumor, calor and rubor
In this 47-year-old woman, the vestibular swelling in the right maxilla is causing a fiery red, painful swelling.

Right: Extraoral swelling of the right cheek, with lower eyelid edema, erythema, and a slightly drooping upper lip are typical clinical signs.

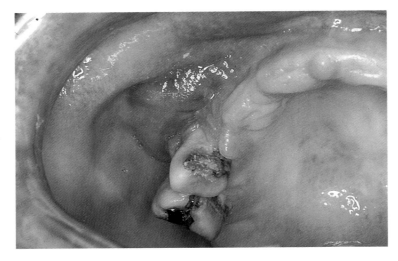
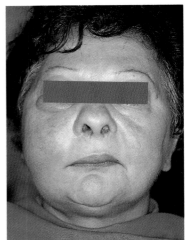

363 Cardinal symptom—*calor*
The heat that always accompanies an inflammatory process can be sensed by placing the palm on the area of swelling.

Right: This thermogram shows the heat of a perimandibular abscess on the right side of the mandible. (Illustration courtesy of N. Hardt.)

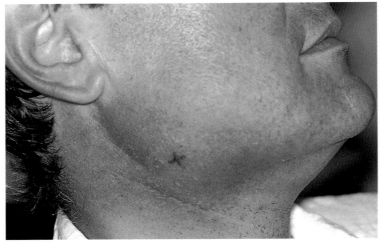
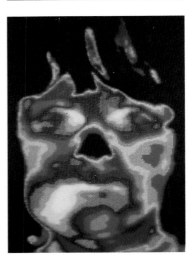

Osteomyelitis

During the course of abscess formation, inflammation of the bone marrow can occur, particularly in the mandible.

The clinical symptoms include pain, fistula formation, osseous expansion, and disturbances of sensation. The course is intermittent, but can be expected to persist for weeks or months, with symptom-free intervals. Possible etiological factors include foreign bodies, chronic dental infection that persists without healing after elimination of the cause, sequestration, and systemic diseases such as diabetes and peripheral circulatory disturbances.

Typical radiographic signs include poorly demarcated osteolysis, which may be detected at some distance from the original focus of infection. The cortical bone may also be involved. In addition, reactive sclerosis, sequester formation, and subperiosteal new bone formation may be observed. Radiographic examination cannot exclude the possibility of a malignant process. Computed tomography and magnetic resonance imaging (Hardt 1991) can provide valuable diagnostic information.

Radiation Osteomyelitis

Radiation osteomyelitis is a special form of osteomyelitis. Often, it is impossible to differentiate between the density of trabecular and cortical bone. The correct diagnosis is based on the medical history. Even years after a course of radiation therapy, radiation osteomyelitis can occur in conjunction with minor surgical procedures in the oral cavity (periodontal curettage or surgery, tooth extraction).

Initial signs of radiation osteomyelitis include areas of mucosa that fail to heal over bone, and nebulous pain in the jaw region (Obwegeser and Sailer 1978, Sailer 1976).

Clinical Tip

The treatment of osteomyelitis should only be undertaken by a specialist.

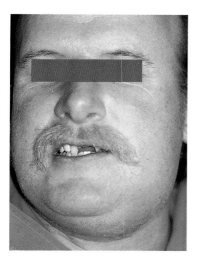

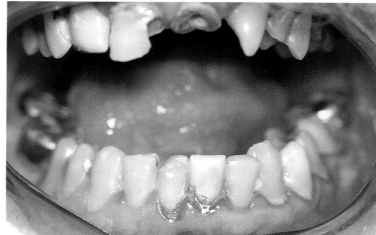

364 Cardinal symptom—*functio laesa*
An inability to fully open the mouth is a typical sign of reduced mobility in the temporomandibular joint.

Left: This 44-year-old man presented with unmistakable symptoms, including swelling, erythema, and limited ability to open the mouth.

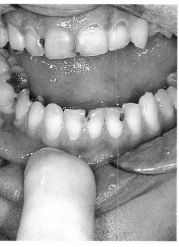

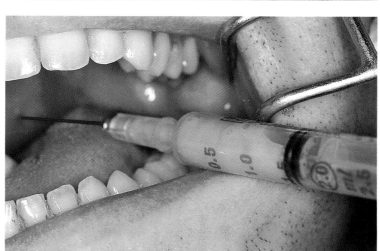

365 Cardinal symptom—fluctuation
Fluctuation in the tissues can be a sign of pus accumulation in an abscess. This can be confirmed by palpation using two fingers *(left)* and by collecting pus on penetrating the area with a syringe.

Identification of the Causative Agent

Further clarification is necessary if there is suspicion of a particularly virulent organism, and if the local symptoms appear threatening. A differential blood evaluation and a white cell count are indicated. An elevated sedimentation rate confirms the presence of an infectious process.

In most cases, bacteriological evaluation is not necessary with dental abscesses. The causative organisms are well known, and respond to penicillin.

If the healing process after surgical intervention appears to be delayed, sensitivity tests should never-

theless be carried out before administering a new antibiotic. If the infection is widespread, blood culture tests should always be carried out to identify aerobic and anaerobic strains.

Clinical Tip

A minor submucosal abscess does not require bacteriological analysis. On the other hand, this test is indicated in cases of recurrent abscesses with unclear etiology, and in patients with poor resistance—for example, those with diabetes or human immunodeficiency virus (HIV) infection.

366 Pus
Light-microscopic image of pus from a dental apical abscess, showing necrotic tissues. The center of the bacterial infection is surrounded by polymorphonuclear granulocytes, several lymphocytes, and cellular debris.

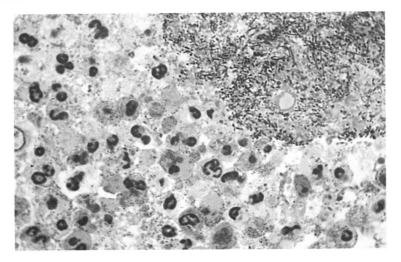

367 Pus
Transmission electron-microscopic image of a typical pus specimen reveals intact and also partly disintegrated polymorphonuclear granulocytes, as well as bacterial infiltration mainly consisting of coccoid forms.

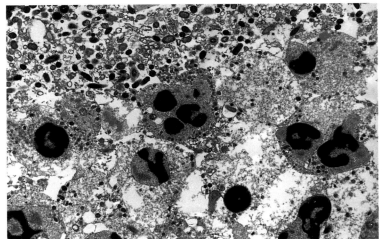

368 Pus
At higher magnification, polymorphonuclear granulocytes and large phagosomes can be identified which contain intact and partially digested bacteria.

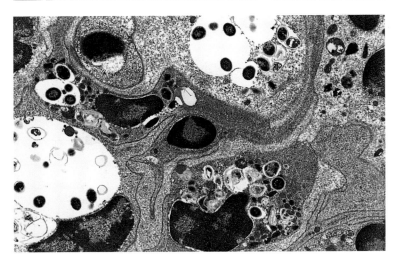

369 Pus
Light-microscopic view of an apical granuloma showing root resorption and accumulation of *Actinomyces*.

(Illustrations courtesy of B. Guggenheim.)

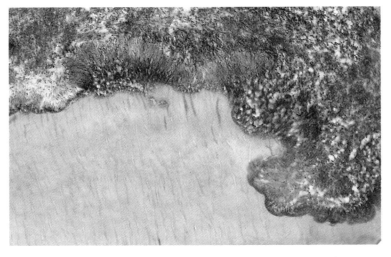

Abscess Incision and Drainage

"Ubi pus ibi evacua." Active surgical intervention is the treatment of choice for virtually any abscess. Differentiating between subperiosteal and submucosal abscesses is of no significance for treatment; it is the anatomical location that is of primary importance.

Antibiotic Therapy

Antibiotics represent a last resort in cases of uncertain symptomatology, life-threatening systemic symptoms, unfavorable dissemination, or if the host resistance is compromised. Antibiotics should be used in as targeted a way as possible in each individual case, depending on the assumed or identified causative bacteria (periodontal, apical, radicular, or specific infection). Antibiotics should not be prescribed as a routine or general procedure (Becker 1968, Rahn 1989, Fleming et al. 1990, Berthold 1993).

General Surgical Procedure

Anesthesia
Nerve block anesthesia with regional infiltration should be used whenever possible. Intraepithelial or subepithelial infiltration of anesthetic solution is mainly used to reduce hemorrhage at the incision site, but is almost never sufficient for opening the abscess itself. If it is not possible to achieve adequate pain reduction using local anesthesia, the patient should be treated under general anesthesia; this is particularly important if mouth opening is severely limited, if the incision site is difficult to access, or if the incision has to be made using an extraoral approach.

Incision
The mucosa and the periosteum are incised with a scalpel (no. 15 blade). The scalpel must be moved perpendicular to the surface of the bone. The point of incision should be at the lowest possible area of the abscess, to enhance natural drainage. With oral abscesses, this is often not possible.

Using a periosteal elevator, the mucoperiosteum is reflected, and a closed hemostat is then inserted into the abscess cavity, opened, and then withdrawn. The amount, color, and consistency of the contents of the abscess should be observed and documented.

The abscess cavity is then rinsed thoroughly with saline solution or neomycin solution.

To enhance drainage, the incision wound is kept open with moist gauze strips, or using a rubber drain.

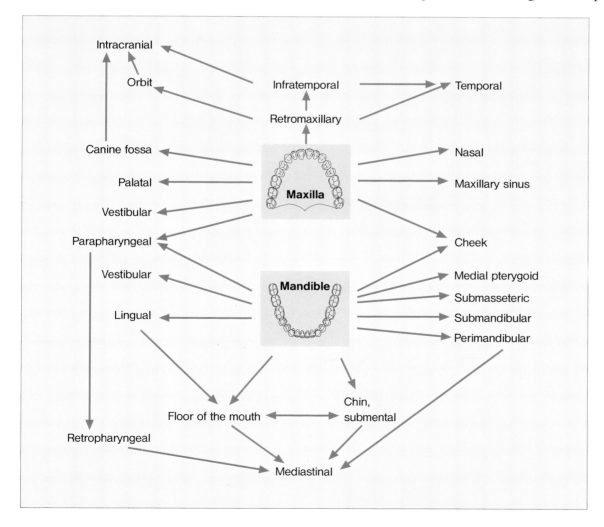

370 Potential spread of dental abscesses
If targeted treatment is not provided, simple abscesses on the alveolar process can spread along natural anatomical pathways into facial spaces. Depending on the virulence of the causative organism and the level of host resistance, life-threatening sepsis may ensue. (Diagram adapted from Obwegeser.)

Surgical Procedure for Mandibular Abscesses

Vestibular Abscess

Usually, a horizontal incision perpendicular to the surface of the bone can be used to sever both the mucosa and periosteum with one stroke. The opened abscess cavity is spread to facilitate pus drainage. Rinsing and drainage are then carried out.

Clinical Tip

The scalpel blade must be guided perpendicular to the bone surface, not obliquely. Care must be taken to avoid the mental foramen.

A vertical incision can be used if subsequent flap reflection is planned—for example, for a root tip resection or cystectomy.

If severe hemorrhage occurs, either vessel ligation or cauterization of the wound margins is effective. Applying compresses should be avoided, as it restricts drainage of the abscess fluids.

371 Submucosal abscess on the mandibular alveolar process
This two-year-old girl had been experiencing pain the region of tooth 44 for several weeks; the pain then subsided, and swelling began to occur three days later on the right side of the mandible.

Right: The periapical radiograph shows the root of tooth 44 and an ovoid area of osteolysis near the apex, surrounded by a partial zone of reactive sclerosis (mesial).

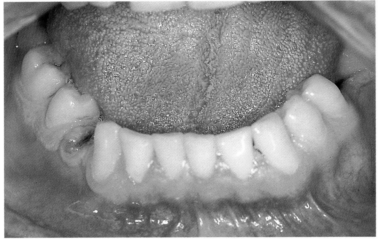
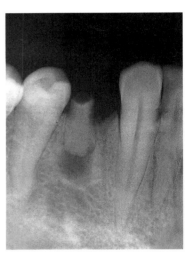

372 Anesthesia
In addition to block anesthesia of the inferior alveolar nerve and the long buccal nerve, topical anesthetic is applied to the mucosa overlying the incision line. This helps to alleviate pain during the incision and also to reduce hemorrhage.

Right: This diagram indicates the planned incision; the blade (no. 15) is positioned perpendicular to the bone surface. As the periosteum is reflected, care must be taken to avoid the mental nerve as it exits from the mental foramen.

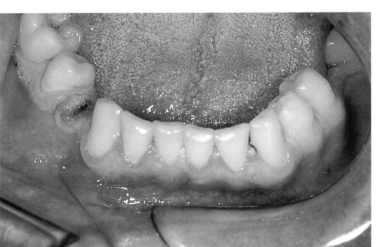
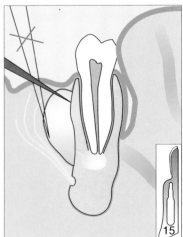

373 Incision
The scalpel severs both the mucosa and periosteum as it is guided perpendicular to the bone.

Right: A periosteal elevator is used to widen the opening to the abscess cavity, allowing complete drainage of the pus.

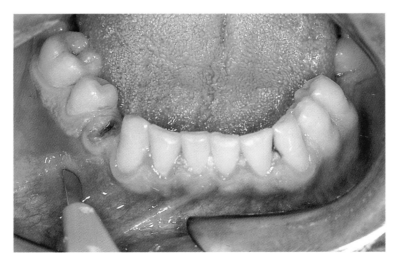
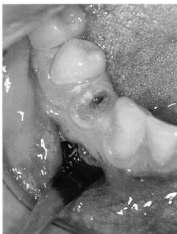

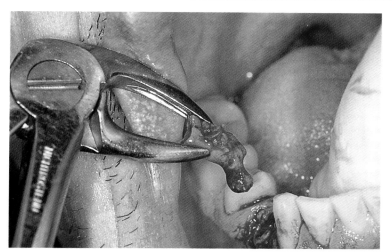

374 Causal treatment
In this case, the causative agent is an infected tooth root, which has to be removed. The extraction is usually performed after incision of the abscess, to prevent the pus from spreading submucosally when pressure is applied to the alveolar process as the tooth is extracted.

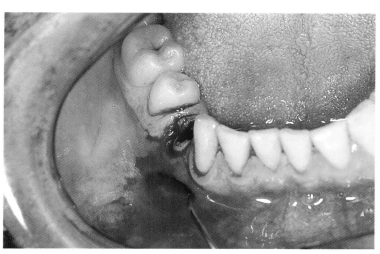

375 Rinsing
The abscess cavity should be rinsed to remove all traces of pus completely.

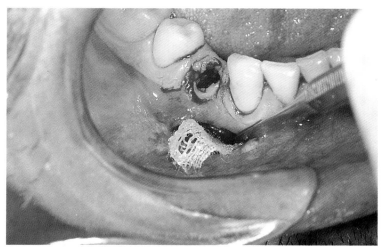

376 Drainage
A strip of gauze is placed in the abscess cavity to keep it open for drainage of any additional secretions that accumulate. The gauze strip is saturated with a disinfecting solution, e.g., Chlumsky solution.

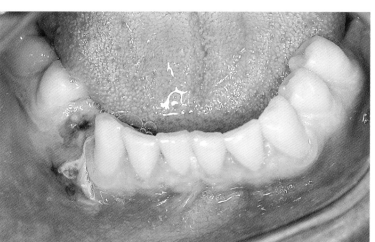

377 Follow-up
The first follow-up appointment should be on the day after surgery, for drainage of any additional secretions. The abscess cavity should be rinsed, and if secretion has continued, another gauze strip can be placed. If this is done, the patient should be seen on the following day, and then regularly until all signs of inflammation have subsided.

Lingual Abscess

The precise location of the abscess should be determined in relation to the position of the mylohyoid muscle. Here, too, the basic rule of using a horizontal incision coursing perpendicular to the subjacent bone applies.

Access in this region may be restricted, especially if the patient's ability to open the mouth is limited; this may require some adaptation of the basic principles. The primary incision through the mucosa and periosteum can be made slightly mesial to the abscess itself at the lingual junction, between the attached gingiva and the floor of the mouth. The periosteal elevator is used to reflect the soft tissues, followed by opening of the incision wound with the forceps, and then rinsing and drainage as usual.

Caution

Anterior: Avoid severing the duct of the submandibular gland.
Posterior: Avoid severing the lingual nerve.

Clinical Tip

With massive swelling of the floor of the mouth, maintain contact between the scalpel and the bone. An incision should never be made into the soft tissues.

378 Lingual abscess on the mandibular alveolar process
A 74-year-old woman presented with pain and increasing swelling under the tongue on the left side, after extraction of tooth 33 one month previously.

Right: This section from a panoramic radiograph reveals poorly demarcated osteolysis in the alveolar process in the region of tooth 33.

Ⓢ

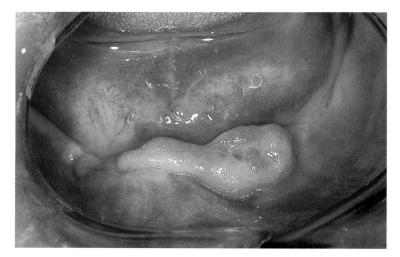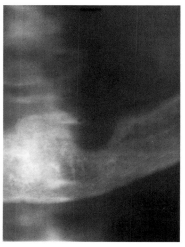

379 Opening the abscess
The scalpel is kept perpendicular to the alveolar process surface while creating a horizontal primary incision to open the abscess.

Right: The primary incision from a lingual approach, using a no. 15 blade.

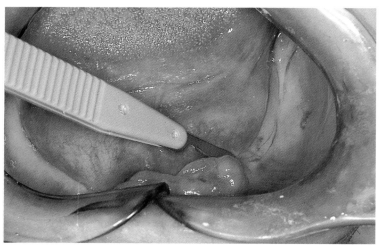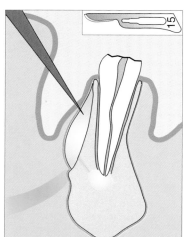

380 Postoperative care
The acute symptoms of infection disappeared after two follow-up appointments for rinsing and changing the drain.

Right: A follow-up radiograph three months later shows osseous regeneration.

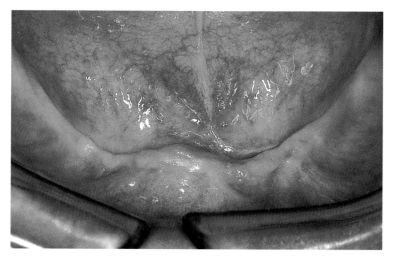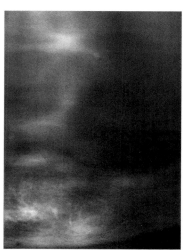

Abscess in the Chin

Abscesses originating from the mandibular anterior teeth may spread beneath the mylohyoid muscle into the submental area directly beneath the skin of the chin. Abscesses of this type are generally well demarcated, and the overlying skin is usually erythematous. If there is not a well-defined abscess cavity, there is a danger that the abscess may spread along the facial planes of the neck and into the mediastinum.

The primary incision should be made from an extraoral approach, into the submandibular fold.

Submasseteric Abscess

These abscesses can originate from infections of the mandibular posterior teeth, particularly the molars, and expand laterally. The border of the mandible can usually be palpated. Patients experience severe difficulty with mouth opening, restricting the access and making administration of block anesthesia more difficult.

The incision should be made vestibularly in the molar region. An elevator is used to reflect the subperiosteal tissues into the submasseteric space, and the forceps or hemostat can be used to spread the wound margins.

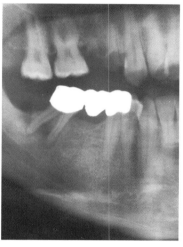 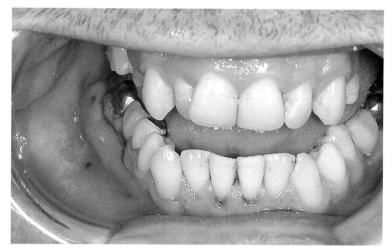

381 Submasseteric abscess
A 36-year-old man had progressive difficulty in opening, and pain on the right side. A firm, swelling was seen at the angle of the mandible, but sensitivity was not affected. Inspection revealed a painful swelling in the posterior segment. Teeth 47 and 48 were nonvital, and there was a 7-mm periodontal pocket distal to tooth 48. Maximum mouth opening was 4 mm.

Left: Note interradicular osteolysis on tooth 47.

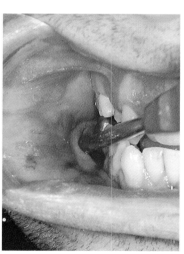 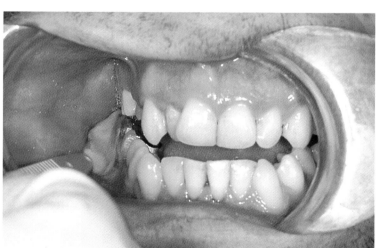

382 Incision and drainage
After block anesthesia and infiltration around the abscess, both buccally and distally, the abscess is incised and the periosteum is reflected distally and caudally using the periosteal elevator. Copious pus immediately flows out. Teeth 47 and 48 were extracted because of their poor prognosis, and because the patient's motivation was inadequate.

Left: Using the elevator to reflect the mucoperiosteum.

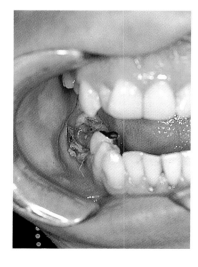 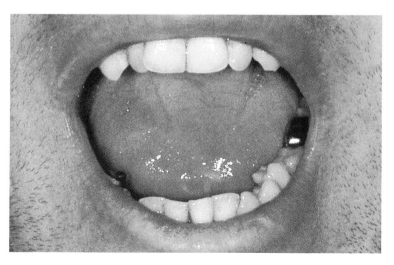

383 Postoperative care
Seven days postsurgically, the acute symptoms disappeared. Mouth opening was measured at 28 mm, and this could be extended to 35 mm with finger pressure.

Left: After daily rinsing and changes of the dressing, the swelling and pain were eliminated by day three, and the patient was able to open his mouth much wider.

Parapharyngeal Abscess

These abscesses usually occur in cases of impaired tooth eruption, or after extraction of third molars when an infected pocket is present. Hematoma formation after administration of block anesthesia may also play an etiological role. Patients may experience difficulty in mouth opening, as well as pain when swallowing.

The primary incision is made vertically in the retromolar trigone, and the wound is opened dorsally on the bone. A hemostat can also be used to open the wound in the parapharyngeal region.

Internal Pterygoid Abscess

This is similar to a parapharyngeal abscess, but derives from an expanding abscess in the mandible. Patients experience extreme difficulty with mouth opening, and this can significantly impede surgical and visual access.

The primary incision is made vertically on the ascending ramus of the mandible, with wound opening on the internal surface of the ramus.

384 Parapharyngeal abscess
This 42-year-old man had been suffering for three days from increasing difficulty in opening the mouth, along with painful swallowing. He had noticed mild discomfort in the right side of the mandible several weeks previously. Tooth 48 had been extracted three months previously because it had failed to erupt properly.

Right: The radiograph shows the empty alveolus of tooth 48, with reactive sclerosis of the mesial wall and osteolysis distally.

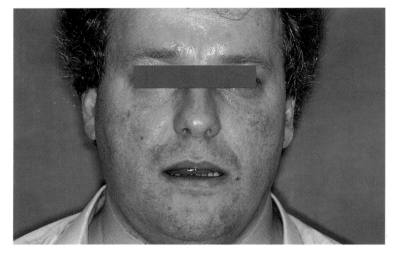

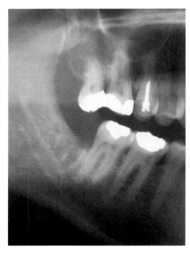

385 Anesthesia
Block anesthesia of the mandibular nerve and local infiltration in the soft palate.

Right: Axial cross-section showing the primary incision site.

1 Mandible
2 Masseter muscle
3 Medial pterygoid muscle
4 Abscess
5 Tonsillar region

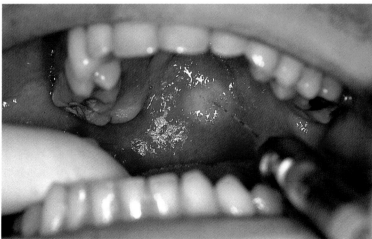

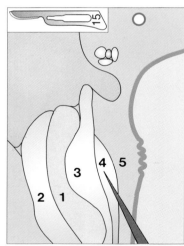

386 Incision
The scalpel is used to make a primary puncture incision and to expand the incision line within the left side of the soft palate.

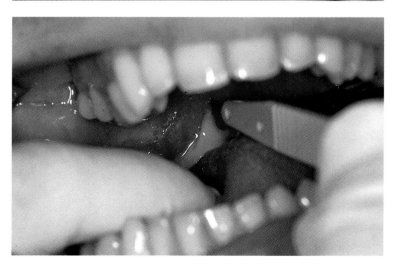

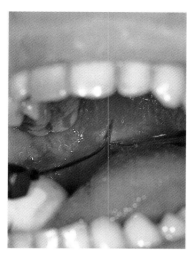
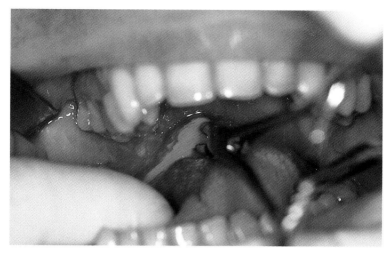

387 Spreading the wound margins

The hemostat can be used to expand bluntly into the abscess cavity on the internal surface of the angle of the mandible. There is copious pus release, and immediate improvement in the ability to open the mouth.

Left: The abscess cavity is thoroughly rinsed.

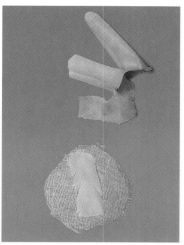
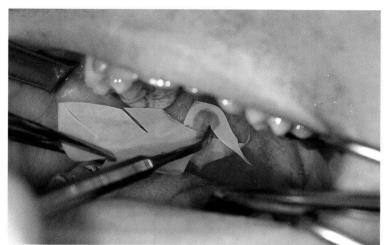

388 Drainage

Due to the depth of the incision, the usual gauze strip does not provide adequate drainage for further accumulations of secretion. A rubber drain is inserted.

Left: A suitable rubber drain can be made simply out of a sterile rubber glove.

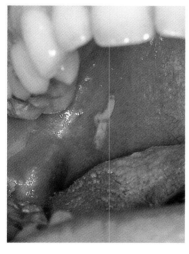
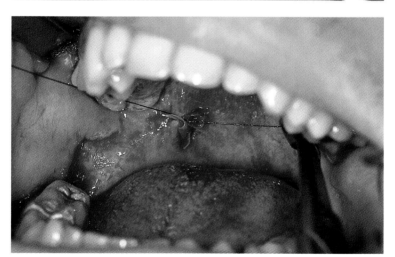

389 Fixation of the drain

A single suture is used to attach the rubber drain to prevent aspiration. The original cause of this abscess was a persistent periodontal pocket on tooth 48; this was treated using a separate incision.

Left: Three days postsurgically, the incision wound is closed by a fibrous covering, and there is no evidence of further secretion.

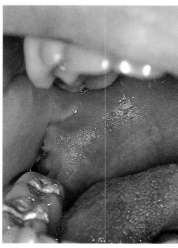
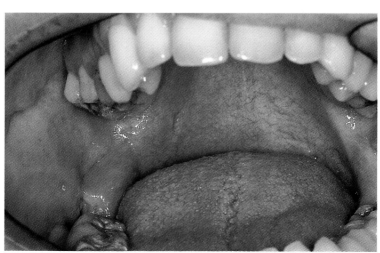

390 Follow-up

Postsurgical check-ups should be made daily until the clinical symptoms of infection have clearly subsided.

When residual secretion has stopped, the drain can be removed in this case on the third postoperative day *(left)*.

Right: The check-up seven days after surgery shows normal mouth opening (48 mm) and virtually complete healing of the incision wound. The treatment plan includes extraction of tooth 48 at the earliest possible opportunity.

Paramandibular Abscess

The most frequent cause of this type of abscess is an apical infection of a mandibular molar that has not been adequately treated. Massive, painful swelling is seen around the mandible, but the mandibular border remains palpable. Patients have difficulty with mouth opening, and this restricts clinical inspection and access, especially if the swelling is lingually oriented.

A paramandibular abscess may develop into a perimandibular abscess with demarcation.

Whether outpatient treatment can be given or the patient should be hospitalized must be decided in each individual case.

Generally, the incision is made using an extraoral approach under general anesthesia. If it is possible to achieve adequate anesthesia locally, a buccolingual or lingual incision can be made. The long primary incision requires a rubber drain to be placed to ensure adequate drainage. The hemostat should be used buccally and lingually to provide broad opening of the surgical site.

Caution

Avoid encroachment on the facial nerve. The incision should be made two fingerbreadths caudal to the margin of the mandible.

391 Paramandibular abscess, vestibular and lingual
This 58-year-old man presented with severely carious and damaged teeth, as well as a pronounced swelling paramandibularly on the right side, including the buccal and lingual aspects of the mandible. It was impossible to palpate the internal oblique line.

Right: The radiograph shows root fragments of teeth 47 and 48, with apical osteolysis but no sclerosis.

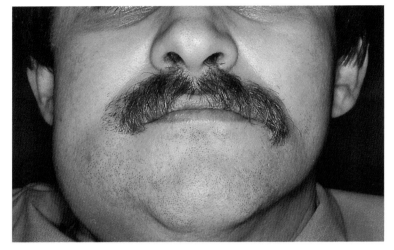
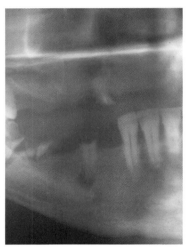

392 Incision
After block anesthesia and local infiltration of the long buccal nerve, the abscess is opened using an incision directed perpendicular to the surface of the bone.

Right: The buccal and lingual incisions. The lingual incision is made horizontally at the transition zone to the floor of the mouth at the level of the first molar.

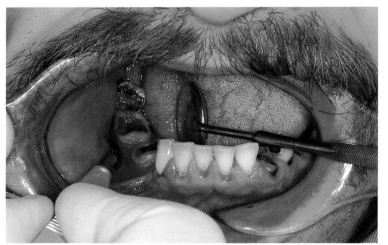
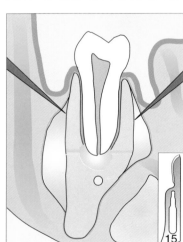

393 Expansion
Both buccally and lingually *(right)*, the hemostat has to be inserted to the bottom of the abscess and withdrawn in the open position to completely open the abscess for drainage. Access from the lingual aspect is achieved in the region of the first molar distally and caudally, with bone contact. This precludes any injury to the lingual nerve.

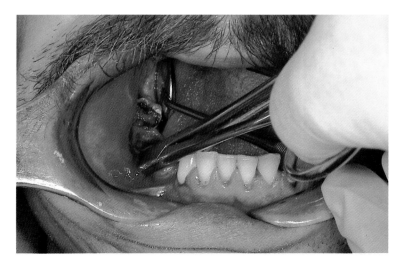
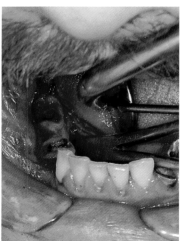

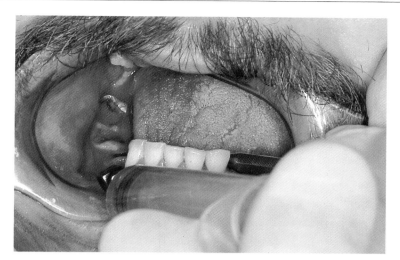

394 Rinsing
A syringe with a blunt tip is used to rinse out the opened abscess cavity thoroughly; gentle massage externally helps to express pus from the intraoral site. The retained root fragments, which are the original cause of the condition, can be extracted during the same procedure.

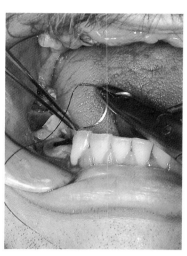 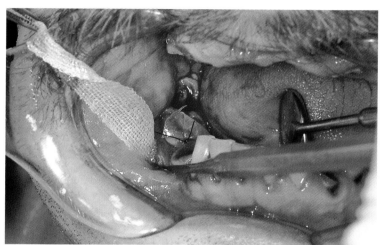

395 Drainage
The long drainage pathway on the lingual aspect is held open using a ligated rubber drain.

Left: Placement of a gauze strip is usually adequate for drainage from the buccal aspect.

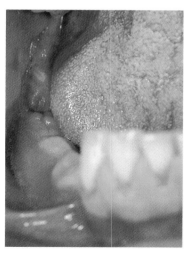 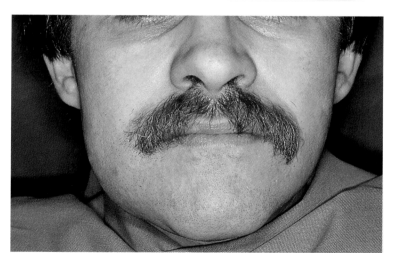

396 Follow-up
After three days of daily dressing change and rinsing on both the lingual and buccal aspects, the active exudation has stopped. Additional drainage is no longer necessary *(left)*.

Right: After a total of five days, there is only an indolent, nonfluctuant swelling on the right side of the mandible.

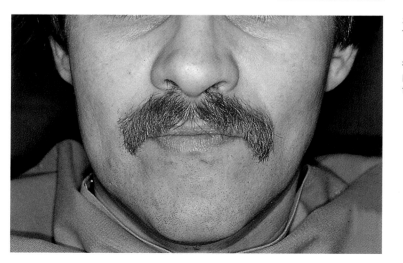

397 Completion of treatment
Ten days later, the symptoms of inflammation have completely subsided; the extraction site is completely covered with granulation tissue and is free of irritation.

Actinomycosis

Actinomycosis usually develops from an incompletely healed infection. The causative microorganism is *Actinomyces israelii*, a saprophytic inhabitant of the oral cavity. This organism becomes pathogenic under anaerobic conditions. The pathogen may come from a necrotic dental pulp, a periodontal pocket, an extraction wound, or even from ulcerated mucosa, and it finds its way into deeper tissues in which there are anaerobic conditions. The pathogenic effect depends on other accompanying agents that produce hyaluronidase. The end result is thus an actinomycotic mixed infection, which derives from a pyogenic dental infec-

tion. This clinical condition is referred to as cervicofacial actinomycosis.

The impressive clinical manifestations include indurated swelling with a bluish-red skin coloring, often associated with fistula formation and subcutaneous spread. Definitive diagnosis is made on the basis of microbiological evaluation using anaerobic cultures.

Treatment includes surgical intervention and a regimen of high-dose antibiotics, and iontophoresis may also be used. Some patients may have to be hospitalized.

398 Actinomycosis
A 47-year-old man presented with a two-week history of gradual, mildly painful swelling and erythema of the skin covering the inferior border of the mandible on the left side.

Right: The radiograph reveals carious teeth, periodontal pockets, and apical osteolysis on tooth 35. The course and the clinical picture suggest actinomycosis.

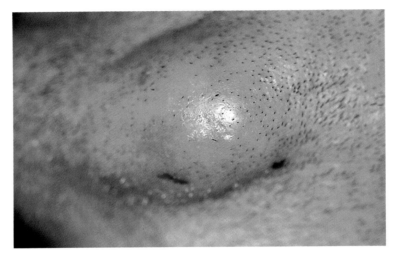 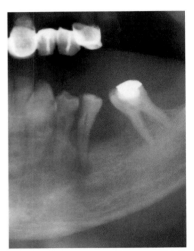

399 Extraoral incision
The abscess is incised both intraorally (vestibular abscess) and extraorally. The incision through the skin is treated with a rubber drain. This provides a relatively irritation-free incision wound. The affected teeth should be extracted during the same appointment.

Right: Aspiration after introducing a syringe tip yields a bloody, opaque secretion. The culture demonstrates *Actinomyces.*

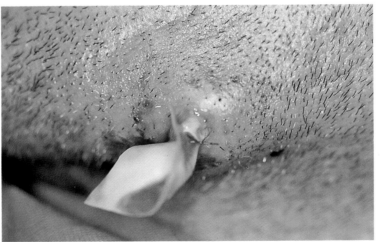 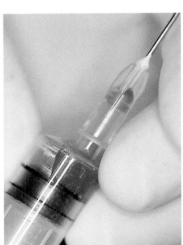

400 Clinical course
After two external drain changes, no further secretion can be detected. The photograph shows the situation after spontaneous healing of the skin wound on the seventh postoperative day. The usual clinical course is short, and free of complications. Swabs of the area cultured anaerobically show no signs of *Actinomyces.*

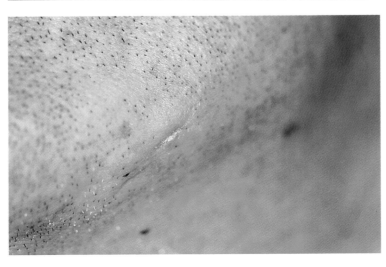

Surgical Procedure for Maxillary Abscesses

Abscess in the Canine Fossa

These abscesses usually originate from the anterior teeth, and less often from the premolars. The most dramatic clinical symptoms include substantial swelling in the upper regions of the cheek, with pain located in the region of the canine fossa. The overlying skin appears stretched, erythematous, and often shiny. Collateral edema often includes the upper lip and the eyelid. The soft tissues of the nose may also be affected. The radiating and very painful indurations toward the median orbital angle are an indication of possible infection via the angular vein. The infection may spread by way of this vein into the cavernous sinus.

Treatment consists of intraoral incision and drainage of the abscess, and elimination of the causative agents. Care should be taken when opening the abscess to avoid injury to the infraorbital nerve where it exits from the skull. Anesthesia is administered extraorally near the infraorbital foramen.

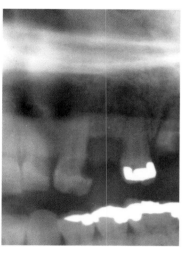
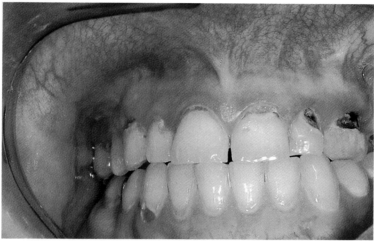

401   Abscess in the canine fossa
Right: Palpation in the vestibulum of the right side of the maxilla revealed a discrete, well-demarcated and indurated swelling.

Left: Radiograph showing a nonvital tooth 15. The clinical and radiographic picture is not typical, and involvement of the anterior teeth has to be excluded.

Ⓢ

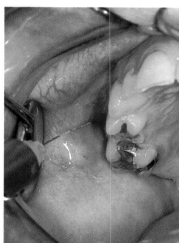
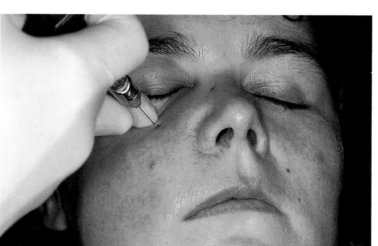

402   Anesthesia
Extraoral infiltration at the infraorbital foramen on the right; this is necessary because intraoral administration would pass through the abscess itself.

Left: Administration of anesthetic solution distal to tooth 16 from the buccal approach.

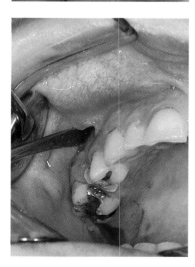
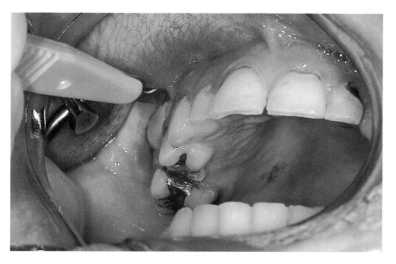

403   Opening the abscess
The primary incision is made at the transition from the mobile mucosa, in a horizontal direction with the scalpel blade perpendicular to the osseous surface.

Left: A periosteal elevator is used to reflect the periosteum. Tissue reflection should be not carried too far cranially, in order to avoid impinging on the infraorbital nerve where it exits from the cranium.

Vestibular Abscess

Vestibular abscess usually originates with the maxillary premolars and molars. Clinical examination normally reveals a firm and painful swelling in the buccal vestibule near the tooth causing the condition.

Treatment consists of opening the abscess, drainage, and elimination of the etiology.

Clinical Tip
The primary incision should be vertical at the site of the anticipated releasing incision; this makes it easier to create an appropriate flap if it is subsequently necessary to close the sinus.

Abscess in the Cheek

Vestibular abscesses from the maxilla, as well as from the mandible, may spread into the soft tissues of the cheek. If an abscess develops in a cranial direction, it meets the adipose tissue in the cheek, with subsequent spread along anatomical planes toward the infratemporal fossa or the pterygopalatine fossa. Further cranial and dorsal spread is possible.

Treatment consists of opening the abscess and blunt enlargement of the abscess cavity. Branches of the facial artery course through the soft tissues. For anesthesia, the buccal nerve is infiltrated along the anterior border of the ascending ramus.

404 Vestibular abscess on the maxillary alveolar process
This 31-year-old man had been experiencing increasing dental pain in the left maxilla for three days. Initially, it had been temperature-dependent, but it had become constant during the previous night, accompanied by swelling in the left cheek, which was beginning to sag.

Right: Periapical radiograph. The CO_2 test on tooth 24 was negative.

Ⓢ

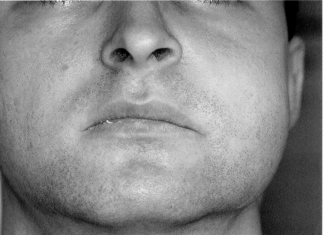
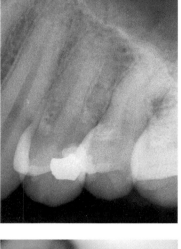

405 Anesthesia
Infiltration within the superficial mucosa.

Right: Infiltration anesthesia near the tuberosity beyond the extent of the abscess.

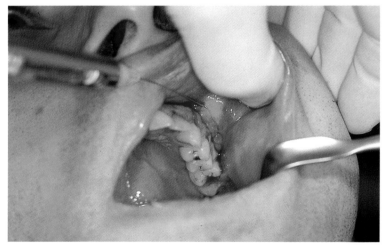
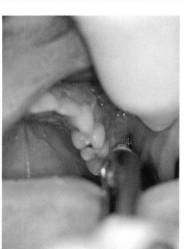

406 Incision
The blade is guided horizontally, perpendicular to the osseous surface, approximately at the mucogingival border.

Right: The correct orientation for the primary incision.

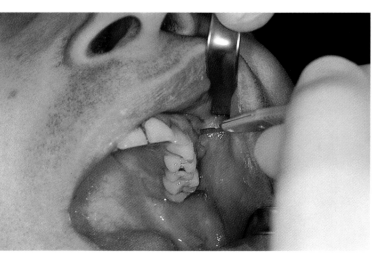
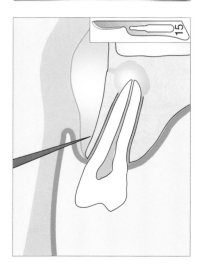

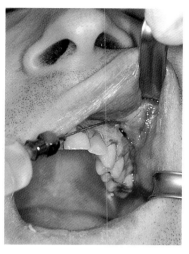
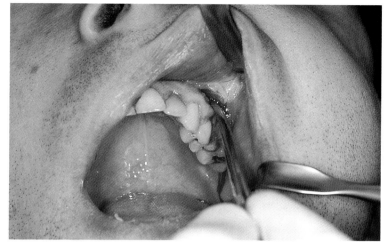

407 Expansion
The entrance into the abscess cavity is widened using a periosteal elevator or a blunt hemostat, and the pus is pressed out.

Left: Rinsing the abscess cavity with saline or neomycin solution.

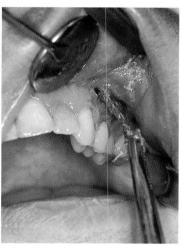
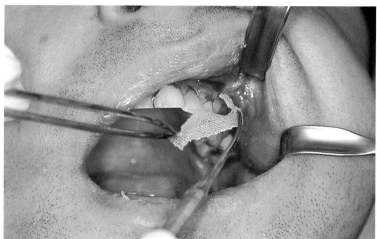

408 Drainage
Drainage of subsequently accumulating secretions is ensured by placing a Chlumsky gauze strip. Treatment of the tooth itself can be initiated during the first appointment. In this case, the tooth is to be preserved.

Left: The drain is changed daily.

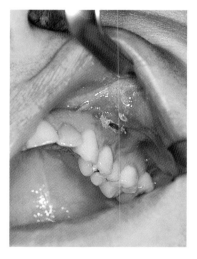
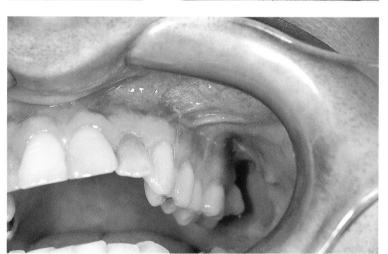

409 Postoperative care
Rinsing and drainage of the abscess cavity are carried out daily until no further secretion can be detected. After three days, it is no longer necessary to change the drain.

Left: Endodontic treatment of the tooth should be initiated before the end of the abscess treatment.

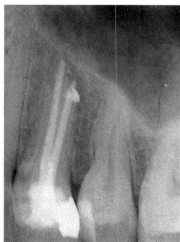
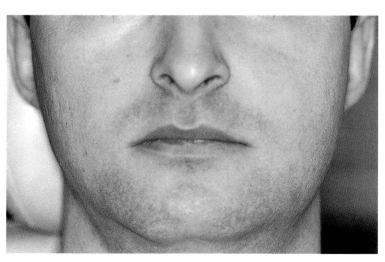

410 Termination of treatment
The oral surgery treatment is complete 14 days postoperatively, with the final postoperative check-up.

Left: The radiograph shows successful obturation of the two root canals of the responsible tooth.

Palatal Abscess

The etiology usually involves the roots of the lateral incisors or the first premolars, as the roots of these teeth often incline palatally. Due to natural hemostasis, the mucosa covering the balloon-like palatal swelling may appear cyanotic and atrophic.

The primary incision is made parallel to the course of the palatine artery. Because of the tautness of the palatal soft tissues, there is a danger that the primary incision will close spontaneously due to soft-tissue pressure. Treatment for palatal abscess should therefore include a double-elliptical incision, with removal of tissue, as shown in the figures below. Drainage and postoperative care should be targeted toward repositioning the firm palatal tissues on the subjacent bone. The period of drainage should not exceed three days.

Clinical Tip

The course of the palatine artery should be noted, and caution should be used. Severe hemorrhage can arise even from the branches of this artery if they are severed. Bleeding can be arrested using ligation at the incision margin or electrocoagulation.

411 Palatal abscess
In this 39-year-old man, tooth 13 had fractured off several weeks previously. During the previous few days, a firm swelling had developed on the right side of the palate. The mass was fluctuant. There was no swelling on the buccal aspect.

Right: The periapical radiograph shows the remaining root of tooth 13, with apical widening of the periodontal ligament space.

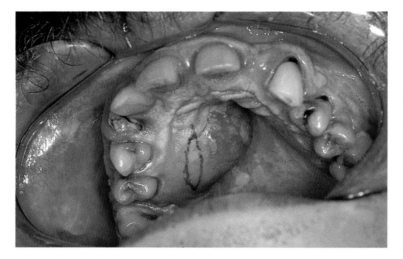
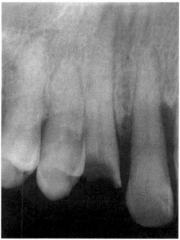

412 Incision with excision
If only a simple incision were to be made, the very firm palatal mucosa would collapse the incision, preventing drainage. For this reason, a double-elliptical incision is made, with excision of palatal tissue to open the abscess broadly.

Right: The position of the palatine artery must be borne in mind.

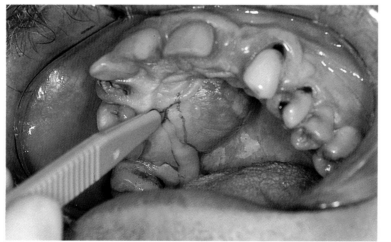
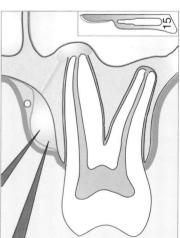

413 Follow-up
The excision opens the abscess cavity broadly. The incision margins collapse, but an opening to drain the secretions remains patent.

Left: In this case, a Chlumsky drain was placed. Daily check-ups are needed until no further secretion is seen. Treatment of the tooth can be started at the first appointment, and continued normally.

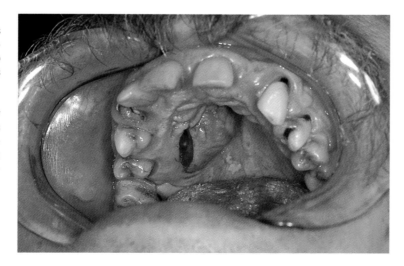
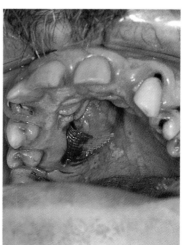

Surgical Procedure for Widespread Infection

Facial space infections

Surgical measures for treating of abscesses within the facial tissue cavities are basically identical to those for abscesses deriving from the alveolar process. As tissue abscesses are deeper, the drainage pathway is longer, and drainage using a rubber tube is usually needed. Surgical access is generally obtained from an extraoral approach under general anesthesia. We prefer short-acting anesthetics administered intravenously. If the patient presents with limited jaw-opening capacity, no attempt should be made to force intubation, as this could result in spontaneous opening of the abscess and the danger of aspiration. In addition, forced mouth opening to allow intubation carries a risk of expressing pus into and along the natural facial planes. Anesthesia for patients with limited jaw opening should be administered only intravenously, or via nasal intubation.

> #### Clinical Tip
> There is a high risk of spreading the infection. The patient should be referred to a specialist.

Temporal Abscess

This type of abscess is usually seen as a sequela of a retromaxillary abscess.

Primary incisions are made from both intraoral and extraoral approaches, and a rubber drain is inserted, passing beneath the zygomatic arch to exit at both aspects. This type of treatment is carried out on an in-patient basis.

Retromaxillary Abscess

Apart from pain in the maxilla and progressive obstruction of mouth opening, there are few clinical symptoms. Possible etiological factors include previous therapeutic measures such as extraction of maxillary third molars, periodontal pocket treatment in the maxillary molar region, or hematoma formation after administration of local anesthesia. The primary incision is made on the buccal aspect of the maxillary second molar, and the abscess is opened by reflection posteriorly and cranially.

Postoperative Care

Clinical treatment of an abscess must continue until all symptoms of infection have disappeared and the etiological factor has been eliminated.

In addition to continuing causal therapy, the abscess cavity must be rinsed and drained daily to ensure that all secretions are drained. Active treatment can only be stopped when no additional secretions are apparent, and when swelling, pain, and trismus are no longer in evidence.

A primary goal of postoperative care is to reestablish normal mouth opening (at least 35 mm). Patients should be instructed to carry out mouth-opening exercises using a wooden spatula.

If firm swelling persists, warm, moist compresses should be applied.

Components of Drains

Sterile gauze, 1 cm broad

Chlumsky solution (ingredient ratios):
—Camphor: 6
—Phenol: 3
—Absolute ethanol: 1

Root Tip Resection

Apicoectomy

Definition

The term "apicoectomy" covers the surgical removal of pathologically altered tissues near the root apex, the elimination of the apical ramifications of the root canal (resection), and simultaneous bacteria-tight closure of the root canal or canals. This surgical technique was first described by Partsch in 1899, and has since been one of the most common procedures in oral surgery.

Indication

The clinical indication for root tip resection may be based on a failure of endodontic treatment, for whatever reasons, or due to the growth and type of a pathological process at the apex of an affected tooth if the tooth is to be preserved in an overall treatment plan (Obwegeser and Tschamer 1957, Nair and Schroeder 1983, Morse and Bhambhani 1990, Negm 1990, Ørstavic 1991).

414 Indications for root tip resection—fistula formation
No periodontal pocket can be detected, and the tooth is not mobile.

Right: The radiograph shows apical osteolysis, which is a sign of chronic infection at the root tip.

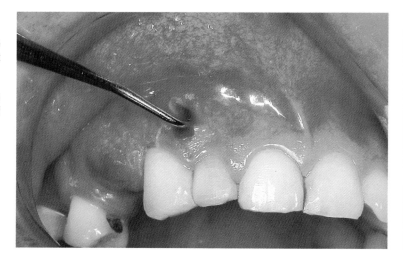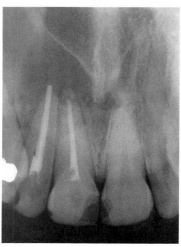

415 Unsatisfactory root canal filling
The widening of the periodontal ligament space in the apical area is a sign of chronic inflammation at the tip of the root of tooth 25. The existing root canal treatment cannot be improved by retrograde approach.

Right: This periapical radiograph depicts tooth 25 with a file in situ. An iatrogenic endodontic failure is suspected.

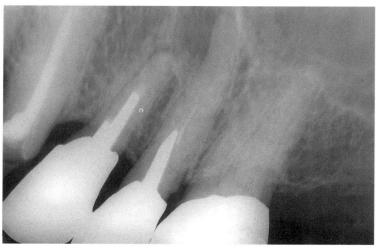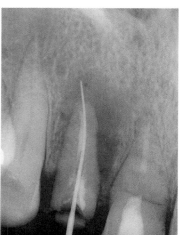

Surgical Procedure

Documentation

The clinical condition of the adjacent teeth should be taken into account, with regard to pocket formation, mobility, and vitality.

The apical region of the tooth to be treated, and the adjacent teeth, must be evaluated radiographically.

—The periapical radiograph provides information about the osseous structures.
—An occlusal radiograph of the anterior segment of the mandible shows the palatal extent of an osteolytic process.
—The panoramic radiograph helps set the surgical indication.

Incisions

The degree and direction of flap reflection are determined by the need to achieve good visualization of the expected surgical field. It is also critical to ensure an adequate blood supply for the flap. If there is scar tissue from previous surgery, a slightly more generous mucoperiosteal flap should be created.

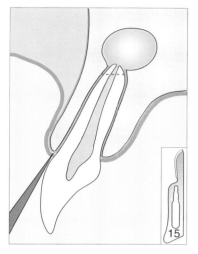
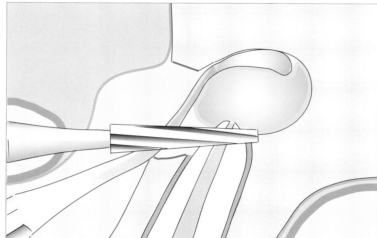

416 Access
Access is achieved by reflection of a mucoperiosteal flap following a primary intrasulcal incision *(left)*.

Right: A tapered fissure bur is used to approach the apex. All granulation tissue is then carefully and completely removed using curettes, and 2 mm at the apex of the root are resected.

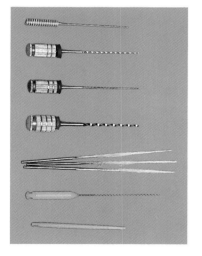
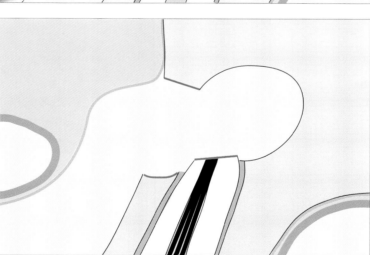

417 Orthograde root filling
During the surgical procedure for apicoectomy, it is often possible to carry out conventional endodontic treatment to create tight closure of the root canal, preventing bacterial invasion. Use of a gutta percha point and radiopaque, nonresorbable cement provides secure closure and a filling that can be checked radiographically.

Left: Instrumentarium for endodontic treatment.

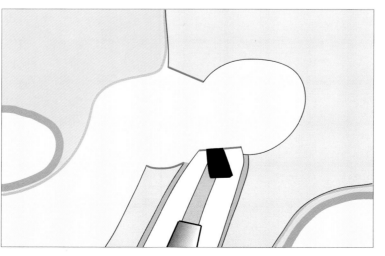

418 Retrograde closure of the apex
If it is not possible to carry out simultaneous conventional endodontic treatment during the surgical procedure, future bacterial colonization of the root apex can be prevented by retrograde filling at the apex. The filling material must be radiopaque, and must be capable of setting completely in conditions that are not absolutely dry. The filling material must not be resorbable. Silver amalgam has now been replaced by glass ionomer cement or composite materials with zinc oxide cement.

Pathogenesis of Apical Osteitis

The precise pathological events that lead to chronic apical osteitis and granuloma formation are still poorly understood. However, there have been some investigations attempting to explain this multifactorial process (Nair and Schroeder 1983). The primary event in the infection is the colonization of the root canal by bacteria from the oral cavity. Because of the local conditions, a selectively anaerobic mixed infection is established. The products of this mixed flora have varying biological characteristics, such as antigenicity, mitogenic activity, chemotaxis, enzymatic histolysis, and the formation of both endotoxins and exotoxins. Within the root canal, these bacteria cannot be eliminated by the normal host response mechanisms, and the lesions therefore have no tendency to heal spontaneously. However, the host defense can prevent spread of the bacteria into the periapical tissues. This is the reason why bacteria are only very rarely observed in a periapical granuloma.

The apical inflammation is caused by bacterial products. This results in tissue destruction and the activation of osteoclasts. These cells are responsible for the apical osteolysis that precedes granuloma formation.

Depending on host defense capacity, the inflammation can appear as an acute infection with abscess formation and external drainage, or as a true osteomyelitis. If the infection becomes chronic, a quiescent phase may ensue, with encapsulation of the inflamed area (granuloma); the spread of bacteria away from the periapical region is prohibited. This condition can persist for long periods of time. The delicate balance between the bacterial flora at the apex and the host defense mechanisms can be tipped at any time by any minute change in the immune response, and the lesion can return to an acute phase. This scenario may also be involved in potential or actual foci of infection.

Chronic periapical osteitis is the pathological process that is most often treated by apicoectomy. Although today's refined endodontic treatment procedures can usually bring apical inflammation under control, there are anatomical and technical problems that prevent elimination of the cause of the apical infection; the result can be permanent bacteriological and toxic effects on the periapical tissues (Lin et al. 1991).

Complete Closure of the Apex

In accordance with these views of the pathogenesis of apical osteitis, complete obturation of the root canal is the most important requirement for success following root tip resection.

Infected periodontal pockets can also lead to apical osteitis in the form of a combined endodontic–periodontal inflammation. In these cases, the primary treatment should aim to eliminate the endodontic infection (König et al. 1994).

Orthograde Closure

If the root canal was not definitively filled before the surgical procedure, this must be accomplished during the operation. The apical region must be completely closed using a gutta percha point or a titanium pin (Ackermann 1951, Berthold 1993, Bhaskar 1966, Ehrl 1990, Rehrmann 1951). For the past ten years, we have used a calcium hydroxide–based cement (CRCS) with gutta percha points for compression and canal obturation (Briseño et al. 1991). Carrying out the root canal filling procedure during the surgical operation provides direct vision during canal instrumentation and rinsing. This increases the likelihood that the entire cross-sectional profile of the canal will be completely filled.

The root tip is resected immediately after endodontic treatment has been completed, directly perpendicular to the cross-sectional profile of the root.

If a titanium pin is used to close off the apex, any excess length of the titanium can be left, and the rest of the root canal can be filled using gutta percha points and cement.

Retrograde Closure

If placement of an orthograde root canal filling is not possible, the canal must be filled using the retrograde approach.

First, the apical 2 mm of the root tip are resected. This resection should be carried out as perpendicularly as possible to the cross-sectional profile of the root, but this is not always feasible. A slightly tangential resection allows the access required for closure in difficult cases. A mini-cavity is prepared using a miniature contra-angle handpiece or an ultrasonic instrument, and filled. The alternative materials which are nowadays used instead of amalgam include glass ionomer cement (Ketac) or zinc oxide-eugenol cement (Super EBA) (Pantschev et al. 1994, Smee et al. 1987). The minimum requirements for any filling material are that it should be able to undergo the final setting reaction in the presence of moisture, and that it should radiopaque (Friedman 1991, Hickel 1990, Halse et al. 1991, Smee et al. 1987).

Possible Problems with Closure

If hemorrhage is a problem during closure of the canal, rinsing with 3% H_2O_2 can be carried out, along with tamponade or application of bone wax.

If the roots of the adjacent teeth are damaged, endodontic therapy, including root tip resection, should be performed during the same appointment.

Opening the Periapical Space

With the exception of apical processes that have perforated through the cortical bone, the inflamed periapical region can generally be located by means of bleeding points. In doubtful situations, a radiograph and a calibrated probe can be used to locate the apical region.

A large round bone cutter is used to remove cortical bone overlying the tip of the root. The tip of the root can be recognized by its color and consistency. A smaller bur is used to expose the root apex, and the surrounding granulation tissue is removed using curettes. If the root tip inhibits the curettage process, it can be immediately resected to facilitate removal of periapical granulation tissues. Removed tissue specimens are normally sent for histopathological evaluation. In straightforward cases with minimal periapical granulation tissue, however, there is usually no need for histological examination.

Failures Following Apicoectomy

Using the techniques described here, the success rate at our clinic has been 85% complete healing over a period of three to six years (Maienfisch 1980). This statistic is based on cases with radiographic evidence of complete reestablishment of the periodontal ligament space in the periapical region, and lacking any clinical symptomatology. Patients who were free of clinical symptoms but nevertheless had a zone of periapical radiolucency were classified under incomplete healing. This category included 11% of all root resections. Failures included those instances in which there was no osseous regeneration, or fistulous tract formation ensued, and those in which inflammatory soft-tissue reactions were recorded. Fewer than 4% of our patients fell into to these categories.

Evaluating Success

The most reliable criterion for successful healing after apicoectomy is the periapical radiograph, along with observations of clinical symptoms. In a report by Halse et al. (1991), only five of 474 teeth that had been treated by apicoectomy failed to show osseous regeneration at the apex one year postoperatively; follow-up examination of these cases failed to reveal any improvement. The conclusion that can be drawn from this observation is that after apicoectomy, there should be evidence of healing within a 12-month period, otherwise the case must be regarded as a failure, with further treatment being indicated.

Primary Incision

Creation of a mucoperiosteal flap after a standard intrasulcal primary incision provides better visualization, and the flap can be repositioned without difficulty (Mühlemann 1963, Pichler 1921). The releasing incisions diverge distally, so that the flap has a broad base. The incisions should not involve the interdental papillae. This technique for preparing a soft-tissue flap virtually guarantees problem-free wound closure, even in cases in which tooth extraction is necessary. The releasing incisions, placed vertically, guarantee an adequate blood supply to the flap.

If healthy periodontal conditions are present, there is no reason to expect gingival recession. If there is extensive restorative work with subgingival crown margins, especially in the presence of pockets deeper than 3 mm, some postsurgical gingival recession can be expected in some cases. If it appears that undesirable aesthetic consequences may occur, the primary incision can be made in the mobile vestibular mucosa. The patient must be advised of the advantages and disadvantages before the operation.

Vestibular Mucoperiosteal Flap (Paragingival Incision of Partsch)

The primary incision is horizontal, with bilateral vertical releasing incisions. The transition from the releasing incision should be approximately a right angle. This allows precise flap repositioning for suture closure. The horizontal incision should course through the mobile vestibular mucosa a few millimeters apical to the mucogingival junction. Before sutures are placed, any areas of mucosa that are adherent should be undermined. This type of flap reflection provides limited direct vision, and does not correspond to the vertical course of vascularization within the gingiva. Repositioning this type of flap is not always precise, and some scar formation can be expected.

Clinical Tip
The location and expanse of the flap must be such that the subsequent suture line will be over bone.

419 Flap design—gingival and paragingival incisions
An intrasulcal primary incision should extend over at least two teeth; vertical releasing incisions into the mobile mucosa can be made unilaterally or bilaterally. The interdental papillae should be included in the reflected flap, and should never be severed. If periodontal pockets are present, some gingival recession can be expected postoperatively.

Below: Paragingival incision. To avoid the danger of gingival recession in an anterior segment in which the crown margins are located subgingivally, a flap can be designed and reflected that does not encroach on the attached gingiva. The vertical releasing incision should be made at a sharp right angle to the horizontal incision; this will be helpful during flap repositioning, for orientation. Disadvantages include difficulty in precise flap repositioning, and scar tissue formation. There is also a risk that the flap will be repositioned directly over an unexpected osseous defect.

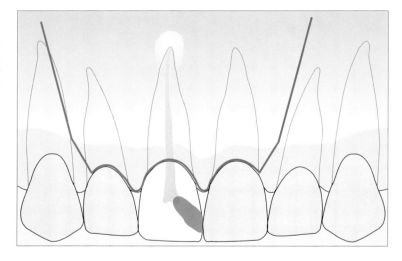

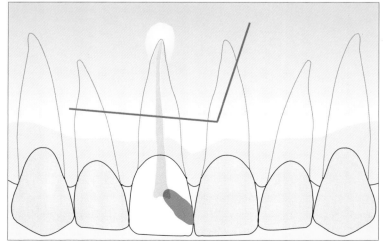

Resection with Orthograde Root Canal Filling in the Anterior Mandible

Anesthesia

Surgical intervention in the anterior mandible requires block anesthesia on the affected side, with local infiltration on the opposite side of the midline.

Anatomy

Care must be taken not to damage the mental nerve where it exits from the mental foramen. During the surgical procedure, this nerve must be shielded from trauma.

Flap Reflection

In the anterior area, the mucoperiosteal flap should be at least as wide as three teeth, and divergent releasing incisions should be placed distally and mesially. Failure to observe these basic principles could result in an inadequate blood supply and limited visual access, or even to trauma of the flap due to tension. In simple situations, it is also possible to work effectively with a single releasing incision.

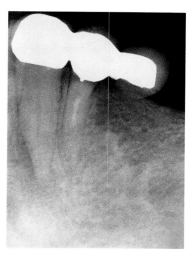
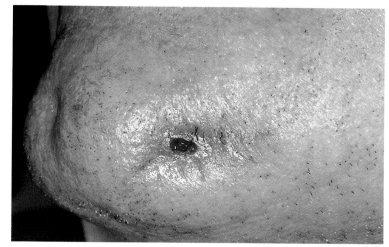
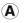

420 Orthograde root canal filling and resection in the mandible

This 42-year-old man had had a persistent fistula on the chin for two years; numerous attempts had been made to close the fistula surgically.

Left: The periapical radiograph reveals an apical radiolucency on tooth 33, which was nonvital, and also on tooth 34, in which inadequate endodontic treatment has been carried out.

Ⓐ

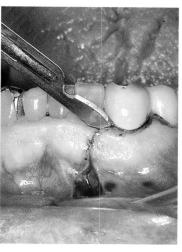
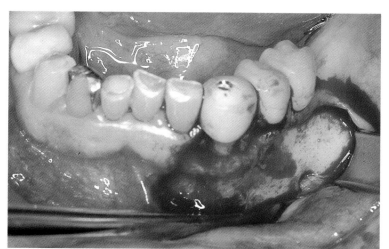

421 Access

The primary incision is intrasulcal, with releasing incisions mesial to tooth 33 and distal to tooth 35. It is necessary to expose the mental nerve where it exits from the foramen. This is the only way of protecting the nerve from injury during the procedure.

Left: Application of the scalpel in the papillary region. The interdental papillae are included in the reflected flap.

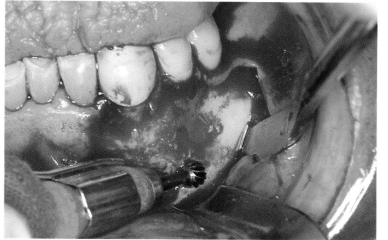

422 Ostectomy

A periosteal elevator is used to protect the mental nerve at the foramen, and a large round bur is used with water cooling to remove cortical bone and expose the apex of the root of tooth 33.

423 Exposing the apex
Careful additional ostectomy reveals the apex of tooth 33, which is then completely exposed by removing granulation tissue.

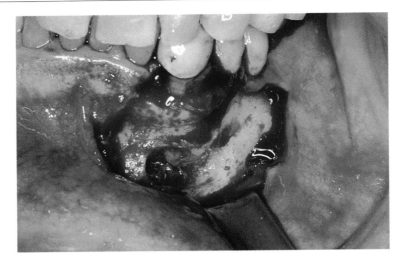

424 Resection
Using a fissure bur, the apical 2 mm of the root tip are resected.

Right: The tip of the root is removed from the osseous cavity.

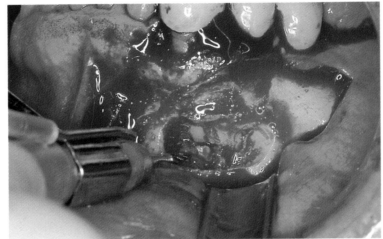
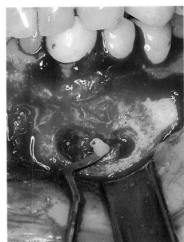

425 Granulation tissue
Granulation tissue is removed and can be sent for histological evaluation (cyst?). The osseous defect is inspected, and any hemorrhage from the bone or soft tissues is arrested by tamponading the wound surface using 3% H_2O_2 solution, or by ligating vessels, or using electrosurgical coagulation. In some cases, diffuse bleeding can be stopped by repeated infiltration of local anesthetic solution, or by compressing bone wax into the area.

Right: Using a Black's excavator to dislodge the granuloma.

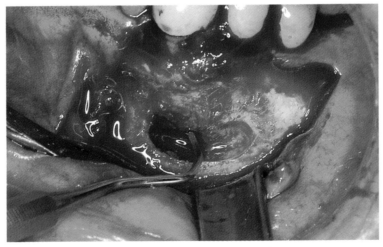
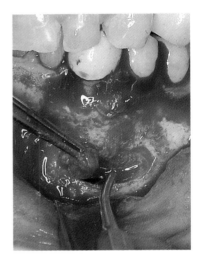

426 Preparation of the root canal
The root canal, which was opened presurgically, can now be cleaned and instrumented.

Right: The root canal is dried using alcohol, applied with cotton wrapped on a steel-barbed broach.

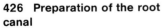
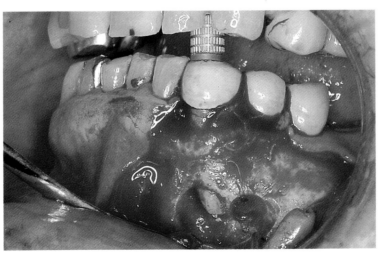
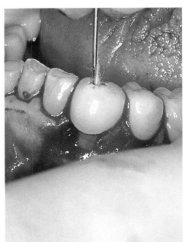

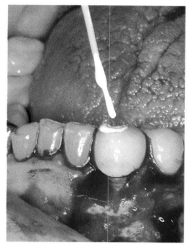
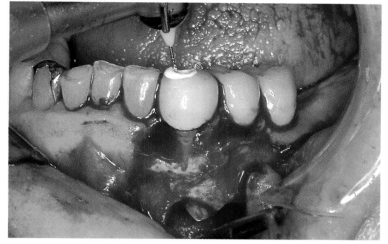

427 Root canal filling
The cement is pressed into the root canal with one or more gutta percha points. The root canal itself, which was opened presurgically, can now be enlarged and cleaned *(left)*.

Right: After drying the instrumented root canal, a lentulo spiral is used to rotate cement into the canal.

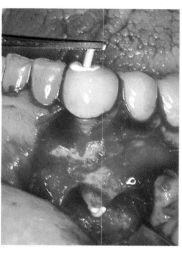
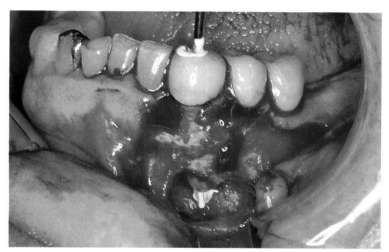

428 Root canal filling
All of the intraoral manipulations are carried out under direct vision, ensuring complete internal coating of the root canal walls *(left)*. The egress of cement and the gutta percha point must be visible at the root apex.

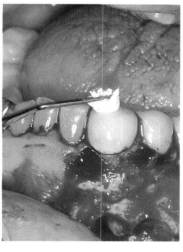
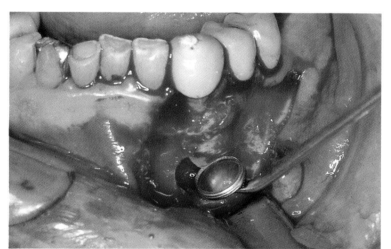

429 Checking for complete closure
A heated instrument is used to remove excess root canal filling material from the root apex.

Left: A check is made for complete closure at the apex by forcefully inserting temporary filling material into the coronal cavity.

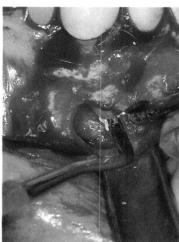
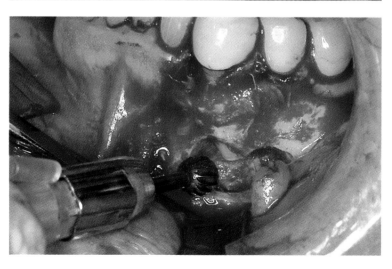

430 Wound treatment and postoperative care
After removal of excess cement from the root apex, the osseous borders are smoothed. The surgical site is then rinsed, and a final inspection is made (to confirm that there has been no injury to the mental nerve), followed by suture closure of the soft-tissue flap. A radiograph should be taken immediately for documentation. Suture removal can be done at seven to ten days, with a check-up after six months.

Left: Removal of excess filling material at the apex.

431 Resection and retrograde filling in the mandible

Same patient as in Fig. 420. Because tooth 34 had previously been treated endodontically, it was not possible to place a new, orthograde root canal filling. After resection of the root tip, a small retrograde cavity is prepared. A miniature contra-angle handpiece is convenient for this purpose.

Right: Resection of the root tip using a fissure bur.

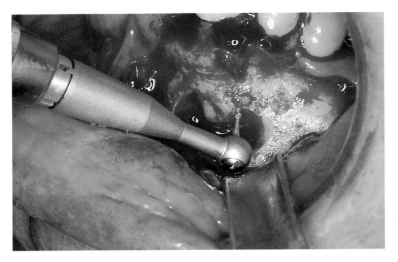

432 Hemostasis

Placing a retrograde filling requires essentially dry conditions in the area. Local hemorrhage from the bone can often be stopped by tapping with a blunt instrument.

Right: Bone wax can be used to stop superficial bleeding from the trabecular spaces.

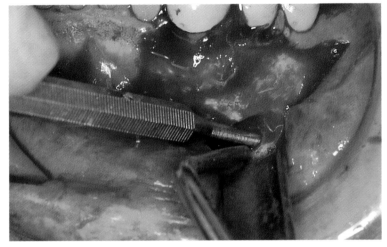
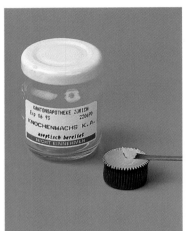

433 Retrograde root canal closure

A special instrument is used to place the filling material in the cavity prepared at the apex of tooth 34. In this case, a modified forceps is being used.

Right: Miniaturized applicator for filling material.

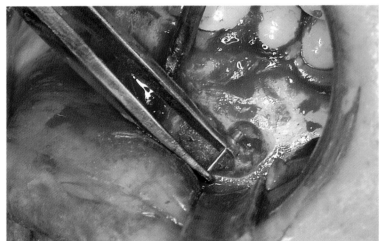
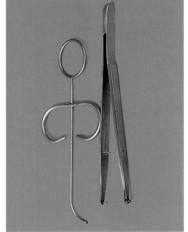

434 Wound treatment

The final filling is checked visually to ensure complete closure of the cavity.

Right: The status of the mental nerve is checked visually before the mucoperiosteal flap is repositioned.

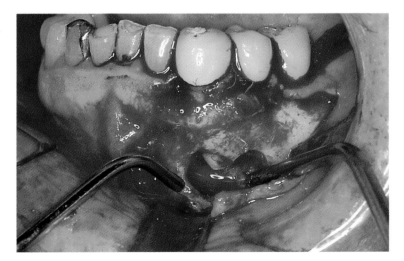
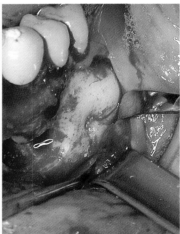

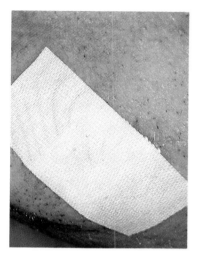

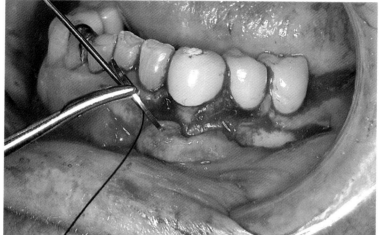

435 Fistulous tract
Before closing the wound with sutures, the external aspect of the fistulous tract is thoroughly curetted, and the external wound is then closed after thorough rinsing.

Left: An adhesive bandage is used to close the external wound.

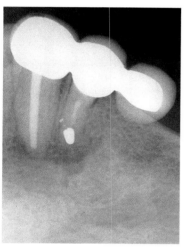

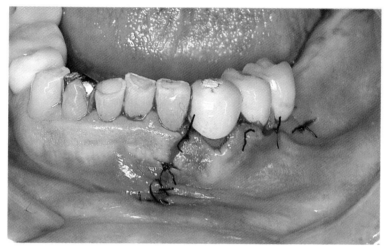

436 Postoperative condition
The tissue flap is repositioned and affixed using interrupted sutures. The sutures can be removed seven to ten days later.

Left: The periapical radiograph taken immediately postoperatively shows an orthograde root tip filling on tooth 33 and retrograde closure of tooth 34.

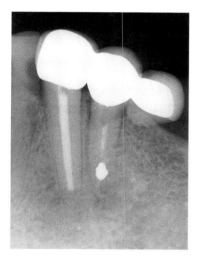

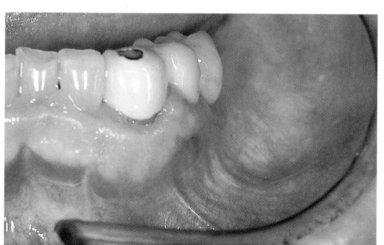

437 Successful course
At the check-up appointment six months postsurgically, the intraoral conditions were clinically acceptable, and the patient had not experienced any disturbances of sensitivity in the region.

Left: The periapical radiograph shows osseous regeneration at the apices of teeth 33 and 34.

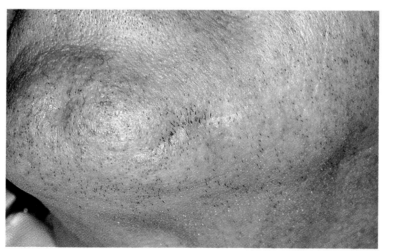

438 Completion of treatment
The external fistula has completely healed without additional treatment, and is scarcely visible.

Resection with Retrograde Root Canal Filling in the Anterior Maxilla

Anesthesia

Local anesthetic must be administered palatally as well as in the vestibule. Infiltration near the infraorbital foramen on the affected side is also normally used, with a terminal depot being placed on the contralateral side. The incisive papilla is infiltrated directly, and infiltration is also given lateral to it toward the affected side.

Flap Reflection

The primary incision should, in almost every case, be intrasulcal to provide unimpeded access. In most cases, two diverging releasing incisions are also placed mesially and distally. In simple cases, it may be possible to work with only one releasing incision.

439 Resection in the maxilla—access
The intrasulcal primary incision courses from tooth 12 to tooth 23, and is enhanced by two releasing incisions.

Right: The occlusal radiograph shows cystic osteolysis in the region of tooth 22, as well as a radiolucency near tooth 11.

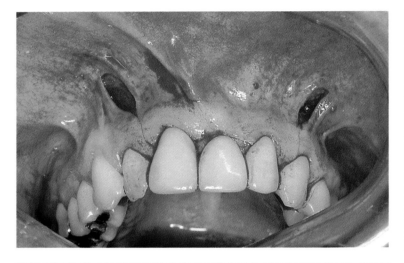
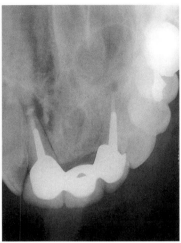

440 Flap reflection
A periosteal elevator is used to reflect the mucoperiosteal flap sufficiently for the apical region of the affected tooth to be viewed directly.

Right: Application of the periosteal elevator near the interdental papillae of tooth 11.

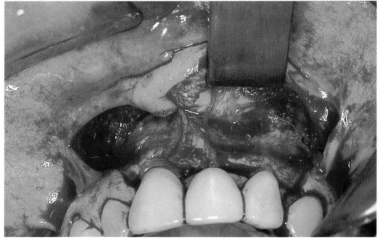
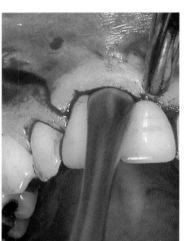

441 Granulation tissue
The bony cavity around the root apex, which has been exposed using a round burr, is carefully probed. A Black's excavator is used to separate the rather compact tissue from the margin.

Right: Exposed buccal surface of tooth 12.

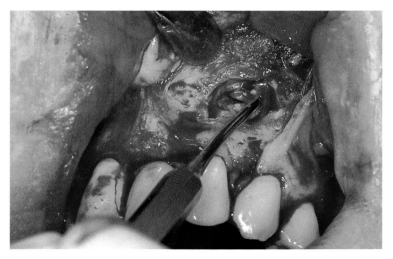
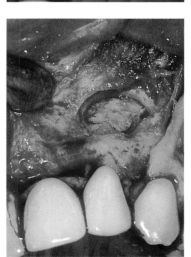

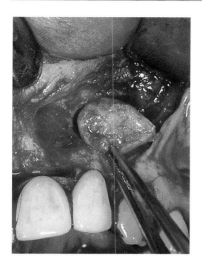

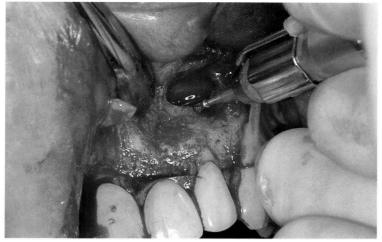

442 Resection
The tip of the root is resected using a fissure bur.

Left: The lining of a cystic formation is removed. Tissues of this type should be sent for histopathological evaluation.

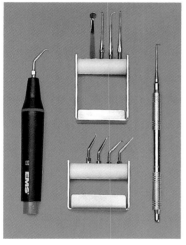

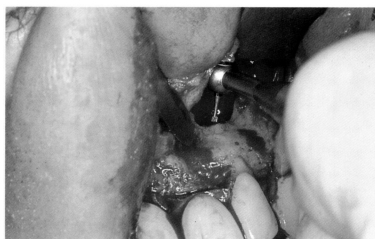

443 Mini-cavity preparation
A miniature contra-angle handpiece is used to prepare a tiny cavity in the root tip.

Left: Cavity preparation can also be achieved using ultrasonic instruments with special tips.

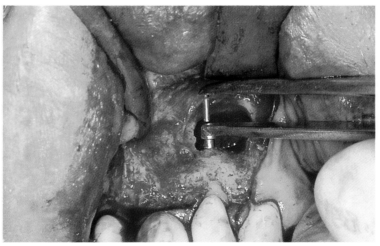

444 Retrograde closure
Retrograde filling, in this case with amalgam. Glass ionomer or zinc oxide cement are now used instead.

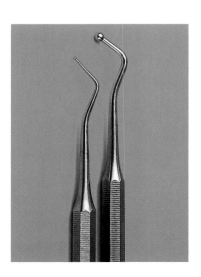

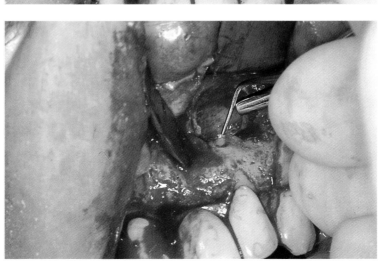

445 Compressing
The freshly-prepared filling material is compressed into the cavity using spherical instruments.

Left: These instruments, with spheres of various sizes, are used for compressing retrograde fillings.

446 Wound treatment
The resection site is checked visually for complete closure of the canal.

Right: The cystic mass that was removed from the apical region should be sent for histopathological evaluation.

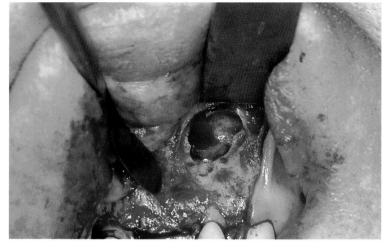
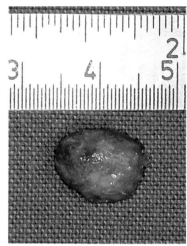

447 Flap repositioning
The soft-tissue flap is replaced and sutured securely.

Right: The postoperative radiograph shows the retrograde closure of the root of tooth 22.

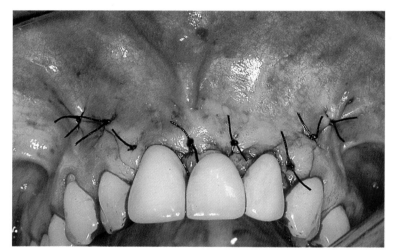
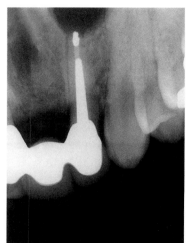

448 Postoperative view
Sutures can be removed one week postsurgically in uncomplicated cases.

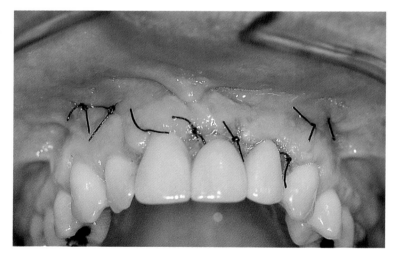

449 Clinical course
The follow-up appointment is scheduled for six months postsurgically. This clinical view reveals symptom-free soft-tissue conditions, and an absence of scar tissue in the surgical area. Note also the absence of any gingival recession at the crown margins.

Right: The radiograph shows complete reossification of the cystic cavity.

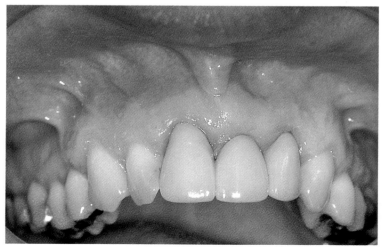
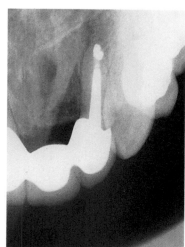

Contiguous Pockets

An osseous defect that extends over the surface of the root cannot always be recognized preoperatively. Even if the patient has not experienced any symptoms, there may be contiguous pocket formation. In such cases, if the primary incision is made in the vestibulum instead of intrasulcally, problems in covering the defect will be encountered. This will be the case regardless of whether the tooth is removed, or if an attempt is made to reconstruct the buccal alveolar wall. If it is decided to retain the tooth, the apical lesion (cyst or granuloma) can be removed, and the cavity can be filled with some replacement material (e.g., lyophilized cartilage chips); the apical part of the root can be covered with the same replacement material. This procedure encourages long-term osseous regeneration as the lyophilized cartilage becomes calcified. If the bony defect is expansive and there is increased tooth mobility, it is advisable to splint the teeth for a period of four weeks.

Whether guided tissue regeneration using barrier techniques can help to preserve the teeth in these rather hopeless cases remains unclear.

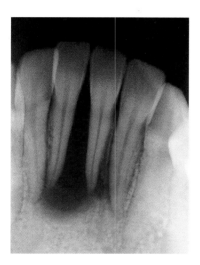

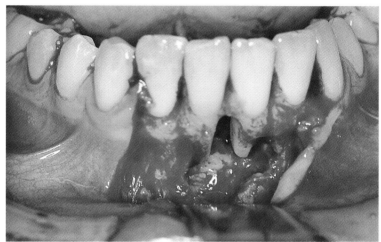

450 Contiguous pocket
Intraoperative view of a contiguous bony defect on the lingual surfaces of teeth 31 and 41. These contiguous periodontal pockets are usually the causative factor in clinical failure. In selected cases, attempts can be made to achieve some osseous regeneration along the root surface if the defect is filled. The best material for this purpose is lyophilized cartilage chips.

Left: The radiograph shows the osteolytic defect at the apex of these teeth.

Ⓐ

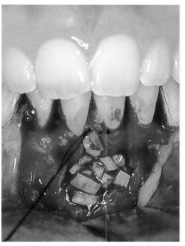

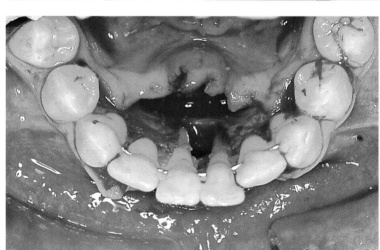

451 Lyophilized cartilage chips
It was necessary to splint the affected teeth, as their bony support was extremely compromised.

Left: The osseous defect is filled with lyophilized cartilage chips, and the wound is securely closed. Postsurgical antibiotic coverage is indicated in these cases.

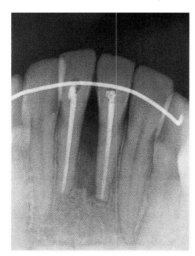

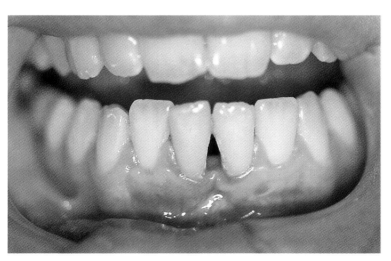

452 Follow-up appointment
Clinically, there is no inflammation, and the periodontal findings are acceptable around teeth 31 and 41 one year after surgery.

Left: The radiograph shows partial reossification of the defect.

Postoperative Care

Immediately after the operation, the results should be documented radiographically.

The patient should apply cold compresses to the region. Good oral hygiene should be supplemented by chlorhexidine rinsing. Anti-inflammatory drugs may be indicated.

The sutures are removed after seven to ten days.

At six months postoperatively, a final clinical check-up should be made, along with radiographic documentation (Rud et al. 1972a, b).

Potential Complications

In addition to the usual postoperative complications, this procedure is associated with a special set of possible difficulties. If the six-month radiographic check reveals persistent apical osteolysis, it is an indication that the closure of the root apex was not complete. A decision must then be taken on a case-by-case basis either to extract the tooth or to attempt repeat treatment with a surgical approach. The possibility of vertical root fracture must also be considered.

453 Complications—persistent osseous defect
The usual cause of this condition is an accessory canal that was not closed off, or continuing bacterial colonization at the root apex with an incomplete closure. Another possible cause is a contiguous periodontal pocket opening into the surgical defect. This series of radiographs taken after apicoectomy on tooth 23 reveals a tunneling defect, which was subsequently filled with lyophilized cartilage chips *(right)* within 18 months of surgery.

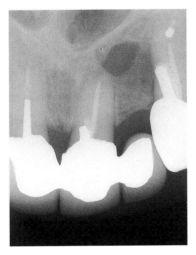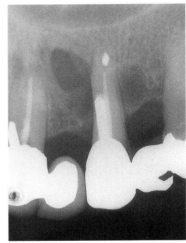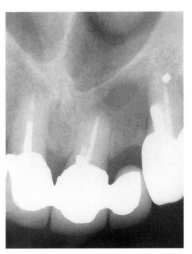

454 Filling a defect
Repeat surgery became necessary in this area due to secondary infection of a periodontal pocket on the mesial aspect of tooth 23. This clinical photograph shows the site after placement of lyophilized chips.

Right: This radiograph, taken 24 months later, shows osseous regeneration in the area.

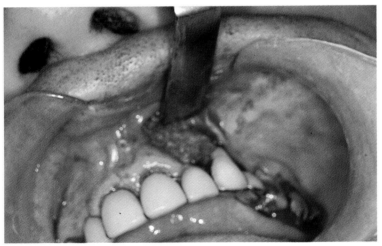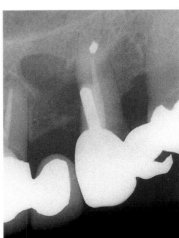

Cysts

Definition

A cyst is defined as a pathological cavity that is lined with epithelium, and which has a centrifugal, expansive mode of growth. The typical shape of a cyst is therefore spherical and balloon-like. The adjacent anatomical structures are often compressed. Root resorption on adjacent teeth is possible.

Cysts contain a serous fluid that contains cholesterol. The etiology varies considerably. Cyst-like cavities without an epithelial lining are called pseudocysts.

Classification

World Health Organization Classification of Cysts

Caused by Developmental Disturbances
Odontogenic cysts:
—Keratocyst (primordial cyst)
—Gingival cyst
—Eruption cyst
—Follicular cyst
—Calcifying odontogenic cyst

Non-odontogenic cysts:
—Nasopalatine duct cyst
—Globulomaxillary cyst
—Nasolabial (nasoalveolar) cyst

Caused by Inflammation
Radicular cyst
Periodontal cyst
Residual cyst

Clinical Classification of Cysts
(Killey et al. 1977, Shear 1992, van der Waal 1993)

Osseous Cysts
Dental cysts:
—Inflammatory radicular cyst, residual cyst
—Inflammatory periodontal cyst
—Follicular cyst
—Periodontal cyst
—Keratocyst
—Eruption cyst

Fissural cysts:
—Median fissural cyst (incisive canal cyst)
—Lateral fissural cyst (globulomaxillary cyst)
—Nasopalatine cyst

Pseudocysts:
—Stafne cyst (lingual cortical defect)
—Traumatic cyst
—Hematopoietic osseous defect

Soft-Tissue Cysts
Salivary retention cyst
Developmental cysts (median and lateral cervical cysts)
Gingival cyst
Dermoid cyst

Development of Cysts

Cysts can always develop in areas in which residual epithelial cells from embryological development processes become lodged in the tissues. Another possibility is pathological development. In the jaws, cysts are especially common because of the presence of ectodermal structures within bone (tooth buds). Epithelial remnants (Malassez rests) sometimes become entrapped after tooth eruption; with appropriate stimulation, these epithelial rests may disintegrate, with central necrosis and development of a cyst. The precise pathogenesis remains unclear. A growth-related cause might result from osmotic internal pressure following epithelial necrosis; in this scenario, the cystic lining represents a semipermeable membrane. This hypothesis serves also explain the shrinkage of the bony cavity after therapeutic fenestration and drainage (decompression) of a cyst.

Odontogenic Cysts

Multiple cyst formation often accompanies the following syndromes:
—Gorlin–Goltz syndrome (keratocyst)
—Dentin dysplasia (follicular cyst)
—Cleidocranial dysostosis (follicular cyst)
—Klippel–Feil syndrome (follicular cyst)

Radicular Cyst

This is characterized histologically by a multilayered, nonkeratinized squamous epithelium. The wall of the cyst may contain aggregations of lymphocytes, cholesterol crystals, *Actinomyces* colonies, macrophages, and goblet cells. The tissues immediately adjacent to the cyst consist of fiber-poor collagen connective tissue.

A residual cyst is in fact a radicular cyst persisting within the substance of the jaw after tooth extraction.

Recent investigations using consistent serial sections of cysts adherent to teeth (Nair and Pajarola 1995) show that with radicular cysts, it is necessary to distinguish between genuine cysts ("true cyst") and "pocket cysts." In addition, residual epithelial cell aggregations have been identified in apical abscesses and granulomas, which is a typical characteristic of cysts as defined by traditional pathologists. This is of clinical significance, because with epithelium-containing abscesses and granulomas, and also with pocket cysts in which the cystic epithelium is in direct contact with the apex, healing can be expected after elimination of the source of infection (endodontic treatment). By contrast, with true cysts, in which the cystic epithelium is enclosed within an isolated cavity, only surgical intervention can bring healing.

Aggressive Cysts of the Jaw

Stoelinga and Bronkhorst (1988) describe the characteristics of certain cystic lesions of the jaws as being aggressive if they exhibit destructive and infiltrative growth, especially high growth potential, and a tendency toward recurrence. This group of cysts includes those from which carcinoma or ameloblastoma can develop, particularly keratocysts and calcifying odontogenic cysts. Such cysts often occupy one-third or more of a jaw, and can even proliferate into the soft tissues.

Follicular Cysts

All follicular cysts contain the crown of a tooth inside their lumen; they are therefore also referred to dentigerous cysts. The cystic epithelium derives from the enamel epithelium after development of the crown of the tooth. The histological picture is one of multilayered, rarely keratinized squamous epithelium, which can also contain mucus-forming cells. Follicular cysts are relatively common, occurring most often in the permanent dentition. They are usually located near impacted third molars in the mandible, or near the canines in the maxilla. There are rarely any clinical symptoms unless the cyst becomes infected. These cysts are usually detected in the course of routine dental radiography, appearing as round, sharply demarcated areas of osteolysis, sometimes containing a large, deformed tooth crown. These cysts can range from a few centimeters in size up to very large, almost grotesque sizes. Follicular cysts in the mandible may impinge on the mandibular canal.

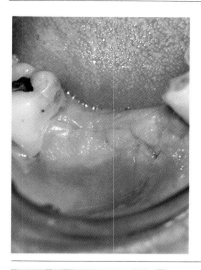
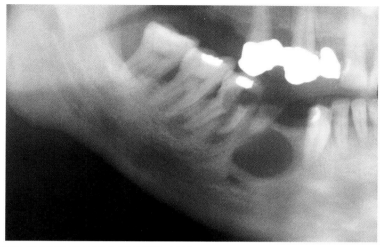

455 Radicular cysts—expansion and osteolysis

The radiograph shows an impressive radicular cyst with a basically round, sharply demarcated structure, which appears to be expanding at the expense of osseous tissues near the apical region of a tooth.

Left: In the non-acute stage, the only clinical symptom may be an indolent expansion of the alveolar process, and if the cortical bone is very thin, it may be possible to detect fluctuation. It is always possible to detect a nonvital tooth (treated or untreated) in the region of the cyst.

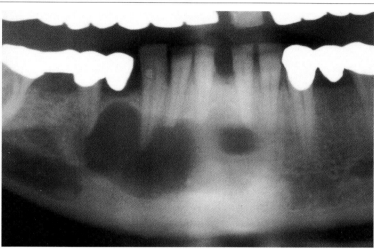

456 Fistula formation

The radiograph clearly shows the source of the fistula. It is cystic osteolysis at the apices of several teeth in the anterior region of the mandible.

Left: A clinical sign may be the presence of an external fistula drainage site that is resistant to treatment.

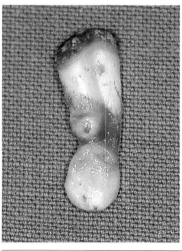
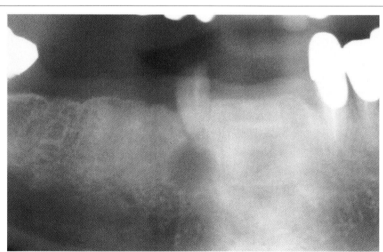
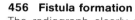

457 Cystic osteolysis

This section from a panoramic radiograph shows the typical appearance of a cyst at the apex of tooth 44.

Left: The extracted tooth brought the attached radicular cyst with it.

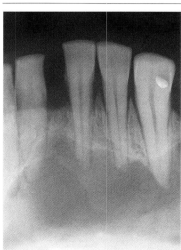
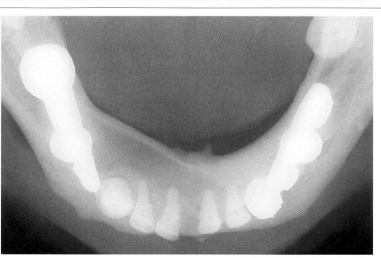

458 Expansion

The extensive growth of the radicular cyst is readily visualized in this occlusal radiograph. The lingual cortical plate is very thin, and appears to be expanded.

Left: This periapical radiograph shows the same cystic development from a different perspective.

Keratocyst

Common synonyms for this include primordial cyst or odontogenic keratocyst. Keratocysts develop either in the alveolar bone proper or distal to the third molar, most commonly in the mandible. Males are more frequently affected than females, the most common ages being the second, third and fifth decades of life. Histologically, the lumen of the cyst is covered by a simple, or more seldom, a multilayered squamous epithelium. The basal-cell layer is typically intensely stained, and the epithelium shows either hyperparakeratosis or hyperorthokeratosis. The cystic wall consists of fiber-poor collagenous connective tissue. The external border of the cyst may show secondary cystic formations. This is probably the reason for the high degree of recurrence. Radiographically, the keratocyst is not easy to distinguish from a follicular cyst. If an impacted tooth is involved, its crown will be located at the margin and not within the lumen of the cystic cavity. In addition, the typical round form of a cyst is usually not seen. The pattern of osteolysis is smooth-bordered, but often multilocular. The size is variable, ranging from a few millimeters to extreme sizes throughout entire jaw

459 Periodontal cyst
Cysts may also develop from periodontal epithelium. This radiograph shows tooth 46 shortly after eruption, with a sharply demarcated radiolucency between the roots.

Right: In this film, a small, spherical cystic development is seen distal to the root of tooth 42.

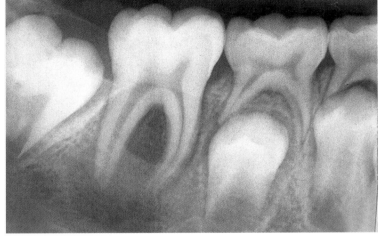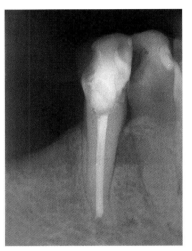

460 Residual cyst
The etiology is identical to that of a radicular cyst. The tooth affected was extracted, but the etiological cyst was not, and its growth continued.

Right: Eruption cyst: as teeth erupt especially the first molars cysts may develop if penetration through the epithelium is delayed. This clinical photograph shows the typical appearance of a bluish swelling of the gingiva at precisely the site at which tooth 26 ought to erupt.

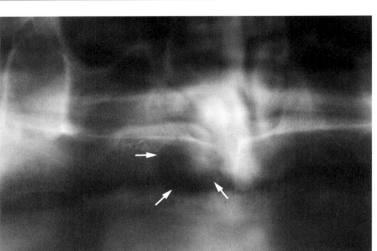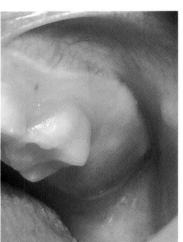

461 Follicular cyst
This cyst develops from the enamel epithelium during tooth development. The crown of the etiological tooth (48) is completely encompassed by the cyst. Cysts of this type can develop massive proportions (arrows).

Right: This section from a panoramic radiograph shows an impacted tooth 38 with an enlarged pericoronal space; this is a typical radiographic sign of likely cystic development.

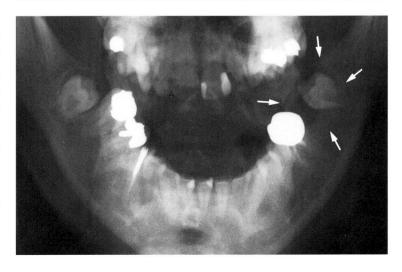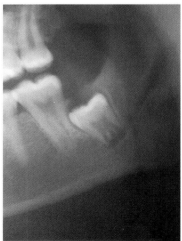

Gorlin–Goltz Syndrome

segments. Within the lower jaw, the mandibular canal is not expanded. Some investigators have suggested that enzyme activity and prostaglandin production, or active growth within adjacent connective tissues and simultaneous epithelial proliferation in numerous centers of growth, might be responsible for the development of keratocysts (Scharffetter et al. 1989, Voorsmit 1990). This hypothesis would also help to explain the high recurrence rate. Many authors have described individual cases with malignant transformation within the cyst.

This syndrome is characterized by basal-cell nevi on the skin, split ribs, and multiple keratocysts; the syndrome is inherited as an autosomal dominant trait. The clinical symptom of multiple keratocysts is almost always present in this syndrome and, in addition to the skin lesions, there are alterations in the eyes, as well as rather typical facial anomalies such as a protruding forehead and hypertelorism (Roth et al. 1989).

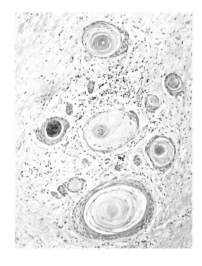 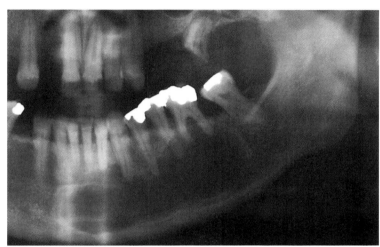

462 Keratocysts
The panoramic radiograph clearly shows extensive cystic osteolysis, stretching from the left molar region of the mandible anteriorly to beyond the midline. The cortical bone is affected in some areas, resulting in the characteristic multilocular appearance. All of the teeth remain vital.

Left: The histological section shows the typical islands of keratin within the cystic epithelium.

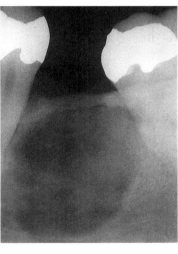 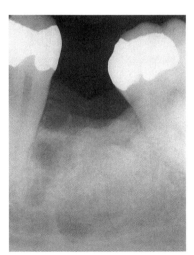

463 Tendency to recur
The radiolucency *(left)* observed in this periapical radiograph was diagnosed as a keratocyst.

Right: Five years after a cystectomy was performed, the radiograph shows extensive osseous regeneration of the cystic defect. However, the osseous structure does not mimic the usual trabecular pattern. A long-term radiographic evaluation is indicated.

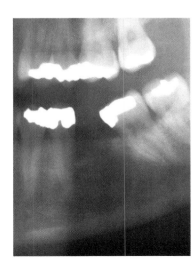 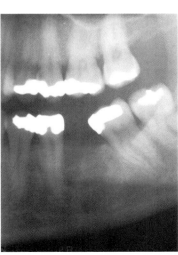 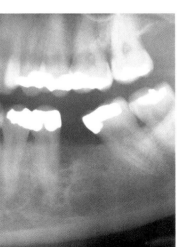

464 Tendency to recur
This series of radiographs, taken over a four-year period, illustrates healing and recurrence of a cystic lesion.

Left: One year later.

Center: Two years later.

Right: Four years later. Near the caudal region of the previous cyst, a new area of osteolysis appears to be developing.

Treatment for Keratocysts

Keratocysts are peculiar because of their high rate of recurrence. Keratocysts can also be categorized as aggressive. For this reason, patients with a diagnosed keratocyst should be included in a recall system that will ensure regular check-ups after treatment of the cyst for a period of six to ten years. Because these cysts are often quite large, the treatment proceeds step by step. Since preoperative diagnosis cannot be definitively established without histological support, the first step is to biopsy the wall of the cyst. This can usually be accomplished when the tooth that is associated with the cyst is extracted. During the procedure, a portion of the wall of the cyst can be harvested as a biopsy, and the cystic cavity itself can be left open. If marsupialization of the cyst is carried out, with removal of the epithelial lining, a six-month waiting period should ensue, with subsequent radiographic evaluation of the degree of reduction in the osteolysis; this will determine the need for additional surgical procedures. In most cases, it is possible to see that the lumen of the cyst has decreased in size due to osseous apposition, and this is a promising sign for complete healing.

465 Dynamics of keratocyst development
Some syndromes are characterized by the development of multiple cysts, as in the case shown here of a patient with Gorlin–Goltz syndrome. The first marsupialization of a cyst was carried out at the early age of seven years, in order to guide tooth eruption. Cystic development can be detected in the region of tooth 45.

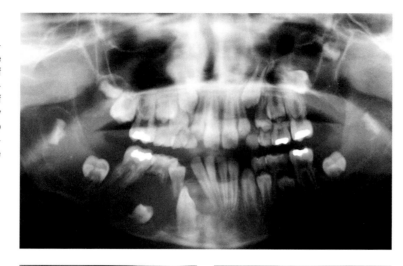

466   Keratocyst development
The cyst adjacent to tooth 45 was marsupialized when the patient was aged 13. Histological examination provided the expected diagnosis of keratocyst. The cystic cavity was rinsed using Carnoy's solution, with every effort being made to spare tooth 45 *(left)*.

Right: As seen in this radiograph, tooth 45 has begun to erupt occlusally. The cyst appears to have been completely eliminated.

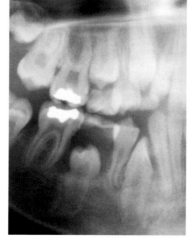
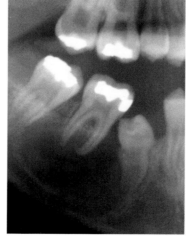

467   Keratocyst development
Six months later, the cyst again became visible at the distal of tooth 45.

Left: When the patient was 17, the situation appeared to have stabilized, but tooth 46 still had to be devitalized and treated endodontically, with an apicoectomy being carried out.

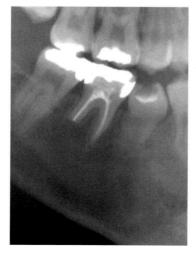
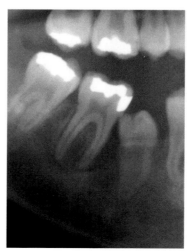

Keratocysts: Follow-Up Care

Clinical and radiographic follow-up at annual intervals may reveal a new radiolucency at sites in which regeneration was previously seen. However, it can be expected in such cases that the osseous apposition will have separated critical anatomical structures such as the

mandibular canal or adjacent vital teeth from any recurrent cyst; therefore, more radical surgical procedures can be instituted. The recurrent cyst can be excised in toto after rinsing with Carnoy's solution and curettage of the bone (pp. 213, 220).

Non-Odontogenic Cysts

The category of non-odontogenic cysts includes aneurysmal cysts of bone, globulomaxillary cysts, nasolabial cysts, incisive canal cysts (cysts of the nasopalatine canal, incisive papillary cysts), median mandibular cysts, median maxillary cysts, and pseudocysts (Stafne cyst, hematopoietic defect). Except for pseudocysts and aneurysmal bone cysts, the other types of cysts can be categorized as developmental cysts. When they are classified in this way, the usual definition of cysts (cavity lined by epithelium) does not apply.

Aneurysmal Bone Cyst

Detection of this type of cyst is usually an incidental finding in a radiograph of the horizontal ramus of the mandible; it appears as a cyst-like area of osteolysis, which may be unilobular or multilobular, and has an irregular border. Histological examination shows some connective tissue with accumulations of erythrocytes, and thrombosis formation. Delicate septa that contain giant cells surround blood-filled regions of various sizes; the central cavity is not typical of a cyst, and contains giant cells of the osteoclast type. From a purely clinical standpoint, this type of cyst may occur as a painless enlargement or expansion of the bone. Treatment consists of gentle curettage and allowing the cavity to fill with blood.

Hematopoietic Defect

This lesion is often an incidental finding on radiographs in young patients. It presents as a circumscribed area of osteolysis in the horizontal ramus of the mandible, generally not sharply demarcated at its mesial extent, and with typical cystic characteristics in the distal portion. The teeth are not involved. On inspection, an empty osseous cavity is found, lined with an extremely thin connective tissue. The inferior alveolar nerve may pass through the cavity hanging like a thread in the space. There is always histological evidence of hematopoietic bone marrow. Treatment is limited to inspection and radiographic follow-up.

If the osseous defect presents unfavorable conditions, it can be filled with lyophilized cartilage.

Clinical and radiograph check-ups should be made twice yearly, and if no recurrence is observed over a two-year period, the check-up interval can be extended to one or two years during the ensuing six-year period (Stefani 1994).

Traumatic Cysts

Synonyms for this pathological entity include solitary bone cyst, hemorrhagic cyst, and extravasation cyst. These pseudocysts are usually seen as symptom-free, well demarcated areas of osteolysis, which seldom cause expansion of the cortical bone in the horizontal ramus of the mandible; they are usually detected before age 20. On inspection, an empty cavity is found, which may sometimes contain a serous fluid. The teeth are not involved. No treatment is actually required, because the cavities usually fill spontaneously with osseous regeneration once they have been opened.

Globulomaxillary Cyst

This type of cyst was once believed to be related to the nasolabial cyst, since they both derive from epithelial rests entrapped during the embryological process of fusion of the nasal and alveolar processes. The globulomaxillary cyst may, therefore, be a fissural cyst. Other authors regard these lesions as manifestations of various other types of cyst (radicular, periodontal, or keratocyst). It is still under debate whether lateral fissural cysts and globulomaxillary cysts are actually more dental in origin. The clinical symptoms include swelling in the vestibulum between the maxillary lateral incisor and canine. The radiograph shows a cystically demarcated, ovoid area of osteolysis, which often appears to be forcing the roots of the lateral incisor and canine apart. The teeth are vital.

Incisive Canal Cyst

These cysts develop in the nasopalatine canal. Median palatal cysts and incisal papillary cysts are different forms of the same type of cyst. It is easy to understand the way in which they develop when one considers the position of the nasolabial canal, in which epithelial rests can be entrapped during embryogenesis, later developing into cysts. The clinical manifestations of this type of cyst include swelling at the corresponding location on the palate. These cysts may be painful even in the absence of inflammation. Radiographically, the cysts appear in the palate as round, oval or heart-shaped areas of osteolysis in the anterior–median area. The teeth are not involved, and are not displaced even if the cyst is extensive. Depending on the origin of the epithelial rest cells, the histological appearance may include multilayered squamous epithelium or respiratory epithelium, or both, and sometimes even nerve tissue (incisal nerve).

468 Nonodontogenic cyst—fissural cyst
These cysts probably develop from epithelial cells entrapped during fusion of the bones of the jaw. The occlusal radiograph shows cystic osteolysis in the region of the incisal canal.

Right: A periapical radiograph shows the area of osteolysis cause by a lateral fissural cyst.

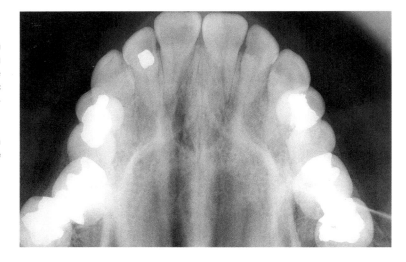
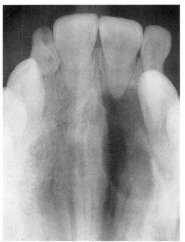

469 Nasoalveolar cyst
Nasoalveolar or nasopalatine cysts are not completely surrounded by bone, and therefore do not always provide reliable radiographic signs. This photograph shows the paranasal swelling caused by the cyst, which is located on the vestibular cortical bone.

Right: After the area has been opened surgically, the well demarcated, protuberant mass is readily visible near teeth 21 and 22.

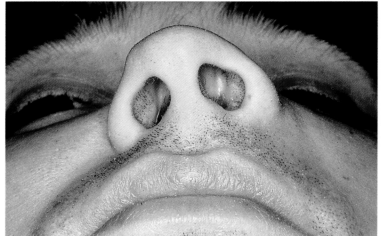
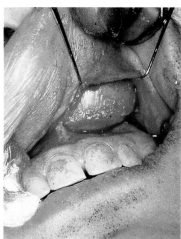

470 Pseudocysts
This type of cyst is limited to the dorsal border of the mandible. Its radiographic appearance is that of a typical, well demarcated cystic defect, which can be clearly seen on this lateral radiographic projection of the mandible.

Right: The CT provides evidence of a lingual depression caused by one lobe of the submandibular gland a typical Stafne cyst.

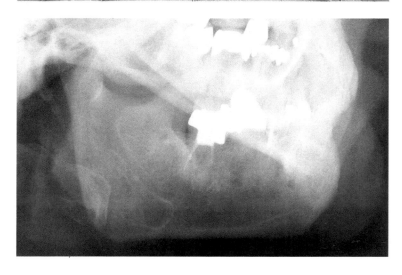
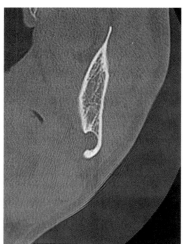

Diagnosis of Cysts

The clinical diagnosis covers a wide range of histological differential diagnoses. Because of the varying pathological behavior patterns of the individual types of odontogenic cysts, a precise histological diagnosis together with thorough clinical data and appropriate radiographic observations are necessary for adequate therapy (Donath 1980).

Clinical Observations

The clinical symptoms indicating the presence of a cyst include changes in tissue contours, especially bulges. Palpation is very important in determining the physical characteristics of the alteration—for example, firm, depressible, indurated, crepitus.

A needle biopsy provides additional information: liquids of various colors and consistencies can be extracted. It is typical to find cholesterol crystals in the cystic fluid.

Radiographic Findings

The absolute extent of the lesion should be calculated from at least two radiographs taken from different projection angles. The cystic process will be visible as a round, sharply demarcated radiolucency, with a delicate border of cortical bone. Adjacent anatomical structures are usually displaced. If the cyst is infected, the cortical bony margin may be lost.

Contrast media may be helpful, especially with soft-tissue cysts. Very precise and detailed information can be obtained from magnetic resonance imaging (MRI) and computed tomography (CT).

Histological Evaluation

The determining factor is the type of epithelium lining the cystic cavity. It is possible to distinguish between radicular cyst, follicular cyst, fissural cyst, and keratocyst, as well as cystic tumors.

Surgical Procedure

Selecting a Surgical Approach

The pathophysiological dynamic of cysts requires considerable experience on the part of the surgeon, who has to select an appropriate surgical procedure. It is critically important to weigh up all the different aspects of the case before deciding on the treatment to be used for the various types of cysts (Baumann 1976, Becker 1971, Berthold and Burkhardt 1989, Berthold and Buser 1982,

Egyedi and Beyazit 1973, Fowler and Brannon 1989, Hardt and von Arx 1990, Holtgrave and Spiessl 1975, Nielsen et al. 1986, Richter et al. 1975, Robinson et al. 1956, Roth et al. 1984, Sailer and Makek 1985, Schmidt et al. 1993, Schroll 1976, Schwimmer et al. 1991, Stoelinga and Bronkhorst 1988, Zetzmann et al. 1955).

The fundamental principle is that the type of treatment chosen must not create functional problems (e.g., defects in the edentulous alveolar process) or aesthetic problems (e.g., in the anterior maxillary region of dentulous patients).

> **Clinical Tip**
> Extensive lesions caused by cysts in the jaw region should be treated only by specialists.

Important Criteria for the Surgical Procedure

Location of the Cyst
Maxilla:
—Maxillary sinus
—Nasal sinus
—Maxillary and nasal sinuses
—Orbit
—Oral cavity or palate
—Incisal canal
—Dentulous or edentulous regions

Mandible:
—Angle of the mandible, ascending ramus, or condylar region
—Mandibular canal, mental foramen
—Lateral or anterior alveolar process
—Edentulous or dentulous region

Size of the Cyst
Determine the stability of the surrounding bone, and determine the danger of possible fracture.

Histological Evaluation
What is the nature of the lesion? Keratocyst, other dental cyst, fissural cyst, cystic tumor, etc.

Time Factor
If the cyst is simply opened, can it be expected to shrink spontaneously?

Patient's General Health
—Systemic condition
—Age
—Patient's expectations
—Patient's degree of compliance

471 Clinical diagnosis
In this case, there was continuous expansion in the vestibulum of the left maxilla, but without signs of infection or any pain. The entire region was deformed, and the teeth appeared to have tipped over.

Right: The radiograph shows a sharply demarcated defect with marginal sclerosis and displacement of the root of tooth 24.

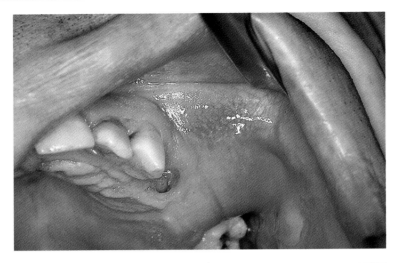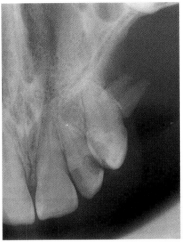

472 Fistula
If a cyst becomes chronically infected, a fistulous tract can develop; these are often difficult to detect clinically.

Right: Using a fine periodontal probe, it was possible to detect the orifice of this fistulous tract.

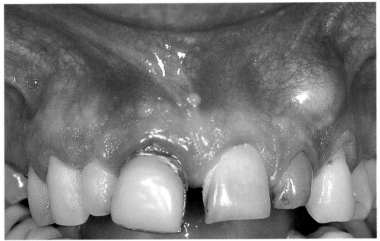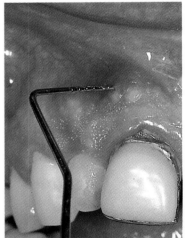

473 Radiographic diagnosis
This occlusal radiograph of the mandible clearly shows the loss of structural integrity on the patient's left side, with marginal sclerosis (arrows).

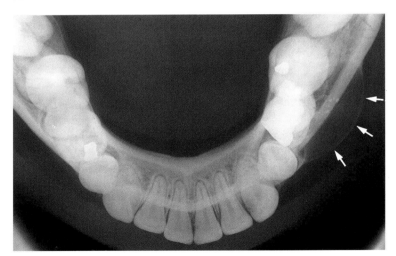

474 Panoramic radiograph
In this panoramic radiograph, it is possible to visualize the cyst distal to tooth 34; it is only partly visible.

Right: The periapical radiograph shows a radicular cyst with osteolysis and marginal sclerosis; however, the radiograph does not reveal the entire expanse of the cyst. In every case, it is absolutely necessary to depict the lesion and its entire extent radiographically.

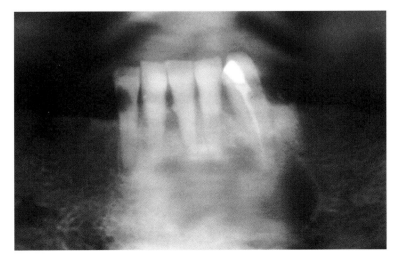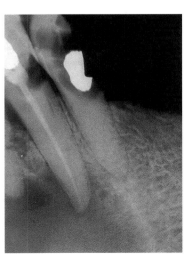

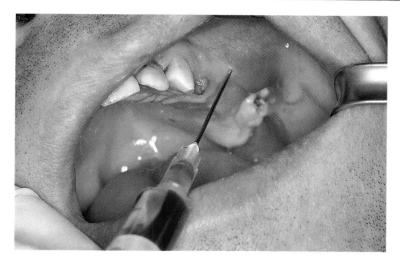

475 Needle biopsy
If cystic fluid can be withdrawn following needle insertion, it is virtually certain that a cyst is present.

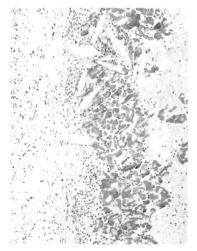
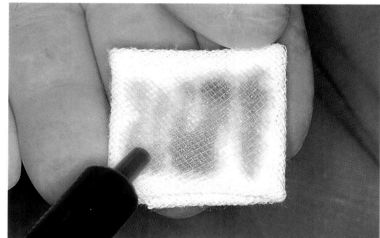

476 Cholesterol crystals
When the cystic fluid contents are expelled onto a gauze square, shiny cholesterol crystals are apparent.

Left: Epithelium of a radicular cyst, with gaps formed by cholesterol crystals.

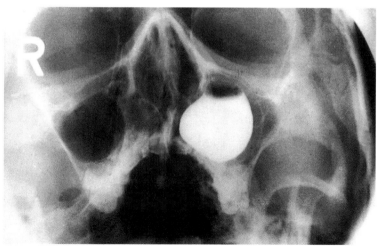

477 Contrast media
The extent of a cyst can be determined radiographically using contrast media and conventional radiography. In this radiograph of the maxilla, a cyst within the maxillary sinus is clearly depicted by the use of an appropriate contrast medium.

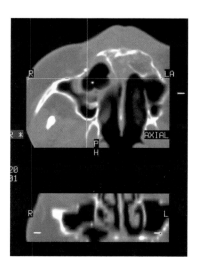
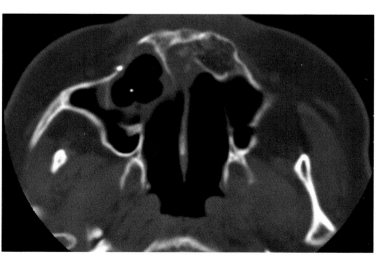

478 Computed tomography
Precise information about the three-dimensional extent of a cyst can be obtained using computed tomography. These images show a cyst in the maxilla, with its border to the maxillary sinus in the axial sections.

Left: Additional information can be obtained from the computed coronal section.

Documentation

A thorough medical history must be taken, and a complete intraoral examination must be carried out. The condition of the adjacent teeth should be recorded in relation to pocket formation, mobility, and vitality. The apical region of the offending tooth and its adjacent teeth must be documented by means of periapical radiographs. A panoramic radiograph should be taken to provide a broad overview. Additional films taken with other projection angles, and possibly also CT or MRI, can be very helpful during the process of reaching a decision concerning treatment.

Armamentarium

The basic surgical set is supplemented with instruments for root canal treatment, similar to the set-up for apicoectomy. Additional clamps can be added to control hemorrhage. It is advisable to have an electrosurgical device nearby, to prevent the need for rush if unexpected hemorrhage occurs. Black elevators are useful for dislodging the cystic lining.

479 Instrumentarium for cystic surgery
The basic surgical kit is supplemented with instruments for endodontic treatment, including a complete series of files for root canal expansion, instruments for retrograde canal closure, excavators for removing the cystic lining, and additional clamps for dealing with hemorrhage. An electrosurgery apparatus should be ready for use.

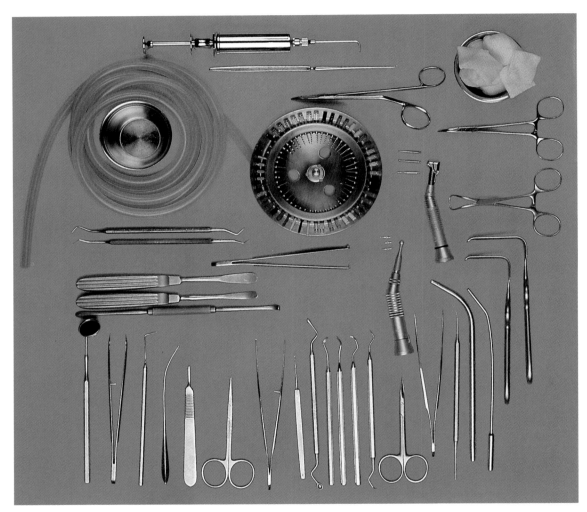

480 Excavators
Black elevators are excellent for enucleating cysts. Using the back surface of the instrument, it is usually possible to remove the cystic lining in toto from the osseous surface.

Right: Double-ended sharp spoon excavators are also suitable for enucleating small cysts.

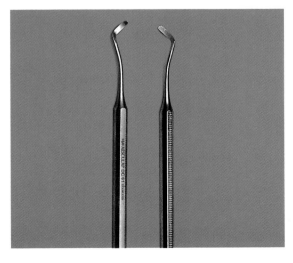
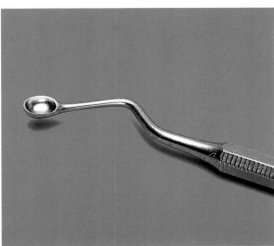

Cystectomy (Partsch I)

Definition

The Partsch I procedure involves opening of the cyst, complete removal of the cystic lining, and primary closure of the cavity. The goal is complete osseous healing of the defect (Becker 1971, Buser and Berthold 1986, Clark and Seldin 1980, Hjørting-Hansen 1970, Roth et al. 1984, Schmutziger 1951, Schulte 1965, Steiner 1965).

Indication

The cystectomy procedure is indicated for the treatment of small cysts with a diameter of up to 2 cm.

Radicular cysts, residual cysts, periodontal cysts (if there is no external connection) and globulomaxillary cysts can be successfully treated by cystectomy.

The Partsch I procedure also provides material for histological evaluation.

Clinical Tip

It is also necessary to provide definitive treatment of the cause , and this may include endodontic treatment, apicoectomy, tooth extraction, and removal of root fragments or foreign bodies.

Cystectomy in the Mandible

During the planning phase, the anatomical location, extent, and adjacent structures must be taken into account. On the basis of the clinical and radiographic findings, cysts that are smaller than 2 cm in diameter are excised in toto. Specimens must always be sent for histopathological evaluation. Access is obtained by reflecting a mucoperiosteal flap and, if necessary, distal releasing incisions. The design and extent of the flap must be such that wound closure can be made over intact bone. Special attention must be given to the point at which the mental nerve exits from the mandible. Special care is required by the possibility of direct contact between the cystic lining and the inferior alveolar nerve, and with the roots of adjacent teeth, particularly the apices. If the apex of a previously vital tooth is accidentally exposed, endodontic treatment should be instituted immediately. The cystic cavity should be allowed to fill spontaneously with a blood coagulum. It is usually not necessary to fill the cavity with any sort of bone replacement material. If there is any danger of a residual osseous defect, the lumen of the cyst can be filled with lyophilized cartilage, or with granular hydroxyapatite (p. 213).

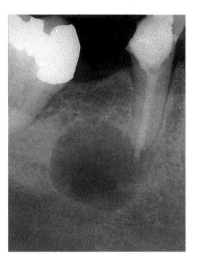

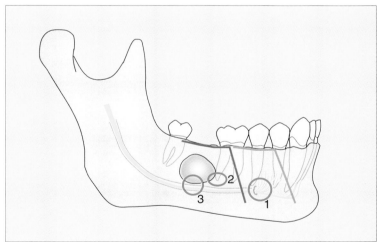

481 Cystectomy–mandibular anatomy
The following anatomical structures require due consideration:

1 Mental foramen
2 Roots of uninvolved adjacent teeth
3 Mandibular canal

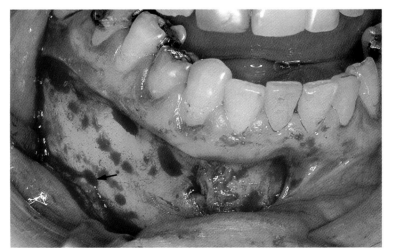

482 Mental foramen
This intraoperative clinical photograph clearly shows the mental foramen (arrow) and the mental nerve, which have to be protected during oral surgery procedures.

483 Cystectomy in the mandible—documentation

The extent of the cyst has to be established in three dimensions, so that a minimum of two projection angles is needed: an occlusal radiograph and a periapical film.

Right: This periapical radiograph provides an incomplete depiction of the radicular cyst on tooth 42.

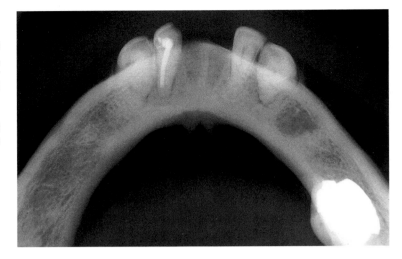
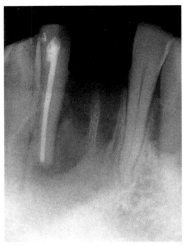

484 Panoramic radiograph

A panoramic radiograph usually provides a good overview, but does not always show sufficient detail of the individual tooth roots.

Right: The cyst that is visible in the radiograph is also associated with the extraoral fistula on the chin.

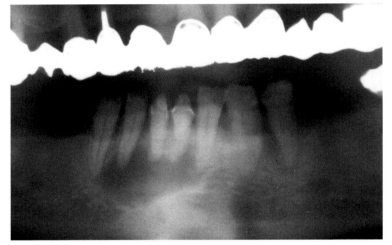
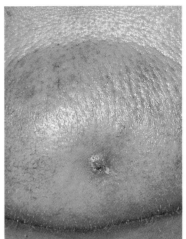

485 Anesthesia

Block anesthesia of the mandibular nerve (1), infiltration at the mental foramen (2), and infiltration in the vestibulum of the contralateral side (3).

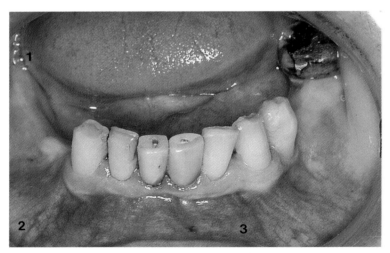

486 Access

Excellent visual access with direct vision is created by flap reflection after a primary incision at the gingival margin and two releasing incisions extending mesially and distally into the vestibule near teeth 43 and 32.

Right: Flap design: the releasing incisions are placed either clearly distal to the mental foramen or mesial to it. The main criterion is that sufficient visual access should be provided.

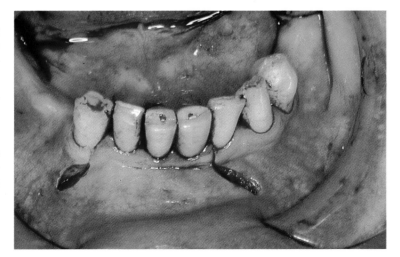
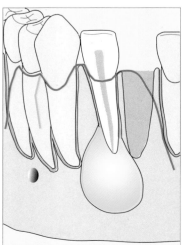

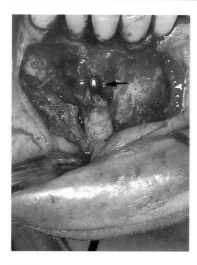

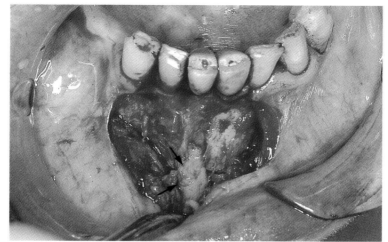

487 Opening the cyst
The cyst is exposed by carefully ostectomy of the cortical bone, with an effort being made to avoid opening the cyst. The fistulous tract (arrows) is visible basal to the flap.

Left: The apex (arrow) of the involved tooth became visible when the cyst was opened.

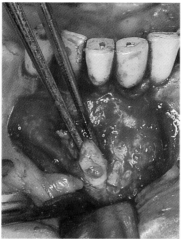

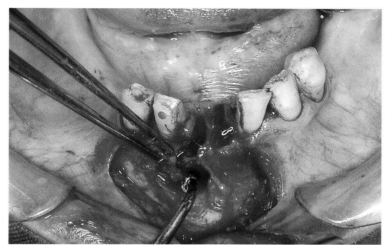

488 Cystectomy
The excavator is used to dislodge the cyst at the margin.

Left: The prepared and probed fistulous tract is severed.

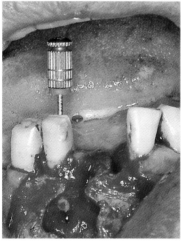

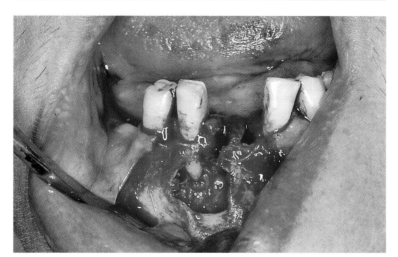

489 Causal treatment
Enucleation of the cyst is followed immediately by treatment of the involved tooth, including root canal treatment and apicoectomy. Because of the massive bony defect, it was necessary to also extract teeth 31 and 41 because they were also associated with the cyst.

Left: Enlarging the root canal following apicoectomy of tooth 42.

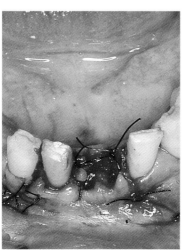

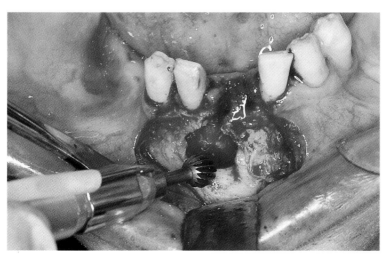

490 Wound treatment
A large round bone cutter is used to smooth any sharp bony margins. The cavity is thoroughly rinsed, and a blood coagulum is allowed to form.

Left: The mucoperiosteal flap is carefully repositioned and sutured securely, with the extraction site being left open.

491 Fistula on the skin
The size of the extraoral fistula required suture closure.

Right: In order to observe the course of healing, the postoperative situation is documented using a periapical radiograph.

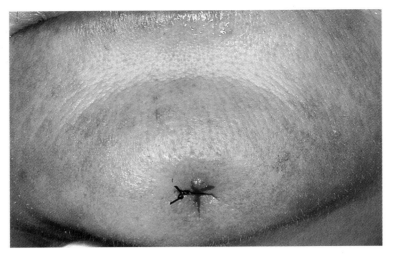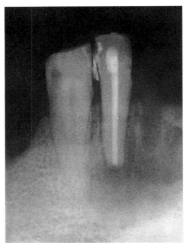

492 Clinical course
The clinical appointment one year later revealed symptom-free, clinically healthy relationships.

Right: The extraoral fistula is no longer discernible.

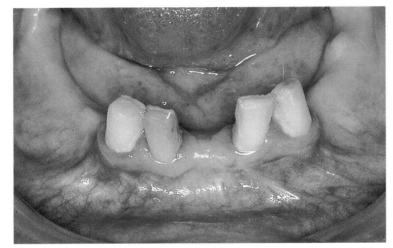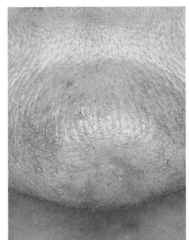

493 Radiographic evaluation
Both the panoramic radiograph and a periapical film show virtually complete osseous regeneration of the cystic cavity.

Right: The periapical film shows an intact periodontal ligament space at the apex of the tooth.

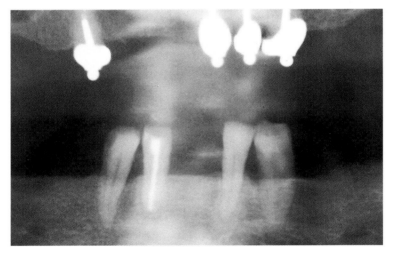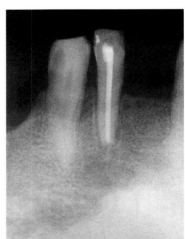

Cystectomy in the Maxilla

When planning the surgical procedure, the structural anatomy of the maxillary bones and any anatomical peculiarities need to be taken into account. The close proximity of the maxillary and nasal sinuses often leads to a connection between the cystic cavity and one of these spaces (see the section on cystostomy, below). As in the mandible, access is best achieved by creating a mucoperiosteal flap, using a gingival intrasulcal incision. Wound closure on an osseous substrate is particularly important if the maxillary or nasal sinus is inadvertently penetrated. Small cysts should be

excised in toto. Histopathological examination is obligatory.

Adjacent tooth roots that are not involved in the cystic process should be carefully protected. The cystic cavities should fill with a blood coagulum. Special measures for treating osseous defects should be implemented only if undesirable aesthetic effects or reconstructive defects appear likely.

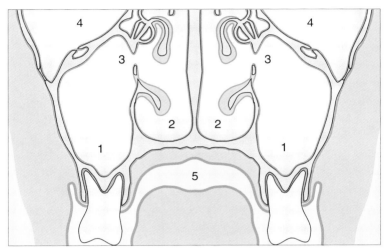

494 Cystectomy in the maxilla—anatomy
A coronal section through the maxillary region.

1 Maxillary sinus
2 Inferior nasal canal
3 Natural foramen
4 Infraorbital nerve
5 Major palatine artery

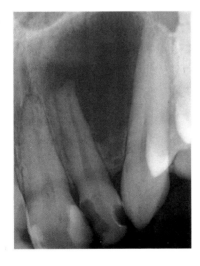

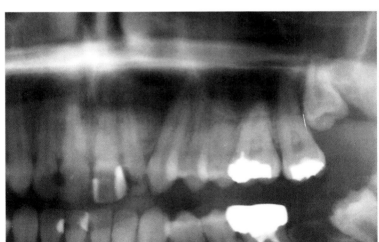

495 Documentation
The radiograph demonstrates the extent of the fissural cyst between teeth 22 and 23. The teeth have been pushed apart. At the clinical examination, a painless discreet swelling in the vestibulum was found. The adjacent teeth have maintained their vitality.

Left: The periapical radiograph shows the cyst apposed to the nonvital root of tooth 22.

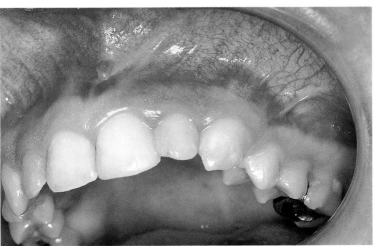

496 Anesthesia
Infiltration at the infraorbital foramen, in the vestibulum near tooth 23 and distal to it, as well as anterior and palatal to the nasal spine.

497 Access
The mucoperiosteal flap is created with an intrasulcal primary incision and a vertical releasing incision near tooth 21. It is not necessary to carry out a distal releasing incision, but if this is used, it allows better visual access.

Right: The interdental papilla of tooth 21 is reflected with the periosteal flap.

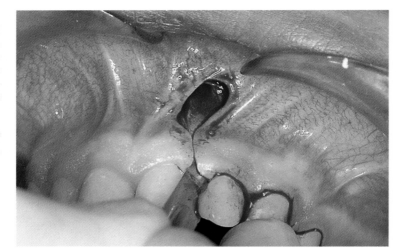
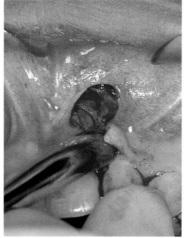

498 Opening the cyst
When the flap is reflected, the slight expansion of the labial cortical plate becomes visible.

Right: An excavator is usually adequate to remove the bony covering.

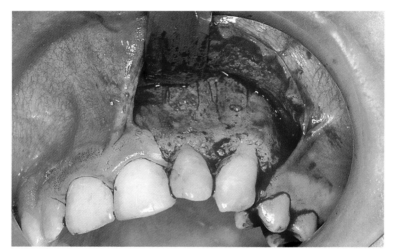
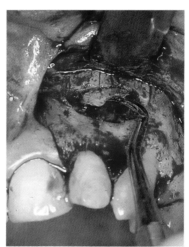

499 Cystectomy
The back of the blade of a Black's excavator is used carefully to dislodge the cyst from its substrate.

Right: The surface of the cystic epithelium becomes visible after removal of the cortical bone.

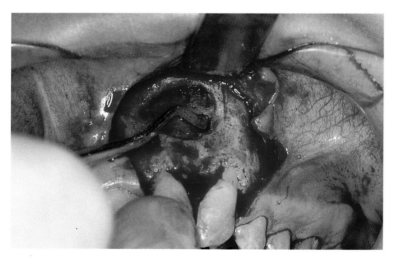
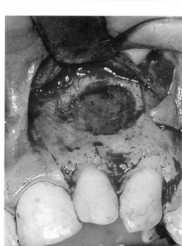

500 Cystectomy
The cystic lining has to be completely removed. The palatal soft tissues can be palpated.

Right: The sac-like cyst should be sent for histopathological evaluation.

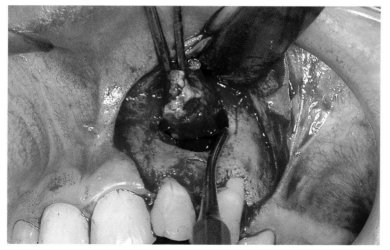
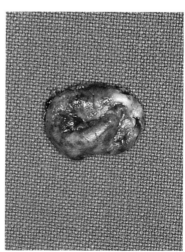

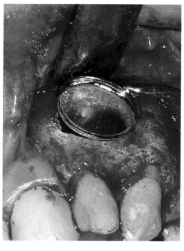

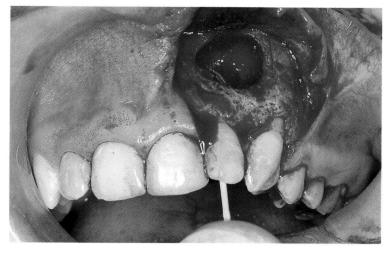

501 Devitalization of a tooth
The apex of the root of tooth 22 has been exposed, and it is therefore necessary to devitalize the tooth. At the same appointment, the tooth is treated endodontically, and the apex of the root is resected; these procedures are carried out after making a second vertical releasing incision to provide better visual access.

Left: A mirror is used to check for complete closure at the resected apex of the root of tooth 22.

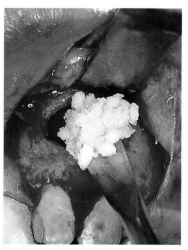

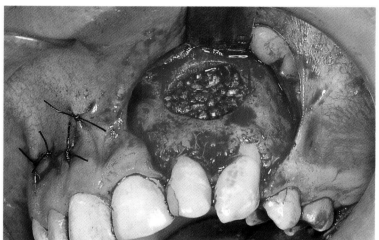

502 Treatment for the cystic cavity
To accelerate healing, the osseous cavity is filled with lyophilized chips and BMP; this is important, because there is only a soft-tissue covering on the palatal aspect. A tunnel-like defect might otherwise be expected. Defects of this kind may cause neural pain.

Left: A spatula is used to insert a paste-like mixture of BMP and lyophilized cartilage into the osseous defect.

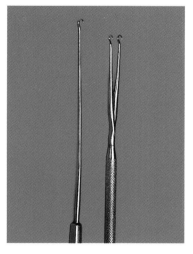

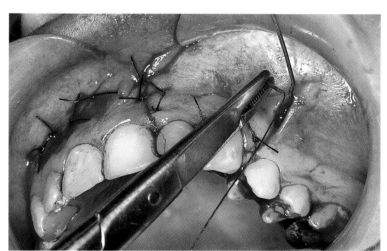

503 Wound treatment
The soft-tissue flap is carefully sutured into place.

Left: It is important to avoid traumatizing the delicate vestibular mucosa. It is advisable to use a Gillies hook instead of a surgical forceps.

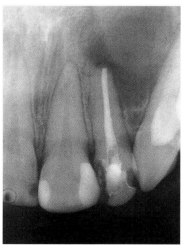

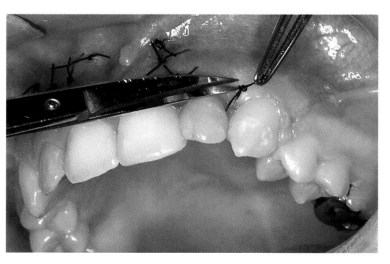

504 Clinical course
One week postoperatively, at the suture removal appointment, the soft tissues are free of inflammation, there is no dehiscence of the wound margins, and there is no infection at the surgical site.

Left: Six months later, the periapical radiograph shows partial osseous regeneration (compare Fig. 495).

Complications

During the Operation
Hemorrhage can be treated by applying pressure, ligation using resorbable suture, coagulation (electro-surgery), or using percussion if the hemorrhage is from bone.

Injury to an adjacent tooth: if devitalization occurs, the adjacent tooth must be immediately treated endodontically. Minor damage to adjacent root surfaces by the burr is usually innocuous. The patient must be informed, however. Delayed complications including root resorption and ankylosis are possible.

Inadvertent opening of the maxillary sinus should not create any particular problem if the mucoperiosteal flap has been properly delineated. The patient should be informed that some bleeding from the nose is possible in the first few hours or days after the operation, and that no forceful nose-blowing should be attempted.

Tunnel-like defect: small defects extending to the mucosa can be left to heal naturally, but larger defects must be filled with bone or with bone replacement material (see pp. 203 and 205).

Postoperative Care
Postoperative infection may occur on the second or third day after cystectomy. This type of infection is characterized by persistent swelling and increasing pain. By removing several sutures, the wound margins can be separated and the wound can be rinsed; a drain can be placed if necessary. Wound rinsing must be carried out daily until the signs of acute inflammation have subsided. This should occur within three days. If the symptoms of acute infection persist, a search must be made for some other causative agent, such as a foreign body, a particular tendency to infection (medical history), pulpal necrosis of an adjacent tooth, etc. If the primary cause is discovered, it must be eliminated. If the patient's immune defenses are in any way compromised, a course of antibiotics is indicated.

If a hematoma has occurred, a preventive antibiotic regimen should be considered. If the extravasation of blood has occurred beneath the flap, a suture can be removed from the releasing incision to allow fluid to drain.

Any wound dehiscence that occurs within three days of the surgical procedure can be corrected by secondary sutures. If the mucosal defect becomes unfavorable, a secondary surgical procedure should be considered.

The formation of a fistulous tract after healing of the intraoral surgical site is evidence of persistent chronic infection. Appropriate diagnostic measures must be taken to rule out foreign-body reaction, perforation of the maxillary sinus, endodontic or periodontal causes, etc. If no causative factor can be identified, a repeat surgical intervention should be considered.

Any recurrence of the cyst can be investigated radiographically after six months. At this point in time, it should be possible to identify a clear reduction in the size of the osteolytic area, even when the original cyst was quite large. The borders of the osteolytic area will appear indistinct, the area of sclerosis may disappear, and the ongoing restructuring of the trabecular bone will show a radial arrangement of the trabeculae. If the osteolytic process persists, a tunneling defect should be considered. Possible treatment options must be discussed in detail with the patient. In almost every case, a second surgical intervention is indicated.

When cysts in the mandible are extensive, the possibility of spontaneous mandibular fracture must be considered. If a fracture has occurred, antibiotic coverage should be prescribed, and the patient should be referred to an oral surgery clinic for emergency splinting.

Recall

The postoperative check-up after healing of the surgical site is generally carried out six months later. It is necessary to follow up the osseous healing until complete regeneration has occurred. The follow-up appointment will be determined by the type of cyst. Keratocyst, for example, must be followed for six to eight years with radiographic check-ups. The dentist should not initiate fixed reconstructive measures until the osseous healing has run its course. It is advisable to reserve time for consultation with the patient during this series of follow-up appointments. The patient should be informed at the outset that a longer-term follow-up will be involved.

Cystostomy (Partsch II)

Definition

The cystostomy procedure involves opening the cyst in order to create a patent connection between the cystic cavity and an anatomical cavity such as the nasal or maxillary sinuses or oral cavity. A portion of the cystic lining is left in situ to cover the osseous defect. Variations include fenestration (small opening) and marsupialization (broad opening at the equator of the cyst) (Baumann 1976, Becker 1971, Brosch 1957, Clark and Seldin 1980, Möbius 1950, Partsch 1892, Schroll 1976, Seldin 1980).

Indication

Large cysts and incisive canal cysts.

Harvesting material for histological diagnosis.

Clinical Tip
If there is any likelihood that the lesion is something other than a radicular or follicular cyst, the patient should be referred to a specialist.

Cystostomy into the Vestibulum

A successful cystostomy procedure requires extensive removal of the oral tissues covering the cyst. Flap design should take this requirement into consideration, along with due regard for the anatomical relationships.

Clinical Tip
The larger the circumference of the cystostomy, the greater the chance of successful osseous healing. With extensive cystostomy, an obturator is generally unnecessary.

If the preoperative differential diagnosis includes suspicion of a keratocyst or a cystic tumor, the surgeon should take the opportunity to carry out an intraoperative histological assessment (frozen section).

Clinical Tip
Leaving parts of the cystic lining behind is only justifiable with squamous epithelial cysts, such as radicular cysts. With all other types of cyst (keratocysts, cystic tumors), a second procedure is required.

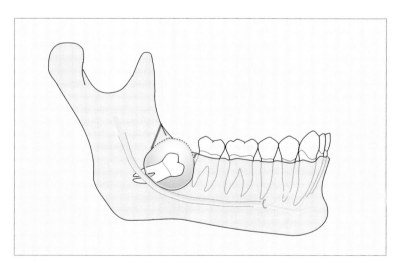

505 Cystostomy in the mandible
The diagram illustrates the principle of creating a patent connection between the oral cavity and a cyst in the mandible. All tissues covering the cyst are removed, creating a situation in which the actual cystic cavity becomes a component of the oral cavity. This allows the internal cystic pressure to become a growth stimulator. Ideally, the lumen of the cyst will decrease in size, and eventually disappear completely. Any residual defect can be corrected during a second surgical procedure if necessary.

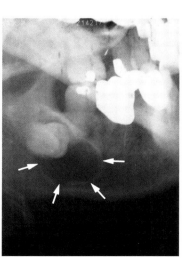
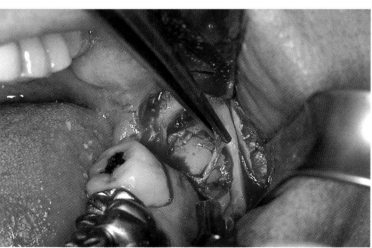

506 Indication
Cysts larger than 2 cm in diameter require cystostomy, particularly when they are immediately adjacent to the oral cavity or to the nasal or maxillary sinuses. The advantage of the cystostomy procedure is that it protects adjacent roots and nerves.

Left: The corresponding radiograph shows a follicular cyst (arrows), with the crown lying inside the cystic cavity.

507 Surgical procedure—periodontal cyst

The marked clinical symptoms are vestibular distension and a deep periodontal pocket on the buccal surface of tooth 46.

Right: The radiograph shows an ovoid area of cystic osteolysis over the roots of tooth 46.

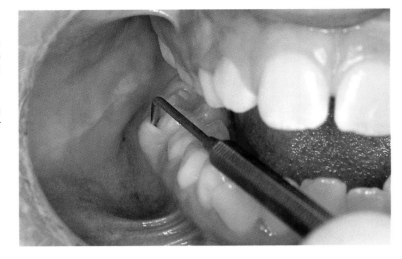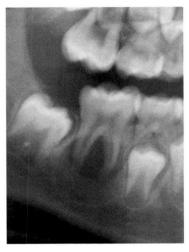

508 Opening the cyst

Without damaging the marginal periodontal tissues, the buccal covering of the cyst is separated and reflected.

Right: Correct technique for the primary incision to open a cyst located on the lingual aspect of the mandible.

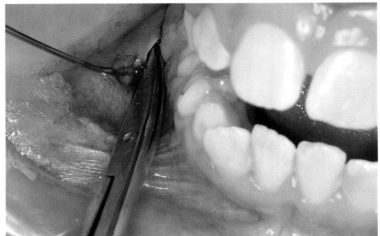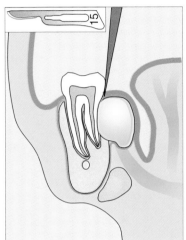

509 Flap maintenance and course of healing

The mucosal flap is reflected caudally, and attached with resorbable sutures near the osseous border of the cystic cavity, which is filled with an iodoform gauze drain.

Center: Clinical view ten days postoperatively.

Right: Clinical view one month postoperatively. The cystic cavity is now much more shallow, and the healing process can now continue without a dressing. The patient rinses the cavity daily using a blunt syringe.

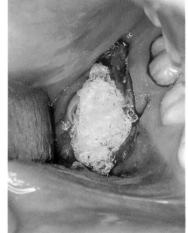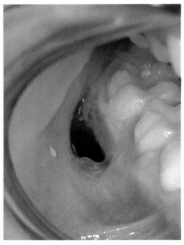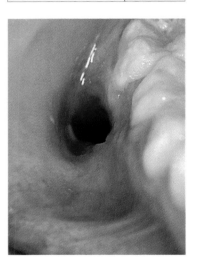

510 Completion of healing

One month after the cystostomy procedure, clinical inspection shows a small scar on the vestibular aspect of tooth 46. The tooth remains vital, and the probing depth on the buccal aspect is only 2 mm.

Right: The radiograph shows that the cystic osteolysis is no longer present, and that the osseous structure has completely regenerated, even interradicularly (compare Fig. 507, right).

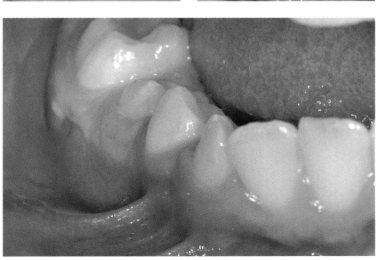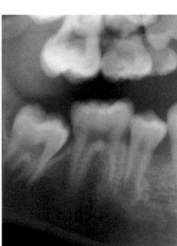

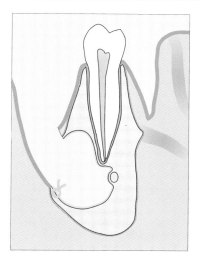

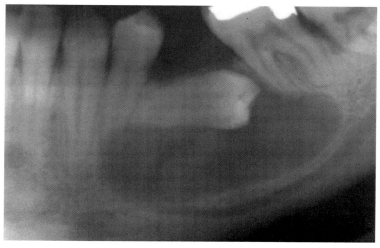

511 Follicular cysts
This section from a panoramic radiograph shows the large area of cystic osteolysis surrounding and distal to the horizontally impacted tooth 35. The mandibular canal has been displaced caudally, and the roots of teeth 36 and 34 appear to lie within the cystic cavity. The teeth are vital, and the sensitivity of the mental nerve is normal.

Left: The principle of surgical opening of the cystic cavity toward the vestibulum.

512 Anesthesia and access
After block anesthesia and infiltration into the vestibulum, a horizontal, slightly arcuate primary incision is made near the mucogingival junction coronal to the cystic protuberance.

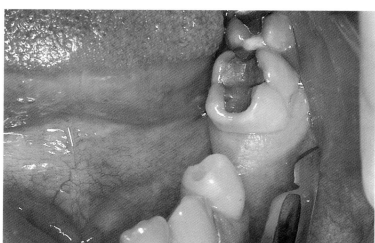

513 Anesthesia and access
The buccal mucosa is reflected away from the very thin bony covering of the cyst.

Left: The mental nerve is exposed at its point of exit from the mental foramen, and an elevator is used to protect it from any inadvertent injury during the procedure.

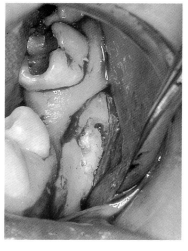

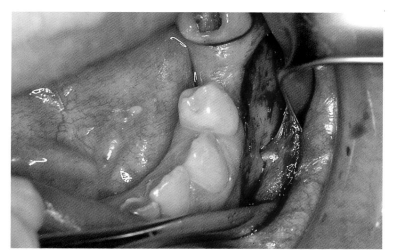

514 Opening the cyst
The osseous covering of the cyst is removed using a Black's excavator, after the creation of several shallow burr holes.

Left: The cortical bone is lifted away using the Black's excavator.

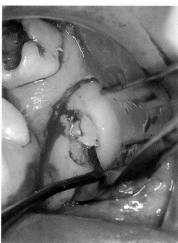

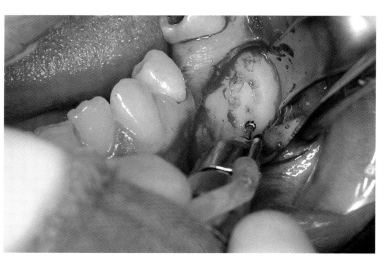

515 Cystostomy

A large, round bone cutter is carefully used to remove the bone covering the cystic cavity. A broad opening is created, but without impinging on the roots of adjacent teeth or the mental foramen.

Right: A scalpel is used to remove a section of the cystic lining along the osseous border, for histopathological examination.

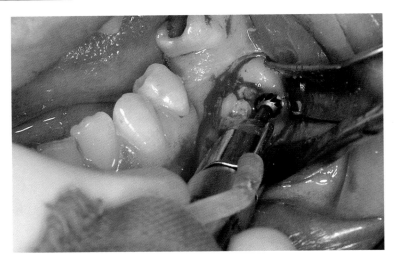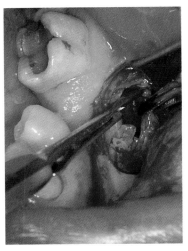

516 Removal of the tooth

The impacted tooth 35 is sectioned and then removed toward the buccal aspect.

Right: Histological section from the follicular cyst, showing a fine, multilayered cystic epithelium with a broad, fibrous sac.

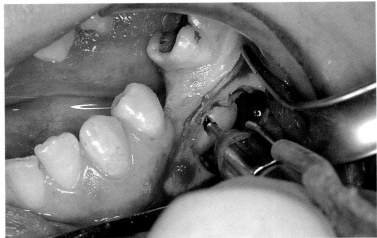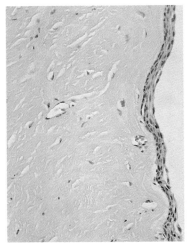

517 Wound treatment

A large, round bone cutter is used to expand the bony opening and create an extensive and patent connection with the oral cavity. Adjacent structures, including teeth and nerves, must be avoided and protected at all costs.

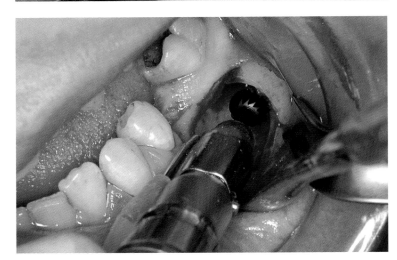

518 Flap fixation

A small, round bone cutter is used to create small holes along the buccal cystic bony margin.

Right: Sutures are placed through these holes to keep the mucosal flap open.

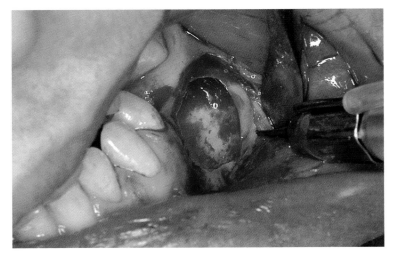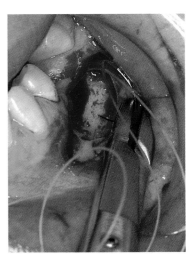

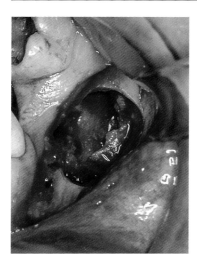

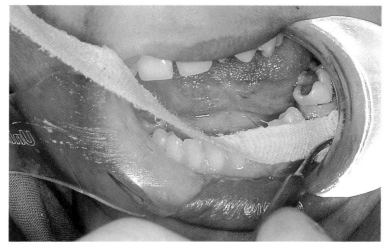

519 Wound dressing

The cystic cavity is broadly opened to the oral cavity, and is filled loosely with an iodoform gauze strip to prevent contamination of the wound by food debris.

Left: The open cystic cavity after suture fixation of the vestibular mucoperiosteal flap, immediately before the iodoform gauze dressing is placed.

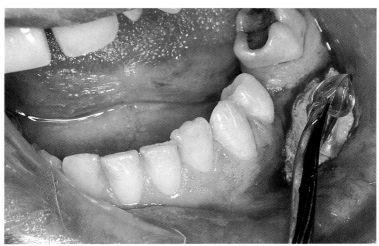
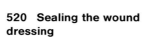

520 Sealing the wound dressing

The surface of the dressing is covered with an acetone adhesive to prevent saturation with saliva.

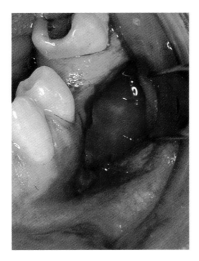

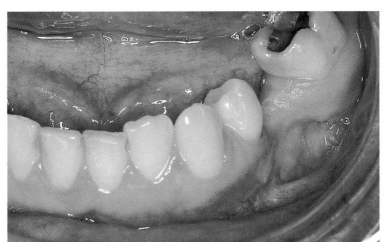

521 Follow-up care

The wound dressing is changed after one week. The clinical photograph *(left)* shows the situation after 14 days, at the second dressing change. Subsequently, two or three appointments at three-week intervals follow the wound healing until the cavity is sufficiently filled with tissue. Final healing can then be left to spontaneous regeneration.

Right: Twelve months postsurgically, the site shows only a slight depression.

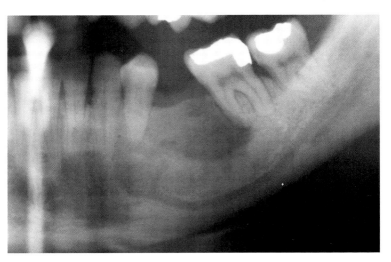
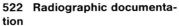

522 Radiographic documentation

This film, taken 12 months postsurgically, shows extensive osseous regeneration, with the formation of a trabecular pattern in the region of the cyst (compare Fig. 511). The arch space created by the missing tooth can now be treated by a general dentist.

523 Follicular cyst near tooth 38

This section from a panoramic radiograph shows the extent of the cyst radiating from the impacted tooth 38; this is a type 4 impaction, with the crown of tooth 38 lying in the cavity of a cyst that is approximately 4 cm in diameter. Note the impingement on the mandibular canal.

Right: An axial (Waters) projection of the mandible, taken with the mouth fully open, shows the cystic expanse lingually and buccally.

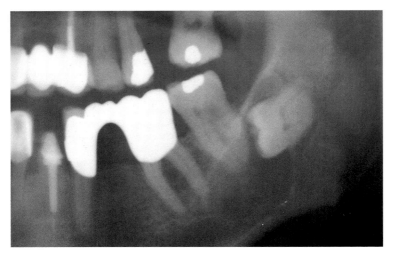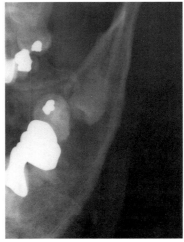

524 Access

The flap design is virtually identical to that used to extract an impacted tooth.

Right: Clinical view after vestibular flap reflection and broad opening of the cystic cavity using an osteotomy with a round bone cutter.

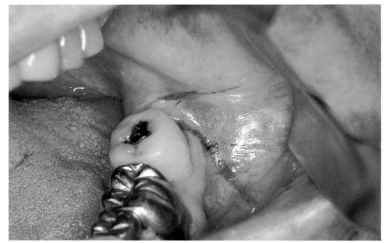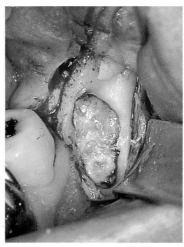

525 Opening the cyst

The large, round bone cutter is again used to expand the osteotomy to remove the impacted tooth. The cystic lining remains intact.

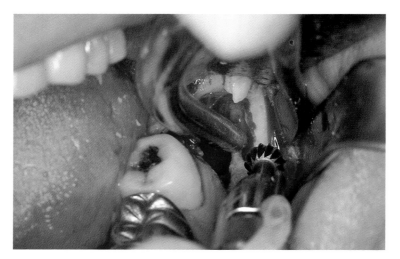

526 Biopsy for histological assessment

A scalpel is used to remove the part of the cystic sac that is visible through the osseous fenestration; the soft-tissue sac is sent for histopathological examination. The remainder of the cystic lining remains in situ.

Right: The tissue is also examined macroscopically. In this case, relatively thin, smooth, skin-like tissue is seen.

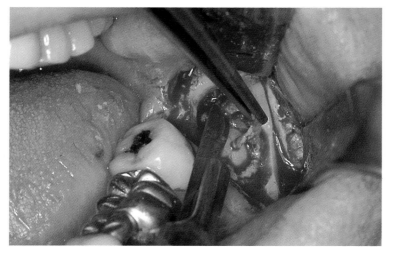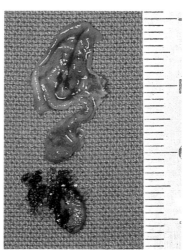

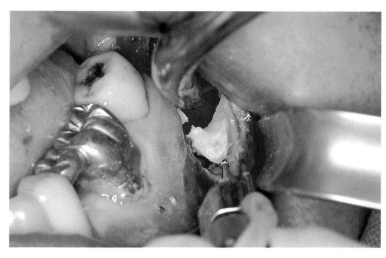

527 Cystostomy
After removal of the tooth, a bone cutter or a chisel is used at the osseous border to create the largest possible connection to the oral cavity.

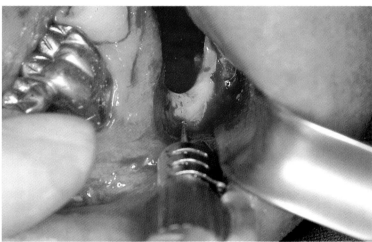

528 Fixation of the mucosa
A small, round bone cutter is used to create several small holes in the basal bony margin, through which sutures can be passed to maintain the mucosal flap in its reflected position.

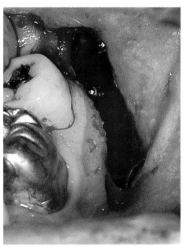

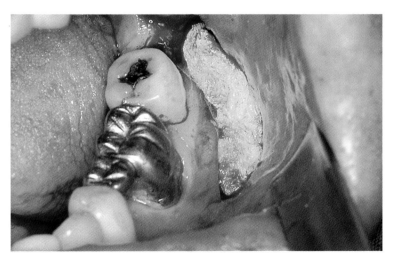

529 Wound treatment and follow-up
Resorbable sutures are used to attach the mucosa to the bone via the small holes, and the cystic cavity is filled loosely with an iodoform gauze strip. This is sealed with a tissue adhesive. Check-ups follow at intervals of 10–18 days, with dressing changes. After approximately three months, the cystic cavity will close sufficiently, and final healing can be left to spontaneous regeneration.

Left: Clinical view of the large cystic cavity after cystostomy and before placement of the dressing.

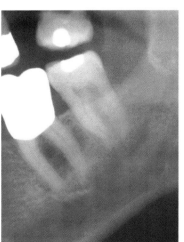

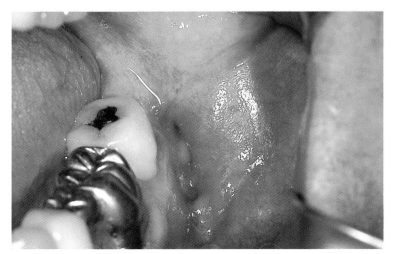

530 Clinical course
This clinical view shows the surgical site eight months postoperatively. Note that a scar-like cleft remains near tooth 38.

Left: The radiograph, taken eight months postoperatively, shows almost complete osseous regeneration of the cystic defect (compare Fig. 523).

Cystostomy on the Palate

In the anterior region of the maxilla, the presence of an osseous covering of a cyst on at least one aspect (palatal or facial) is important. If the bony covering is lacking on both surfaces, a tunnel-like defect can be expected. In cases such as this, cystostomy toward the palate should be considered.

Broad cystostomy toward the palatal aspect is the method of choice in the treatment of incisal canal cysts. With radicular cysts that have developed palatally near the anterior teeth, especially the lateral incisors, cystostomy is often the simplest treatment.

In difficult cases, if it is necessary to carry out an apicoectomy during the same procedure, it may be necessary to gain access from the buccal aspect. It is important to note, however, that in such cases the buccal osseous wall has to be reconstructed. This can be achieved using an osseous pedicle graft from the periosteum.

In the interest of patient comfort, a removable palatal stent may be inserted after marsupialization of cysts on the palate.

531 Maxillary cystostomy—radicular cyst in the anterior segment
This maxillary occlusal radiograph shows a 3-cm cystic osteolysis in the region of teeth 11 and 12. Clinically, a fluctuant mass was palpated on the palate. Teeth 11 and 12 reacted negatively to vitality testing.

Right: Fistulous tracts were evident both vestibularly and palatally. At the time of surgery, there were no symptoms of acute infection.

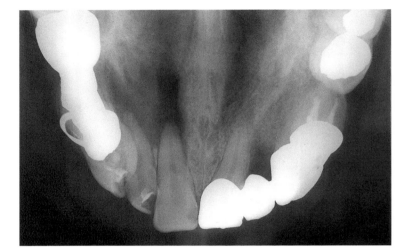
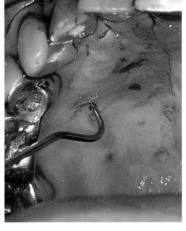

532 Access
With a palatal entry, the teeth must be treated endodontically, with an apicoectomy at the same appointment, but this is virtually impossible from a palatal approach. Thus the cystic cavity was opened from both the vestibular (**A**) for root tip resection and palatally (**B**) to remove the cyst. The bony plate on the buccal aspect was left attached to its periosteum, so that it could be replaced postsurgically.

Right: The two approaches.

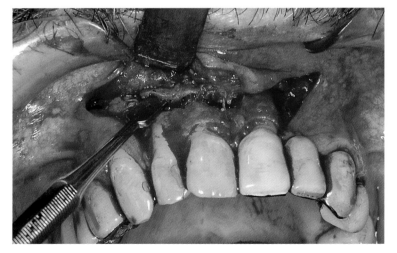
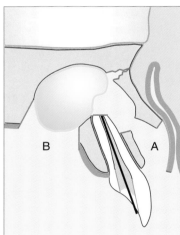

533 Wound closure
The mirror is used to check for complete closure of the root canals of teeth 12 and 11.

Right: After root canal filling and apicoectomy of both teeth, the vestibular access site is closed with the bony lid and the mucoperiosteal flap, which must be securely sutured.

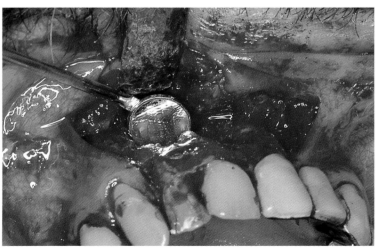
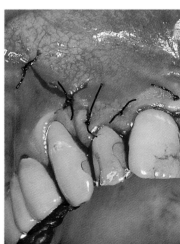

Tunnel-Like Defect

Any surgical procedure that perforates the alveolar process facio-orally creates what is known as a tunnel-like defect. Depending on the geometry of the defect, osseous regeneration in the central area of the tubular defect may be incomplete when healing occurs. This will be the case when new bone formation from the margins of the osseous defect does not keep pace with the ingrowth of connective tissue from the soft-tissue covering. The center of the wound thus retains scar tissue, which quite often leads to weather-related discomfort or even constant pain.

All of the possible methods of achieving osseous regeneration may be indicated for treatment of a tunnel-like defect, including autologous bone, lyophilized cartilage, hydroxyapatite, and membrane techniques (guided tissue regeneration or guided bone regeneration).

The surgical procedure for dealing with this type of osseous defect is described on p. 304.

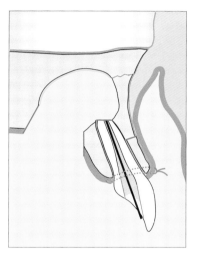
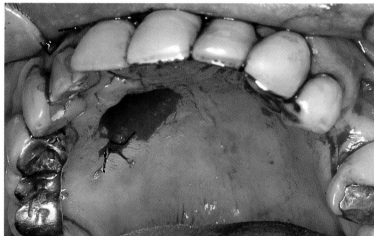

534 Marsupialization
After probing of the osseous defect, an appropriate mucoperiosteal flap on the palate is reflected. A band of soft tissue at least 2 mm wide must be left undisturbed to provide a continuous bridge of gingiva. The mobilized palatal soft tissue is excised so as to create the widest possible opening of the cystic cavity. This provides tissue for histological examination; the remainder of the tissue flap is repositioned and secured with interrupted sutures.

Left: The surgical principle after closure of the vestibular access.

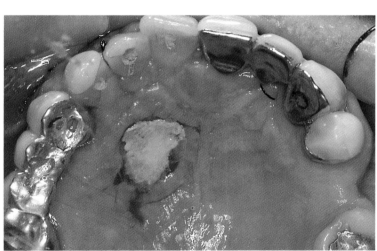

535 Wound treatment
The palatal defect is filled loosely with iodoform gauze and coated with a tissue adhesive. The dressing is changed after one week, and then at intervals of two or three weeks until the defect has filled sufficiently.

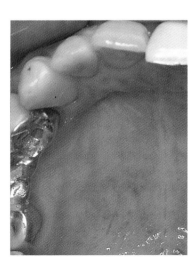
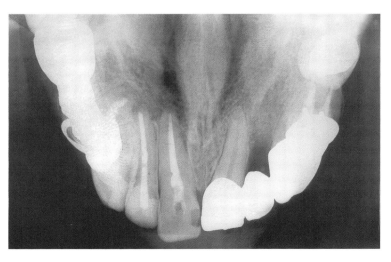

536 Course of healing
The check-up six months later, with a radiograph showing a much smaller defect due to the circumferential apposition of new bone (compare Fig. 531).

Left: The clinical view shows a slight depression at the surgical site, but this was not causing the patient any problems. All of the teeth are stable, and there is no periodontal pathology.

Cystostomy to the Nose

Indication
This procedure is usually indicated for cysts adjacent to the incisor teeth that can enlarge to such an extent that the floor of the nose is approached. Cysts adjacent to the canine teeth can develop either toward the nose or toward the maxillary sinus. Using a nasal speculum, it is clinically possible to detect expansion in the anterior portion of the nasal floor.

Anesthesia
Topical anesthesia is used.

Surgical Procedure
From a vestibular approach, the cyst is opened, tissue is harvested for histopathological examination, and a broad connection to the floor of the nose is created. A piece of iodoform gauze is placed via the nasal cavity, with the end wrapped round a gauze square, and inserted into the anterior part of the nasal cavity. The patient is recalled after three days, and the gauze strip is shortened. Subsequent appointments are at ten-day interval. The course of osseous regeneration is documented radiographically after six months.

537 Cystostomy to the nose or maxillary sinus
The panoramic radiograph provides an overview of the cystic osteolysis near the roots of teeth 12 and 13; the lesion, a lateral fissural cyst, has expanded to the floor of the nose. The roots of the teeth have been displaced, but vitality is maintained. Visual inspection of the anterior part of the nasal floor shows a slight protuberance in the right nasal canal.

Right: Cystostomy to the floor of the nose and maxillary sinus.

 ©

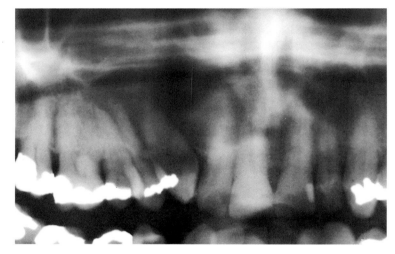
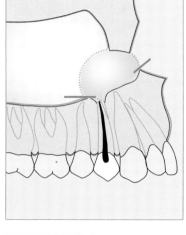

538 Anesthesia
Nerve block anesthesia is administered at the right infraorbital foramen, with infiltration at the palatal foramen and the incisal foramen, as well as near the anterior nasal spine and in the vestibulum on the left side.

Right: Administration of anesthesia to the floor of the nose is achieved using a topical anesthetic placed within the nasal cavity on the right side, using a tetracaine-soaked gauze square.

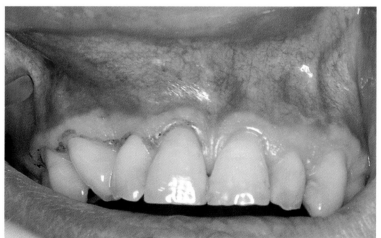
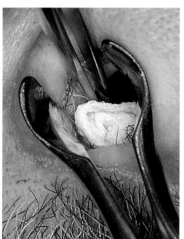

539 Opening the cyst
The cystic cavity is exposed by ostectomy using a round bur. Once exposed, the cyst can be opened.

Right: A scalpel is used to excise a portion of the cystic lining from the buccal approach.

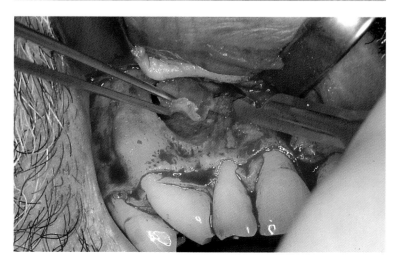
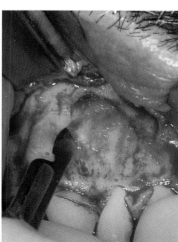

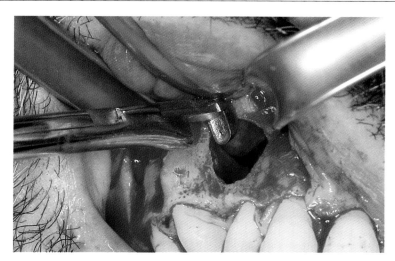

540 Cystostomy
The size of the osseous orifice is carefully enlarged by removing bone at the margin until sufficient visual access from the caudal aspect is achieved. In some cases, a bone punch can be used to advantage for this enlargement procedure.

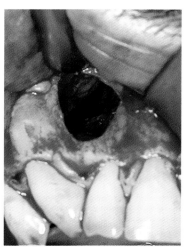
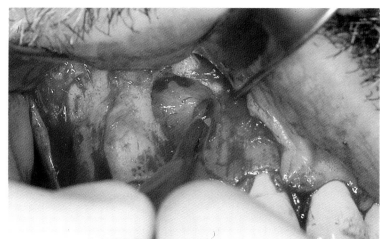

541 Connection to the nasal cavity
After inspection and palpation of the remaining soft tissue that is closing off the floor of the nose, the scalpel is used under direct vision to create a connection with the nasal cavity.

Left: Clinical view into the nasal cavity after removal of the soft-tissue interface.

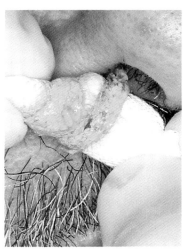
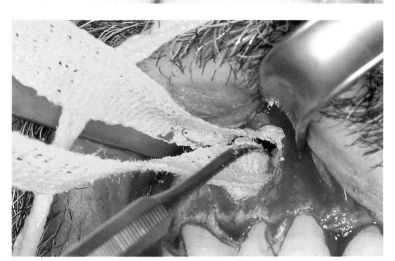

542 Wound treatment
A suitable length of iodoform gauze is inserted through the external nasal canal. The strips are layered to allow subsequent removal via the nose in reverse order.

Left: The end of the gauze strip is wound round a gauze square to prevent loss of the free end into the depths of the nose.

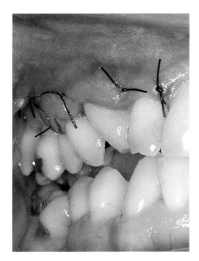
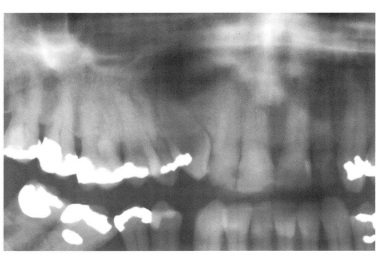

543 Follow-up
At three days, the wound is examined. The iodoform gauze dressing can be shortened. Additional appointments should be made at one week and at ten days. The soft tissue flap can be repositioned interrupted sutures *(left)*.

Right: Note the osseous condition at one year: The cyst is much smaller. The teeth were vital and the patient had no symptoms.

Cystostomy to the Maxillary Sinus

Indication
The indication for this procedure is based on the proximity of the maxillary sinus to the cystic cavity and the adjacent but uninvolved vital teeth, which will be at risk if the entire cystic lining is removed. The patient should be informed of the possibility of postoperative hemorrhage from the nose, and to avoid sneezing.

Anesthesia
Infiltration near the infraorbital foramen and the tuberosity, and on the palate.

Surgical Procedure
Access is achieved by reflecting a vestibular flap. After the cyst is opened, sufficient material is removed for histopathological examination, and apicoectomy is performed as necessary. The cystic cavity is then opened to the maxillary sinus. A test is carried out to demonstrate uninhibited movement of air in the maxillary sinus, and then the access can be closed. With small cysts, it is usually not necessary to incorporate a nasal fenestration.

544 Cystostomy to the maxillary sinus
This half-axial projection of the maxilla shows an arcuate line of sclerosis (arrows) in the right maxillary sinus; this is a typical sign of cyst formation (residual cyst) toward the maxillary sinus.

Right: The surgical principle in marsupialization to the maxillary sinus.

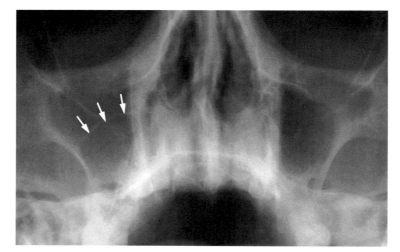 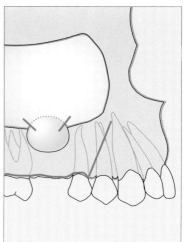

545 Access
It was possible to palpate a firm distension in the area of the right maxilla clinically. Access was achieved by a primary incision along the edentulous ridge, with vertical releasing incisions near teeth 17 and 13.

Right: The mucoperiosteal flap is carefully reflected, with care being taken to avoid cutting into the cyst.

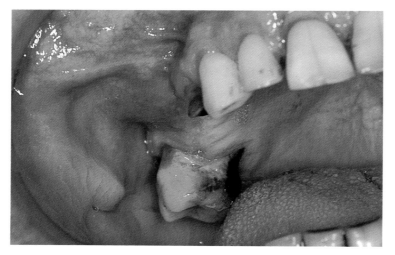 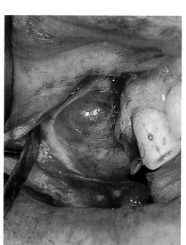

546 Opening the cyst
The buccal portion of the cystic lining is removed; this allows direct visual inspection of the extent of the cyst in the direction of the maxillary sinus.

Right: The balloon-like cyst is poorly adherent, and can be carefully teased away from the bone.

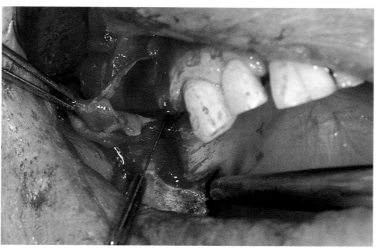 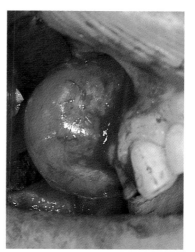

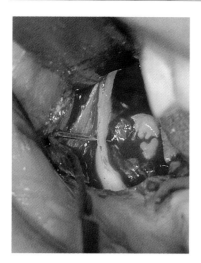
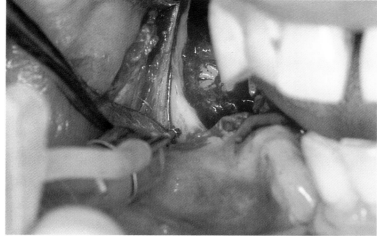

562 Maintaining an open site
Several drill holes are placed along the buccal cortical margin to accept sutures for securing the soft-tissue flap.

Left: The inserted probe demonstrates the drill holes in the buccal cortical bone.

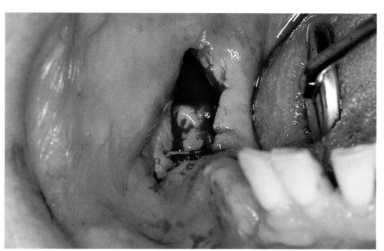

563 Wound treatment
The soft-tissue flap is sutured buccally and caudally using resorbable material.

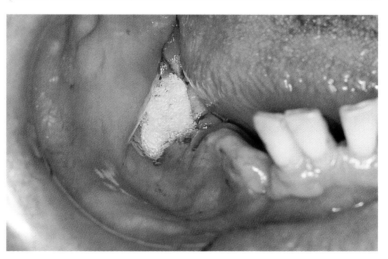

564 Wound treatment
The exposed area is filled with iodoform gauze, which is coated with a tissue adhesive.

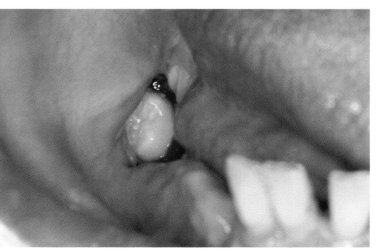

565 Follow-up
The dressing is changed on the tenth postoperative day, and can usually be removed completely after three weeks. This photograph, taken ten days after the procedure, shows irritation-free conditions at the surgical site. The crown of tooth 48, which was left in situ, is visible.

566   Clinical course
This panoramic radiograph, taken six months postsurgically, clearly shows that osseous apposition has occurred in the region of the follicular cyst; note also the osseous regeneration in the alveolus of tooth 47.

Right: The clinical photograph shows the collapsed soft tissue above the impacted tooth 48. At this point, the second surgical procedure can be initiated.

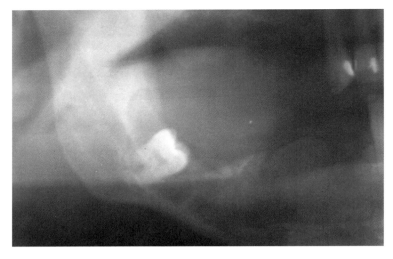 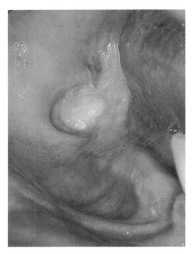

567   Second operation
Access is achieved in the same way as in the first operation; additional ostectomy is carried out as required to expose the impacted tooth 48 and section it into two pieces. This helps to protect the mandibular nerve. The surgical wound is treated in the open fashion.

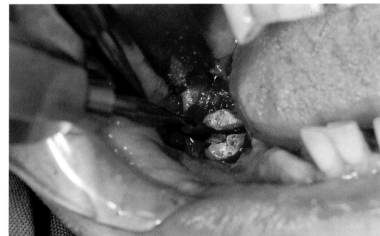

568   Final clinical view
In this case, there were no complications of any kind. The patient's ability to eat was never compromised. This photograph was taken 18 months after the second surgical procedure. The contour of the alveolar process is acceptable. A partial denture to replace the missing teeth should present no difficulties for this patient.

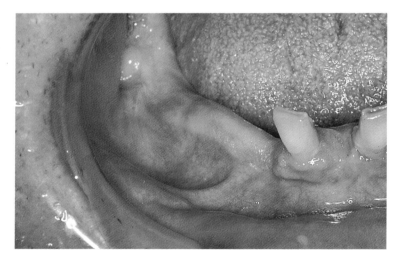

569   Radiographic documentation
This section from a panoramic radiograph taken 18 months postoperatively shows virtually complete regeneration of the osseous defect, with a regular trabecular structure of the new bone. The sensitivity of the structures supplied by the mandibular nerve was completely preserved.

Right: The initial radiographic view, for comparison.

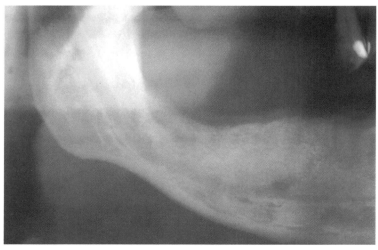 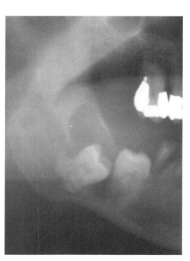

Treatment of the Cystic Cavity

Decision-Making Criteria

Small cystic cavities (up to ca. 1 cm in diameter) do not usually require any special treatment after cystectomy, unless a functional or aesthetic problem has developed.

Filling of a defect is always indicated if functional or aesthetic problems are anticipated as sequelae of cyst treatment; this is particularly true of extensive cysts in the alveolar process. It also applies to cystostomy and marsupialization.

Treatment of keratocysts often requires special interventional strategies.

Clinical Tip
Attempts to direct the healing of a cystic cavity should be considered long before the time of surgery. The local situation, as well as long-term planning, are the major factors in choosing appropriate surgical methodology. It is absolutely necessary that the patient should be completely informed and should fully understand the choice of a method for compensating osseous defects and irregularities.

Special Procedures Associated with Keratocysts

Necrosis of the Cystic Lining
The major determinant of keratocyst recurrence after surgical therapy is the presence of fragments of the cyst that have not been completely eliminated. In order to remove the cystic lining completely, including the connective-tissue capsule and all epithelial components, the cyst must be treated before and after its removal using Carnoy's solution (pp. 181, 213, and 220). This treatment should be carried out twice for five-minute periods. No lasting damage to any exposed nerves is caused (Frerich et al. 1994, Voorsmit et al. 1981, Voorsmit 1990).

Eradication
For keratocysts, we recommend radical removal of the cystic lining followed by thorough grinding out of the cystic cavity as far as the immediately adjacent anatomy allows.

Bone Replacement Materials for Filling Defects

Requirements
Materials for use in filling osseous defects have to meet certain requirements. The material must:
—Not cause inflammatory reactions in adjacent tissues.
—Not lead to encapsulation of connective tissue.
—Not cause immune reactions.
—Not initiate malignant transformation.
—Not produce toxic by-products.
—Not have any electrolytic or galvanic properties.
—Not provide a transfer mechanism for infections.

Or, stated positively, bone replacement materials must:
—Stimulate osseous regeneration and consolidation.
—Provide physiological resistance.
—Provide long-term, functional resistance and resilience.
—Remain observable (radiographic contrast).
—Be readily obtainable.
—Be easy to apply.

Special Terminology
Autogenic = autologous = host-derived.
Allogenic = homologous = derived from the same species.
Xenogenic = heterologous = foreign-body material derived from a different species.

Biologically Active Bone Replacement Materials

—Autologous bone transplant: trabecular or cortical bone.
—Sterile, lyophilized, allogenic bone.
—Sterile, lyophilized, allogenic cartilage.
—Combinations with bone morphogenetic protein (BMP).

These various types of bone replacement material are either incorporated into host osseous tissue or replaced by host osseous tissue.

Lyophilized Cartilage Chips

Lyophilized cartilage is replaced by endogenous bone after a period of calcification. This biological phenomenon can be exploited in attempts to correct various osseous defects. The importance of this material was referred to above in the discussion of contiguous pockets in relation to apicoectomy, and again in the discussion of tunnel-like defects. If unfavorable osseous defects in the alveolar process persist after cystectomy, lyophilized cartilage can substantially reduce or eliminate many problems associated with such defects. Antibiotic rehydration of this material allows it to be used even in situations in which there is infection.

The procedure is simple. Before closure of the wound, the rehydrated chips are placed in the osseous defect. Systemic antibiotic coverage is unnecessary. Careful wound closure prevents the ingress of saliva and the development of an inflammatory process. Use of this material is also indicated when cysts larger than 2 cm are removed, and no postoperative complications can be expected; this is in contrast to other methods using foreign substances and systemic antibiotic administration.

570 Treating the cystic cavity—contiguous pocket
In this case, the osseous defect in the alveolar process was extensive, with exposure of the root of tooth 12 after removal of a large radicular cyst. In a case of this type, spontaneous osseous regeneration via granulation tissue cannot be expected.

Right: This occlusal radiograph shows the osseous defect distopalatal to the root of tooth 12.

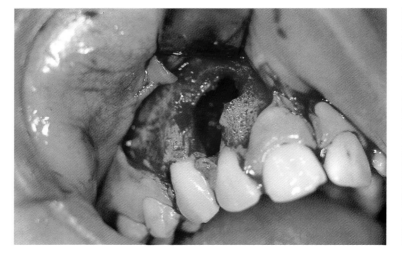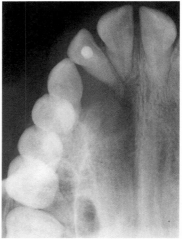

571 Lyophilized cartilage
After cystectomy and apicoectomy, the cystic cavity was filled with lyophilized cartilage chips. In this case, systemic antibiotics were prescribed for a one-week period.

Right: This radiograph was taken immediately after the procedure; the lyophilized cartilage cannot be visualized in a radiograph.

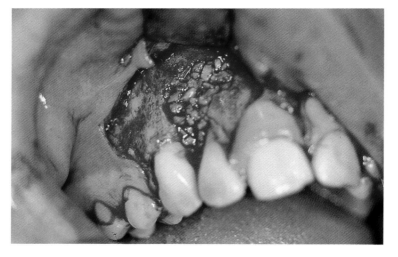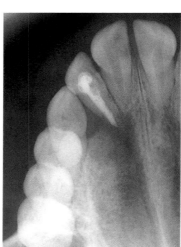

572 Clinical course
The clinical view 24 months after the surgical procedure revealed healthy clinical conditions, and there was no pocket formation on tooth 12.

Right: The radiograph shows virtually complete osseous regeneration.

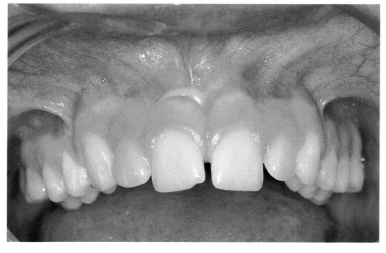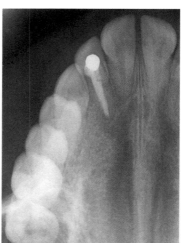

The postoperative course after filling a cystic defect with lyophilized cartilage is identical to that after cystectomy alone. Osseous regeneration of the cystic cavity can be observed radiographically after a certain period of time. If the cyst was larger than 2 cm in diameter, the area of osteolysis will remain visible in the radiograph up to and beyond one year postoperatively.

However, the marginal demarcation will no longer be sharp, and ossification may not be readily evident. Complete conversion of the filling material into autogenous bone can be expected only after a period of two years. The regenerative process in the mandible can be expected to last slightly longer than that in the maxilla.

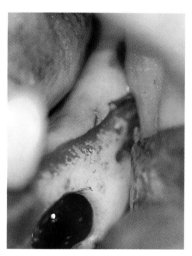
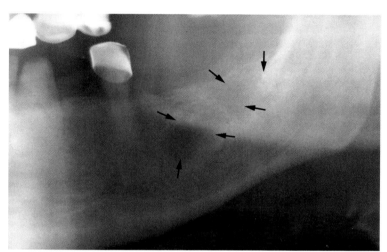
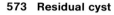

573 Residual cyst
The radiograph shows an extensive residual cyst in the horizontal ramus of the mandible (arrows). Cystostomy is not the treatment of choice, primarily for prosthodontic reasons.

Left: This clinical photograph was taken immediately after the cystectomy procedure.

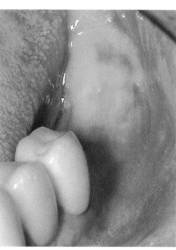
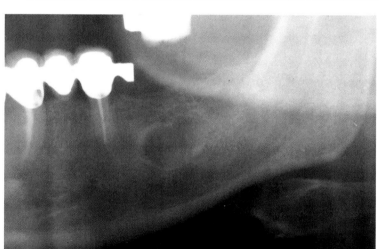

574 Clinical course
Almost complete reossification in the distal area is seen in the radiograph taken 18 months postoperatively, but in the anterior segment the reossification process is not yet complete.

Left: The alveolar process has been completely maintained, and is capable of supporting a prosthesis.

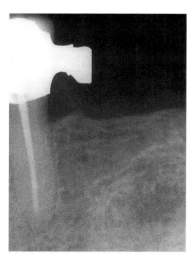
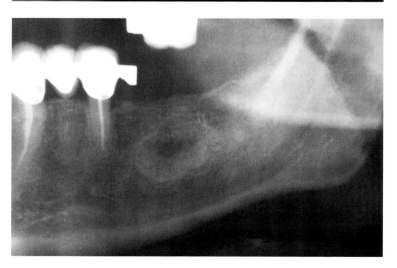

575 Late follow-up
Three years postoperatively, the panoramic radiograph shows complete osseous regeneration of the previous cystic defect.

Left: A periapical radiograph shows the trabecular structure of the newly formed bone.

Lyophilized Chips and BMP

Bone morphogenetic protein (BMP) activates the differentiation of immature connective-tissue cells into osteocytes. The combination of lyophilized cartilage chips and BMP causes an acceleration of osseous regeneration in the cystic cavity after cystectomy. The combined use of these two materials can lead to a significant reossification of the former cystic cavity within six months.

Larger Lyophilized Cartilage Pieces

For either esthetic or functional reasons (e.g., denture bed), there is sometimes a need to enhance the alveolar process in areas in which there are defects. Autologous bone, hydroxyapatite, and larger pieces of lyophilized cartilage can be used for this purpose. The physical properties of lyophilized cartilage—its slight tendency to shrink and its resistance to infection—are significant advantages. The cartilage pieces are approximated to the defect as inlays or onlays. Complete immobilization is a prerequisite for complication-free healing; the other factor is complete coverage by the soft tissue flap.

576 Lyophilized cartilage and BMP
This section from a panoramic radiograph clearly shows an extensive follicular cyst near tooth 38, as well as involvement of the roots of the endodontically treated tooth 37.

Right: The clinical photograph shows the defect after cystectomy and removal of tooth 38. The entire length of the distal root of tooth 37 became exposed, i.e., its bony covering was lost. The tooth should really be extracted.

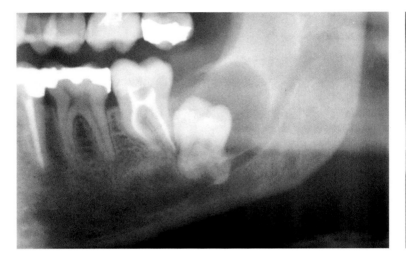
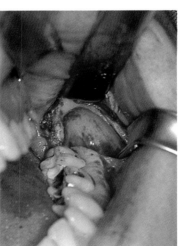

577 Clinical course
This detail of a panoramic radiograph taken immediately postoperatively will provide a baseline for assessing the course of healing of the osseous defect. An extensive area of osteolysis at the angle of the mandible is clearly visible.

Right: The cystic cavity was filled with a mixture of lyophilized cartilage chips and BMP.

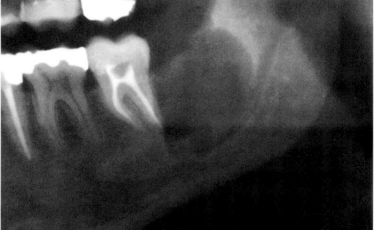
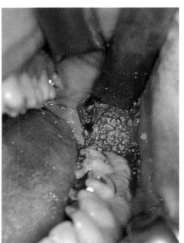

578 Completion of treatment
The radiographic follow-up seven months postoperatively shows extensive osseous regeneration, but the trabecular structure remains poorly organized.

Right: The clinical view shows irritation-free conditions, and there was no pocket formation on the distal aspect of tooth 37.

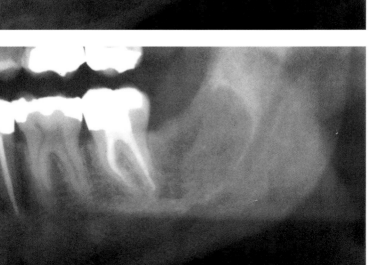
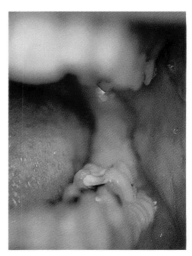

Biologically Inert Bone Replacement Materials

—Tricalcium phosphate
—Synthetic and biological hydroxyapatite
—Glass ionomer

These materials are partly inert, and some of them are absorbed at various rates (phagocytosis, hydrolysis). The materials have a certain osteoinductive potential, i.e., new bone tends to grow into them. However, they only partly meet the important criteria listed on page 213. The use of these materials is restricted by the local anatomy; in areas of the alveolar process that will be loaded occlusally, use of such material is questionable. The effects may only be observed many years after placement.

The only advantages of these materials is their availability and ease of use.

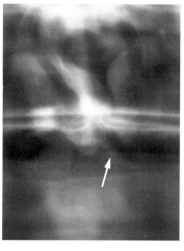
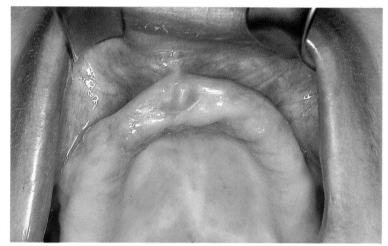

579 Lyophilized segments of cartilage
The radiograph shows a 1-cm residual cyst in the region of the right maxillary anterior segment *(left)*.

Right: An osseous defect in this region might compromise the stability of a complete denture.

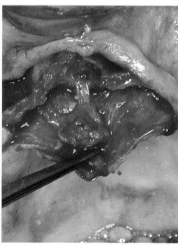
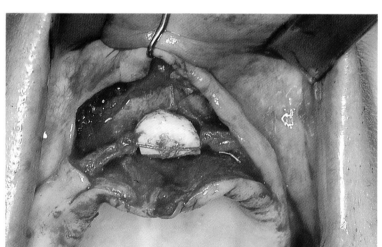

580 Correcting the defect
The osseous defect on the anterior maxillary ridge is filled using a cartilage onlay, which is affixed with resorbable sutures.

Left: This clinical photograph shows the exposed residual cyst.

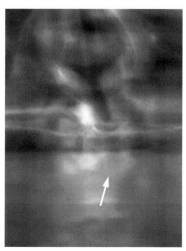
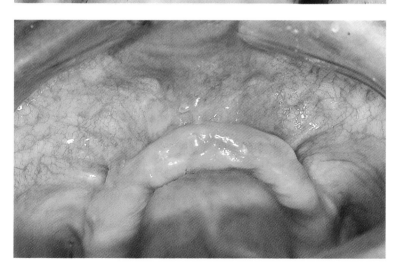

581 Clinical course
Reossification in the area of the cystic cavity is clearly seen in the radiograph taken 18 months after the surgical procedure *(left)*.

Right: The clinical photograph shows the excellent ridge profile of the maxillary alveolar process. This photograph was taken one year after the surgical procedure.

Hydroxyapatite

Hydroxyapatite-based bone replacement material (p. 305) is a practical method of filling osseous defects. However, only a limited area of the replacement material will actually become ossified; osseous integration is normally limited to the margins. Hydroxyapatite is tolerated as a harmless foreign body. Depending on the particle size, resorption can be anticipated to a greater or lesser extent. Hydroxyapatite has no anti-infectious properties, and should therefore only be used in areas that are free of inflammation. An advantage of hydroxyapatite lies in its unrestricted availability.

In some instances, granular hydroxyapatite will be recognized as a foreign body, and will be encapsulated by connective tissue. When this material is used, it must be understood that the area will remain as one of limited biological resistance over the long term. In areas of the alveolar process that are loaded (e.g., by a denture base), if the mucosal covering is thin, the material can become infected and eventually be evulsed as a result of the persistent inflammatory process. The clinical removal of implanted hydroxyapatite is very difficult, and complete elimination of the hydroxyapatite is hardly possible.

582 Granular hydroxyapatite—palatal cyst
The occlusal radiograph shows the cystic cavity, which incorporates a mesiodens, in this 35-year-old woman.

Right: The clinical view shows the situation after a palatal approach to open the follicular cyst.

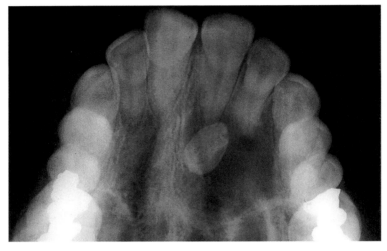
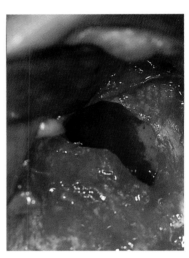

583 Surgical procedure
The tooth is removed along with the cystic lining, and the osseous defect is filled with granular hydroxyapatite that has been saturated with an antibiotic solution *(right)*.

Left: The radiograph shows the situation six months postoperatively. Note the indistinct borders of the defect of the cystic cavity, and the barely visible granular areas that are incipient areas of recalcification.

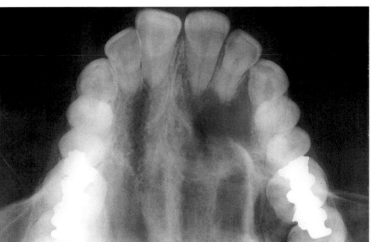
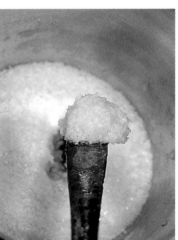

584 Clinical course
Eighteen months later, these occlusal radiographs show an almost completely restructured osseous picture.

Right: The clinical photograph shows irritation-free conditions in the surgical area, and the teeth are vital.

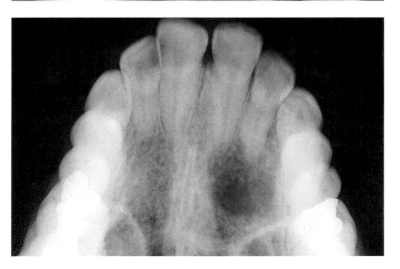
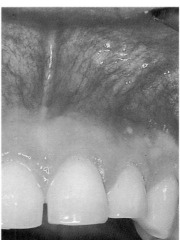

Guided Tissue Regeneration (GTR)

The underlying biological principle of this treatment technique consists of creating a cavity by forming a ceiling above an osseous defect, to provide an area for undisturbed differentiation of mast cells into osteoblasts and osteocytes. A secondary goal is to inhibit the replacement of osseous tissue by soft connective tissue.

In our experience, we have found no particular indication for the use of membranes or barriers in the treatment of cystic cavities.

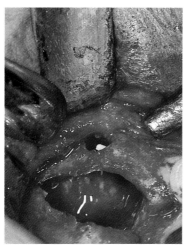
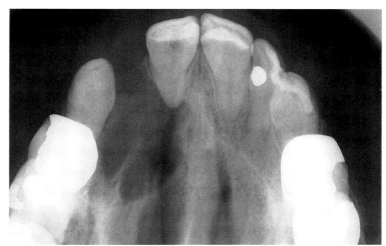

585 Cyst in the alveolar process
In this 26-year-old woman, the radiograph shows the osseous situation after trauma with loss of tooth 22 and a cyst adjacent to the nonvital tooth 21.

Left: The clinical photograph taken during the operation shows the defect, which extends into the alveolar process.

Ⓢ

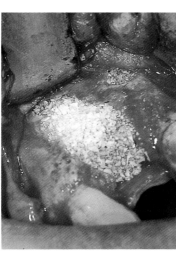
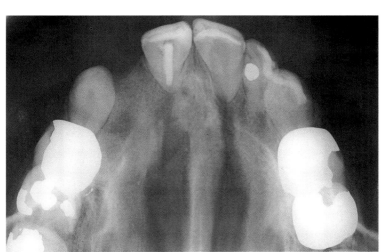

586 Clinical course
The postoperative radiograph shows the hydroxyapatite material that was used to fill the bony defect.

Left: Clinical view of the osseous defect filled with granular hydroxyapatite.

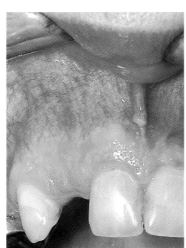
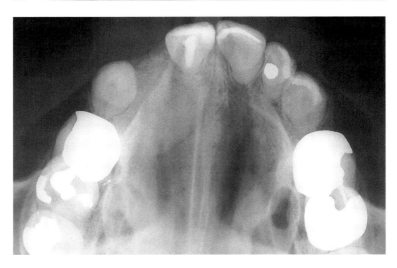

587 Completion of treatment
This radiograph, taken six months postoperatively shows the clear demarcation between the filling material and the surrounding new bone within the previous cystic osseous defect. The radiolucent zones surrounding the granular filling material indicate a connective-tissue encapsulation without further ossification.

Left: The clinical photograph has an irritation-free appearance and an optimum edentulous ridge profile.

Treatment Using Carnoy's Solution

In his studies of the behavior of keratocysts, Voorsmit (1990) proposed the use of a tissue fixative. This procedure was intended to reduce the frequency of recurrence with this type of persistent cyst. Experience at our own clinic in the treatment of keratocysts supports Voorsmit's approach. The cauterizing solution is placed in the lumen immediately after opening the cyst, and remains there for five minutes. Care must be taken to prevent contact between the cauterizing solution and mucosal surfaces or with teeth. After the area has been rinsed with physiological saline, the procedure is repeated. Only now is the lining of the cyst completely removed. Treatment of the cavity with Carnoy's solution (see p. 213) is then repeated.

If the procedure is correctly carried out, no adverse side effects will be encountered. In particular, exposed nerves (e.g., the inferior alveolar nerve) are not injured by the procedure.

Composition of Carnoy's solution:
600 ml absolute alcohol
300 ml chloroform
100 ml 98% acetic acid.

588 Carnoy's solution
A keratocyst with an impacted tooth 38 in a 20-year-old woman.

Right: Clinical photograph after opening of the cyst and extraction of the tooth. After complete removal of the cystic lining and freshening up of the osseous surface, the cystic cavity is treated twice for five minutes with Carnoy's solution. Because Carnoy's solution is a powerful cauterizing agent, it should not be allowed to come into contact with other teeth or adjacent mucosa.

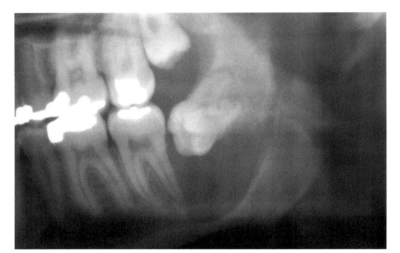 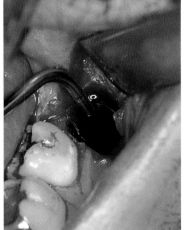

589 Clinical course
The postoperative panoramic radiograph for purposes of comparison.

Right: The cystic cavity is left to heal in the open method, as with cystic marsupialization.

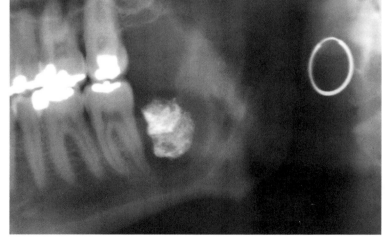 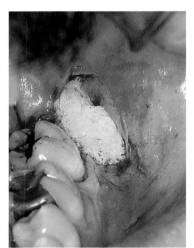

590 Postoperative view
Clinical follow-up after treatment for a keratocyst should continue for up to ten years. This detail of a panoramic radiograph shows the condition after four years, with osseous regeneration and no signs of cystic recurrence.

Right: The clinical photograph shows scar tissue at the surgical site, but the patient is completely free of symptoms.

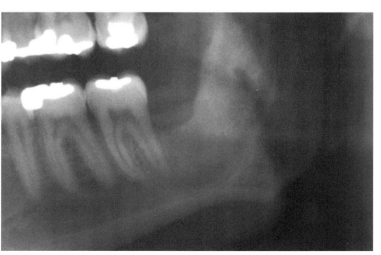 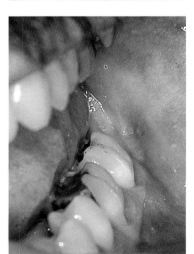

Soft-Tissue Cysts

Cysts in soft tissue are similar to cysts in the jaws, both with regard to their structure and appearance and in their behavior. These cysts are readily accessible for inspection and palpation; aspiration with a syringe tip usually confirms a diagnosis. Soft-tissue cysts can show increases in size and fluctuation. The initial differential diagnosis may include abscess, and this can be excluded by the medical history, since cysts are painless and mobile.

Four types of soft-tissue cyst are distinguished:
— Retention cysts
— Developmental cysts
   (nasolabial cyst, nasal orifice cyst)
— Gingival cyst
— Dermoid cyst

The most common cysts in the mucosal regions of the oral cavity are salivary retention cysts (mucocele). The ranula, a retention cyst of the floor of the mouth, has a special place in oral surgery.

The other types of soft-tissue cyst are relatively rare, and should be treated by specialists (Galloway et al. 1989, Skouteris and Sotereanos 1987, van den Akker et al. 1978).

Surgical Procedure

Retention cysts are either excised in toto or, in the case of ranula of the floor of the mouth, marsupialized. Because the cystic lining is delicate, it is easy to puncture the cyst during preparation for surgery. If this occurs, surgical extirpation is usually not possible. Injecting the cystic cavity with a rubber impression material will help to prevent this complication.

Small retention cysts can also be treated by cryosurgery.

Postoperative scar formation at the surgical site may provoke further stenosis. Recurrence of a retention cyst is therefore always possible, and the patient should be informed about this.

Caution
Care must be taken to protect the sublingual duct and the lingual nerve during surgery for treatment of ranula.

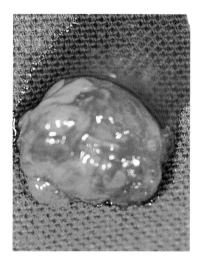
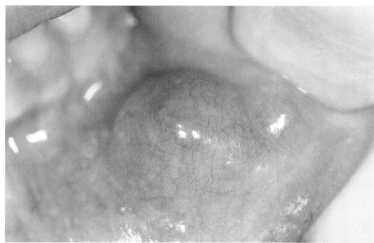
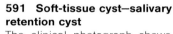

591 Soft-tissue cyst—salivary retention cyst
The clinical photograph shows a painless, taut swelling in the lower lip of a 17-year-old boy. Note that the mucosal covering is intact.

Left: The excised cyst presents as a glassy mass that is filled with thick mucous.

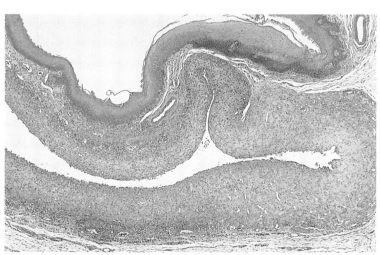

592 Histology
The section stained with hematoxylin and eosin shows the oral epithelium (above) and the salivary duct with inflammatory infiltrate within the surrounding connective tissues (below).

Retention Cyst of the Lip

The lips are a frequent site for the development of salivary retention cysts. These are usually several millimeters in diameter, often bluish in color, and present as taut swellings on the oral aspect of the lip. During surgical removal of this type of cyst, the configuration of the vermilion border of the lip must be taken into account. The cyst is either teased out from underneath the mucosa (extirpation) while maintaining the epithelial covering, or excised in toto. The excised material should always be sent for histopathological examination.

Excision should not be carried out too deeply, because an incision into the lip musculature will sever small vessels, leading to unexpected hemorrhage. All bleeding has to be arrested before suture closure, to prevent hematoma formation within the lip. Small retention cysts of less than 3 mm in diameter can also be treated using cryosurgery. The disadvantage of this procedure is that no material for histopathological examination is obtained.

593 Retention cyst on the lower lip—anesthesia and excision
Local infiltration in the vestibulum is sufficient. The small retention cyst located beneath the labial mucosa is prepared for excision by holding the lip with two hands and pressing the cyst outward. The finger pressure lateral to the cyst on both sides also reduces bleeding.

Right: The surgical principle: removal of the cyst in toto, preserving the covering mucosa.

 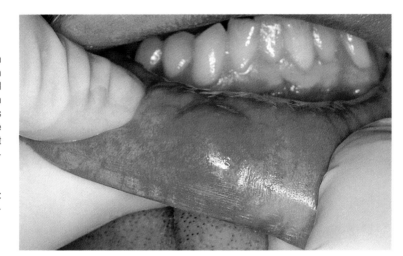 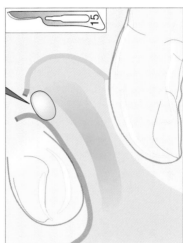

594 Exposure of the cyst
The primary incision is made horizontally on the oral aspect of the labial mucosa, and blunt scissors are used to separate the mucosa from the underlying cyst. It is important that the cyst should not be touched, since if the cystic fluid is expelled, it will no longer be possible to differentiate the cystic tissue from the surrounding tissue.

Right: A tissue retractor is used to retract the mucosa, and blunt dissection is used to expose the cyst.

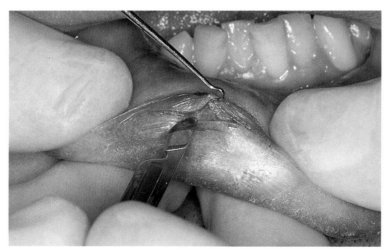 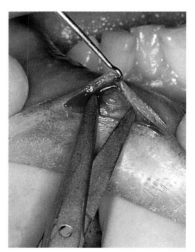

595 Removing the cyst
The taut cyst is teased free of its attachment to the tissues under the mucosa.

Right: Retention cysts are very delicate. Grasping the cyst with a surgical forceps is likely to burst the cyst, making subsequent procedures more difficult.

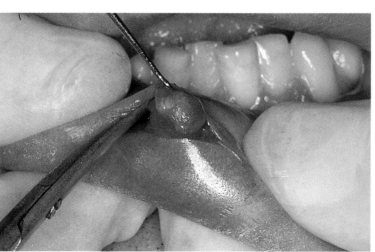 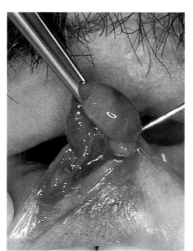

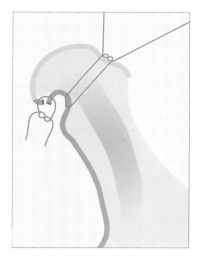

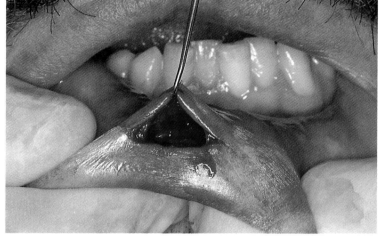

596 Wound treatment
Removal of the cyst creates a soft-tissue cavity within the substance of the lip, with a tendency toward hematoma formation.

Left: The translabial suturing technique to eliminate the soft-tissue cavity.

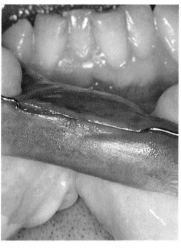

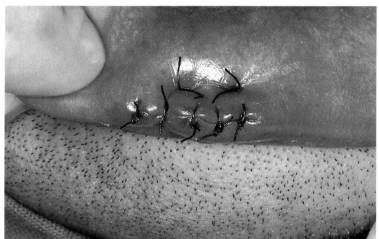

597 Suture closure
The margins of the wound are carefully adapted, and then apposed using interrupted sutures. Final closure is achieved by placing two translabial sutures.

Left: Precise wound margin adaptation is achieved by placing two tissue retractors as shown in the photograph, and applying slight tension.

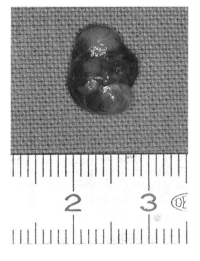

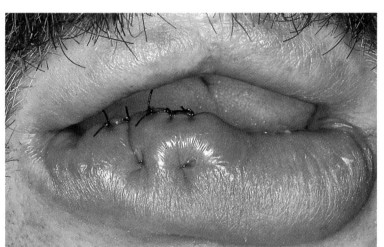

598 Course of healing
The translabial sutures are removed three days later. The remaining sutures are removed after an additional five-day period.

Left: The extirpated cyst is sent for histopathological examination.

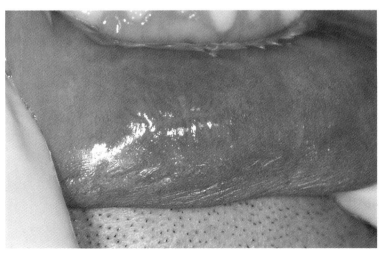

599 Completion of treatment
Eight months postoperatively, there was only a discrete scar, with no defect in the lip contour.

Retention Cyst of the Oral Mucosa

Two arcuate incisions can be used for the excision of retention cysts located in the extensive oral mucosa, e.g., in the cheek. Blunt scissors are used to free the taut cyst from its surrounding tissues. The scalpel and scissors must be used very carefully, since the thin cystic lining is very easily damaged; if this occurs, the cyst will collapse, and it becomes very difficult to carry out precise and controlled excision. All hemorrhage must be completely stopped before suture closure, to prevent hematoma formation. The wound is closed with interrupted sutures.

Adaptation of the wound margins after extensive incisions will be easier if blunt scissors are first used to undermine the mucosal layer.

In small cysts, cryosurgery may be indicated. However, in these cases it is not possible to obtain a histopathological diagnosis.

Clinical Tip
Salivary retention cysts have a tendency to recur. The patient should be appropriately informed.

600 Excision of a retention cyst on the cheek
This 66-year-old man had noticed an indolent swelling on the interior surface of the left cheek; it had a tendency to disappear and then reappear several weeks later. Clinical inspection revealed a 0.5-cm, soft, well-demarcated swelling with an intact mucosal covering.

Right: The surgical principle is excision of the cyst, including its covering mucosa.

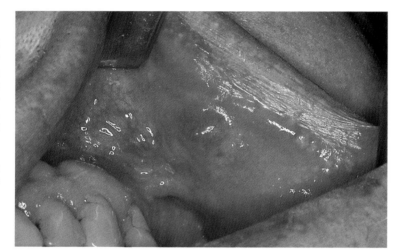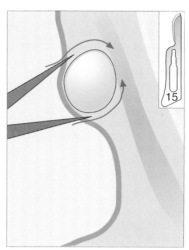

601 Excision
After administration of infiltration anesthesia, two arcuate incisions are made to encompass the excision site.

Right: The scalpel is guided in such a way that a wedge-shaped tissue incision is prepared.

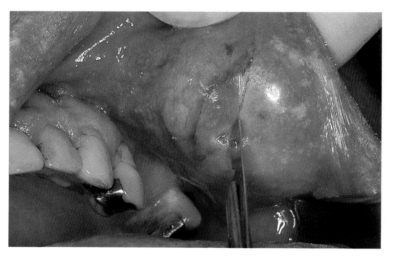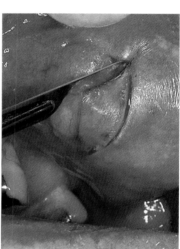

602 Excision
Blunt scissors are used to displace tissues adjacent to the cyst.

Right: To avoid traumatizing the small cyst, it is engaged securely using a tissue retractor.

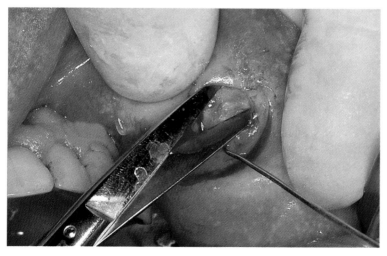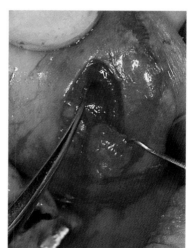

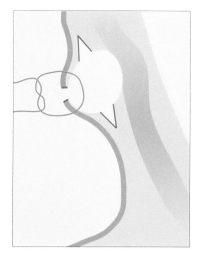

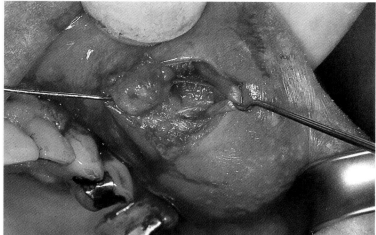

603 Protection of vessels
Careful dissection has revealed a vascular bundle, which can be protected.

Left: Suturing of the mucosa after the excision.

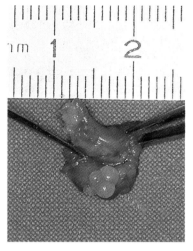

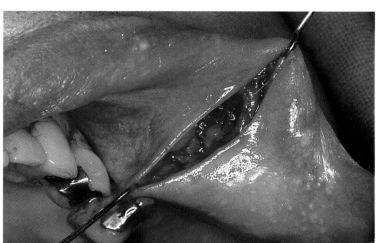

604 Wound closure
The elliptical wound is closed by applying tension with two tissue retractors, resulting in good approximation of the wound margins.

Left: The excised cyst is approximately 1 cm in diameter; several small fat cells are attached to it.

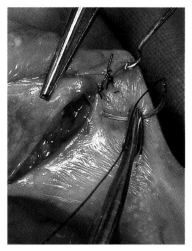

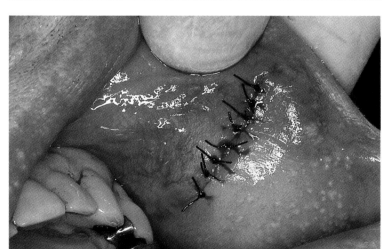

605 Wound closure
The mucosa is securely closed using individual sutures.

Left: Without impinging directly on the wound margin, surgical forceps can facilitate suture closure.

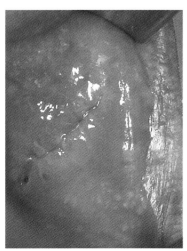

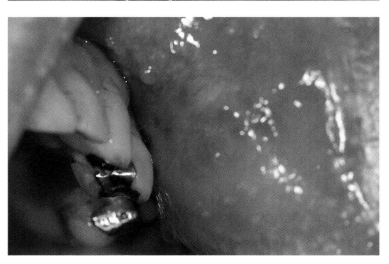

606 Clinical course
The sutures are removed one week postoperatively *(left)*.

Right: At the follow-up appointment two months later, a normal appearance of the cheek mucosa was seen at the surgical site, without no symptoms of recurrence.

Excision after Filling the Cyst

Large retention cysts, which often have very thin walls, are easily punctured during surgery. This can be avoided if the cystic lumen is drained before the operation and then refilled with a thin rubber impression material. This also provides visual control of the boundaries of the cyst, even if there are small perforations, making precise extirpation possible.

The procedure is simple: after applying a local anesthetic, a large-caliber needle is inserted into the cyst, and the cystic contents are aspirated; the shrunken cystic sac is then filled via the same needle with thin impression material. It is now possible to carry out the excision whether or not the mucosal covering remains intact.

607 Filling a large retention cyst
In this ten-year-old girl, a firm, well-demarcated swelling occurred on the left side of the lower lip; it had developed within the space of a month.

Right: The surgical principle: the cystic contents are aspirated and replaced with a thin rubber impression material.

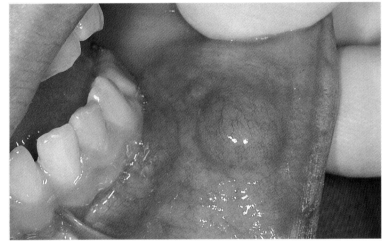
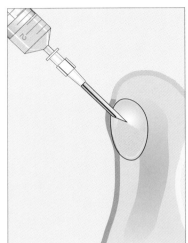

608 Filling the cyst
After aspiration of the thick mucous contents of the cyst, the cystic cavity is carefully filled with the rubber impression material.

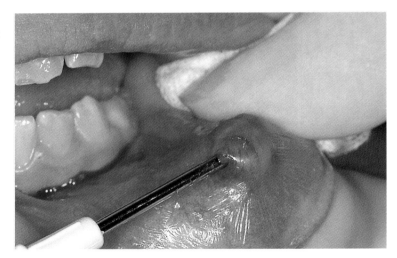

609 Primary incision
The primary incision follows the vermilion border of the lip.

Right: The scalpel must be guided carefully and not too deeply, in order to avoid damaging the cyst.

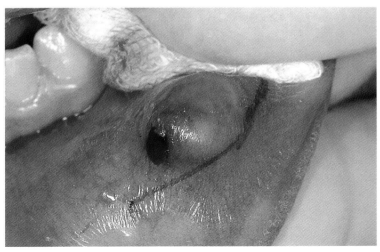
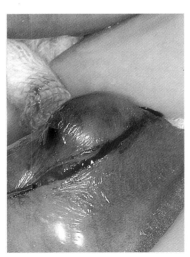

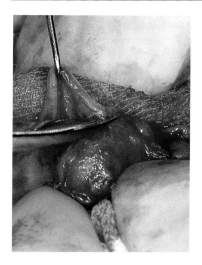

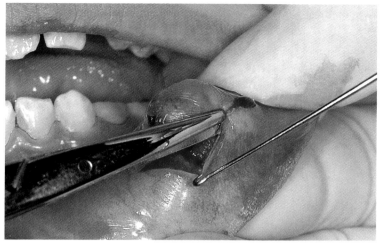

610 Cystectomy
Blunt scissors can be used to free the rubber-filled cystic mass from its surrounding tissues.

Left: The tissue retractor can be used to advantage for retracting the delicate mucosa away from the cyst.

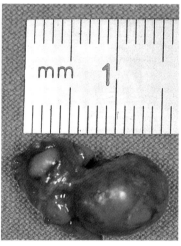

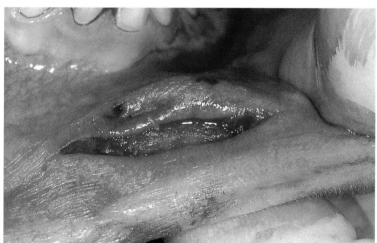

611 Cystectomy
Applying pressure to the external surface of the lip makes it easier to tease out the ovoid cystic mass.

Left: The cyst that was removed had two chambers. Thanks to the rubber impression material filling, the cystic sac remained intact.

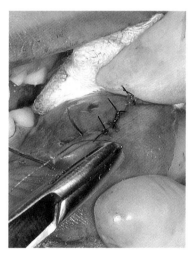

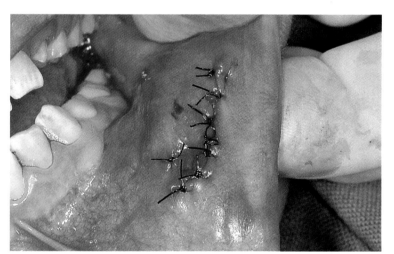

612 Wound treatment
The incision in the lip is closed by interrupted sutures.

Left: Since it was possible to enucleate the retention cyst completely, the mucosal covering remained intact and was easily repositioned and closed.

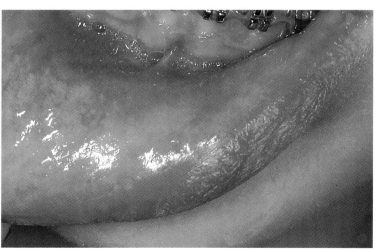

613 Clinical course
Suture removal was carried out one week postoperatively. The next follow-up appointment was at one month (photograph); there were no signs of cystic recurrence.

Ranula

Because of their peculiar appearance, large retention cysts in the floor of the mouth are termed ranula ("small frog"). They usually occur unilaterally, and are characterized clinically by a smooth-surfaced, spherical swelling under the tongue, which is very often noticed by the patient. Ranulas are usually located superficially, but in rare instances may perforate the musculature of the floor of the mouth and advance in a cervical direction.

The most common treatment for retention cysts of the floor of the mouth is marsupialization. Care must taken to avoid injury to the submandibular duct and the lingual nerve. Anatomical orientation can be enhanced by placing a probe in the submandibular duct. Sutures are placed in a circular arrangement before removal of the roof of the cyst. This makes it possible to carry out the extensive marsupialization before the cystic contents are spilled and the tissue collapses. Filling the cystic cavity presurgically with a rubber impression material can simplify the operation and improve visual access.

614 Marsupialization of a ranula
In this 17-year-old girl, a swelling had developed on the left side of the floor of the mouth over a one-year period. The swelling, within the sublingual plica, was taut, immobile, and painless, and its mucosal covering was intact and glassy in appearance. Expiration with a syringe retrieved thick saliva.

Right: The surgical principle: marsupialization after removal of the covering mucosa and previous filling of the cystic cavity.

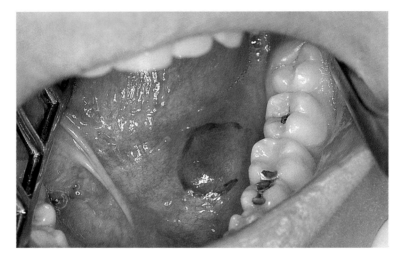
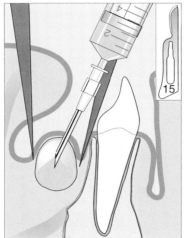

615 Cystostomy
Before making the primary incision through the cyst's mucosal covering, circular retentive sutures are placed. This prevents the cyst from collapsing if there is accidental puncture and its contents are released.

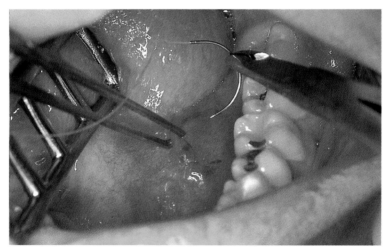

616 Keeping the cyst open
The primary incision was circumferential inside the series of retentive sutures; once opened, the cyst immediately collapsed. To prevent recurrence caused by scar tissue shrinkage, the lumen of the cyst is kept open by placing an iodoform gauze strip.

Right: The clinical photograph shows the situation six months postsurgically, with no evidence of recurrence.

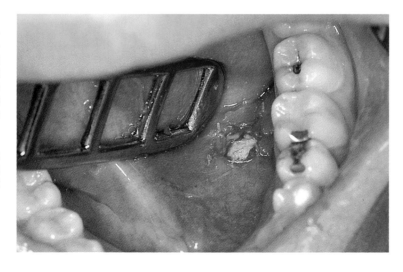
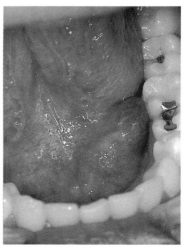

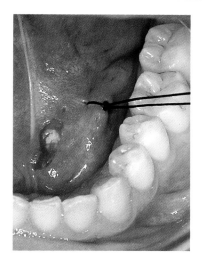
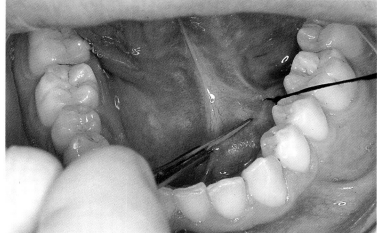

656   Opening the duct
A probe is inserted into the duct, and a scalpel is used to open the duct along the probe.

Left: The sialolith now becomes clearly visible.

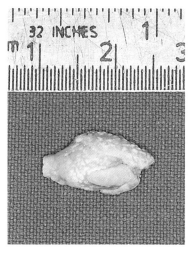
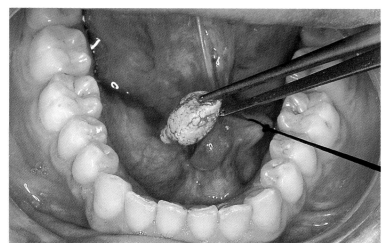

657   Removing the sialolith
A surgical forceps or clamp is used to tease the sialolith out of its bed.

Left: This stone was over 1 cm in extent. The sialolith should be carefully inspected macroscopically.

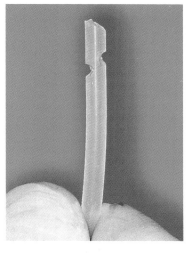
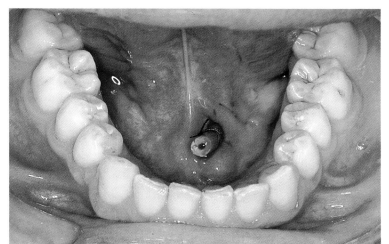

658   Wound treatment
To avoid stenosis of the duct due to scar formation, a small rubber tube is inserted into the new orifice and left in situ for eight days.

Left: To enhance saliva drainage, lateral perforations are made in the rubber tubing. The end of the tube inserted into the duct should be slightly rounded.

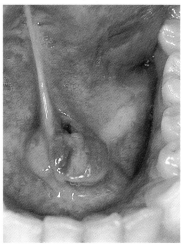
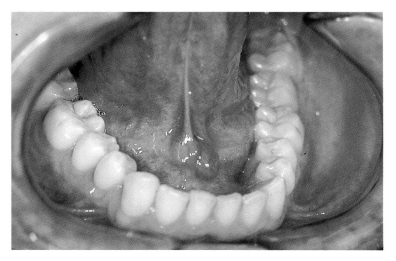

659   Postoperative care and completion of treatment
The tubing is removed one week later. The patient is advised to eat foods that encourage saliva flow, or to suck on sour tablets (*left*).

A follow-up appointment one year postoperatively showed normal salivary flow from the "new" orifice of the submandibular duct (*right*).

Sialolith in the Parotid Duct

Clinical Findings

Unilateral swelling of the parotid gland coinciding with stimulation of saliva suggests a sialolith in the parotid duct. The differential diagnosis must exclude other diseases, and the sialolith should be identified radiographically with a sialogram. In rare cases, oral parafunctions involving hypertrophy of the buccinator muscle or masseter muscle can cause temporary stenosis of the salivary duct.

Surgical Procedure

A sialolith can be removed from the peripheral segment of the parotid duct by inserting a probe into the duct and incising the duct along the length of the probe. Sialoliths that are located more deeply should only be diagnosed and treated by a specialist.

660   Sialolith in the parotid duct
This 31-year-old woman had been suffering recurrent swelling at the angle of the mandible, with pain in the region of the ear. These symptoms occurred mainly during eating. Extraoral inspection revealed a relatively dense, pressure-sensitive swelling in the area of the parotid gland on the right side.

Right: The papilla at Stensen's duct is erythematous, palpation is painful, and only a few drops of saliva can be massaged out. The saliva is initially slightly cloudy.

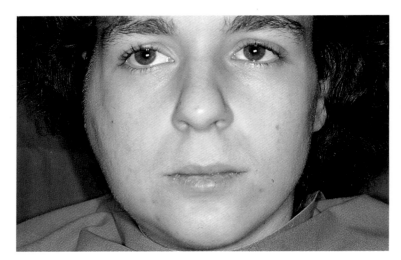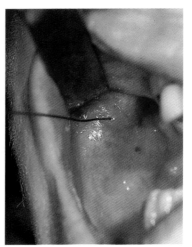

**661   Surgical procedure—
ductal ligation**
Before any further probing of the duct, a ligature is placed distal to the palpable sialolith. The mucosa is then incised until contact with the stone is made.

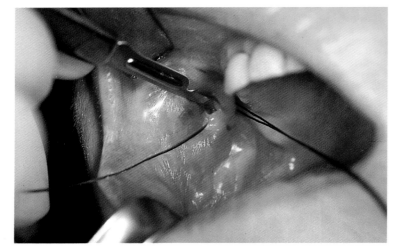

662   Sialolith removal and postoperative care
A forceps can be used to remove the sialolith from the duct easily. The incision is quite short, and healing is left to occur spontaneously. The patient is advised to use lemon-flavored chewing gum to maintain the patency of the orifice.

Right: The small incision wound, held open so that the saliva flow can be observed.

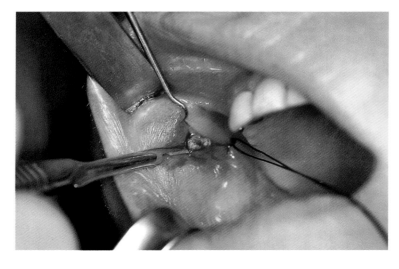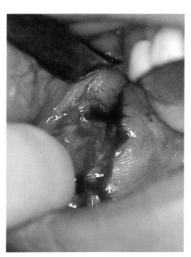

Tumors

Definition

A tumor is a neoplasm—a mass of new tissue growing independently of its surrounding structures, and which has no physiological purpose.

Pathology and Diagnosis

Recognition of a tumor disorder, and differentiation between tumor and common inflammatory processes, requires a thorough medical history and a careful clinical examination. If any doubts persist, a specialist should be consulted (Mittermeier et al. 1980, Schroeder 1991, Shafer et al. 1974, Van der Waal 1993).

Diagnostic Table

	Benign	Malignant
Medical history		
—Pain	Yes/No	No
—Period of observation	Long	Short
—Weight Loss	No	Possible
Clinical findings		
—Demarcated swelling	Yes	No
—Mobile swelling	Yes	No
—Mobile surface	Yes	No
—Intact surface	Yes	No
—Regional lymph nodes	None	Possible

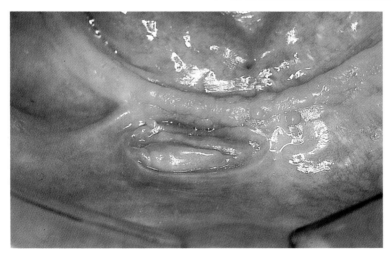

663 Benign tumor
Benign alterations of this type usually have a clear etiology, and are well demarcated. The ulceration is painful, and application of topical measures is effective. This painful ulceration in the mandibular vestibulum is well demarcated, and the borders can be palpated. The etiology involved trauma from the denture base. After shortening of the base, the lesion healed within ten days.

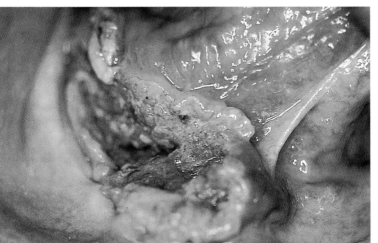

664 Malignant tumor
Malignant lesions often have no recognizable etiological factors, and are usually poorly demarcated. The ulceration is painless, and local application of therapeutic measures is ineffective. The sublingual area here shows a lesion that the patient had noticed one month previously and had treated with topical iodine. The lesion was painless, poorly demarcated from surrounding structures, and had a verrucous ulceration pattern.

Surgical Treatment

Small, benign tumors are removed in toto whenever possible. In most cases, this procedure is carried out as an excision or extirpation biopsy. The removal of benign tumors may justify localized nerve damage, with possible attendant disturbance of sensitivity or motor function. In the case of extensive lesions of the oral mucosa, only a partial biopsy is usually harvested (p. 254).

Patients who have undergone biopsy should be placed on a regular recall schedule. If the histopathological evaluation shows that the lesion is, in fact, benign, additional follow-up visits can be canceled if no recurrence is seen within one year.

Clinical Tip
Any oral lesion that raises a suspicion of tumor must be appropriately diagnosed. The diagnosis must be based upon a pathologist's evaluation of the biopsy. Questionable cases must be referred to a specialist, who should also carry out any subsequent treatment.

665 Excision biopsy—indication
Lesions that are smaller than 1 cm in diameter, and which raise no suspicion of malignancy, can be excised in toto.

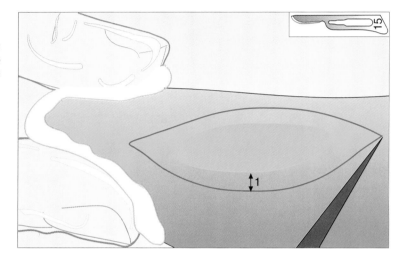

666 Partial biopsy—indication
Lesions that are larger than 1 cm in diameter and raise no suspicion of malignancy should be subjected to partial biopsy for further clarification. The excision should be performed as a wedge procedure extending from the center of the lesion to the bordering healthy tissue. If there is any suspicion of malignancy, further evaluation should be referred to a specialist.

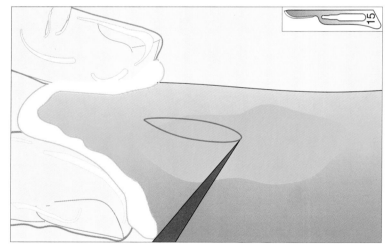

Anesthesia

If possible, do not infiltrate near the excision site. The anesthetic solution will permeate the tissue, which can lead to difficulty in histological interpretation due to artifacts.

Surgical Procedure

Tissue removal should be carried out using a scalpel or scissors. Using electrosurgery or laser surgery can burn the tissue margin and create artifacts.

The clinical report sent with the biopsy to the pathology laboratory should include:
—Patient data, age and sex.
—Relevant medical history, including clinical symptoms and duration of the lesion.
—Specific clinical observations: symptoms, peripheral reactions, extent, tissue surface characteristics, mobility, location.
—Details of the radiographic appearance (include radiographs with the submitted specimen).
—Differential diagnosis.
—Specific questions, e.g., type of epithelium, degree of dysplasia.

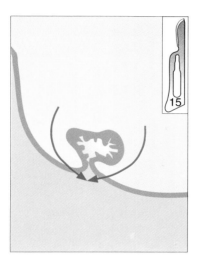
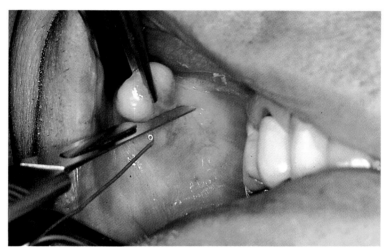

667 Excision of a pedunculated fibroma
After administration of block anesthesia in the affected region, the fibroma is grasped with a surgical forceps and severed at its base with a circular incision. Shown here is a probe that has been inserted into the duct of the parotid gland; this provides a visual cue to avoid damage to the duct.

Left: Excision at the base of an exophytic tissue proliferation.

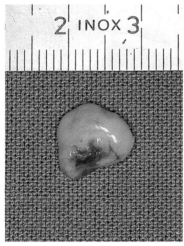
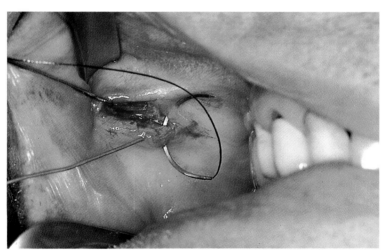

668 Wound treatment
The relatively broad tissue wound is closed using interrupted sutures.

Left: This tissue biopsy is sent in toto for histopathological examination.

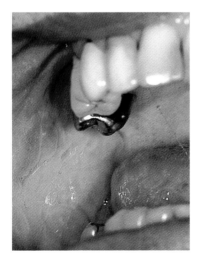
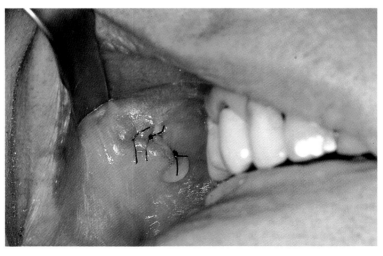

669 Clinical course and completion of treatment
Sutures can be removed one week postoperatively. Note the free flow of saliva from the duct.

Left: Clinical view after the surgical procedure.

670 Leukoplakia on the lateral lingual border

Recurrent leukoplakia was detected 6 months later.

Right: In this 62-year-old woman, a smoker, verrucous leukoplakia had been observed on the right lateral border of the tongue four years previously. The pathology report at that time indicated hyperplasia with hyperkeratosis of the oral mucosa, with severe dysplasia of the epithelium, and carcinoma in situ. The patient was a cigarette smoker.

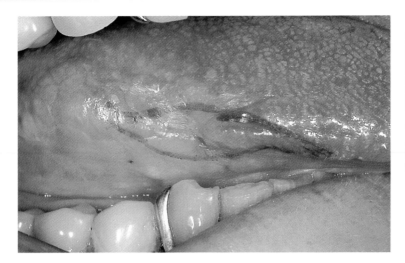

671 Excision

After anesthesia of the lingual nerve on the right side and infiltration into the distal border of the tongue, the lesion is excised as a wedge biopsy from the border of the tongue.

Right: The excisional biopsy was approximately 2 cm in extent.

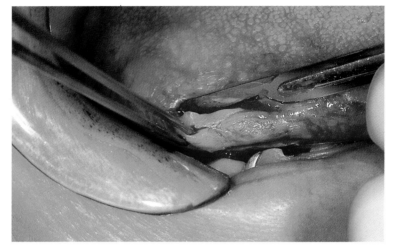
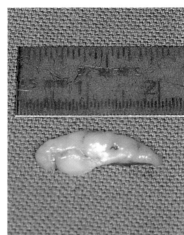

672 Wound treatment

Clinical view immediately after the excision biopsy.

Right: Interrupted sutures are used to close the elliptical wound after slight undermining of the wound margins.

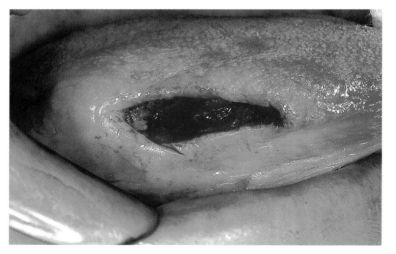
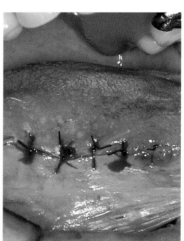

673 Clinical course

Follow-up with this patient was carried out every six months. This clinical photograph shows the situation one year after the last excision. At this point, the patient had stopped smoking.

Right: The histological examination shows moderate epithelial dysplasia.

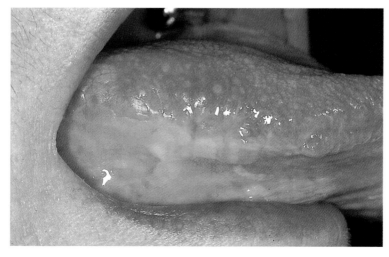
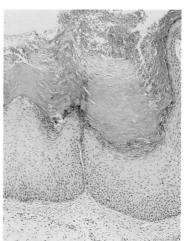

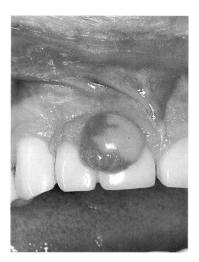

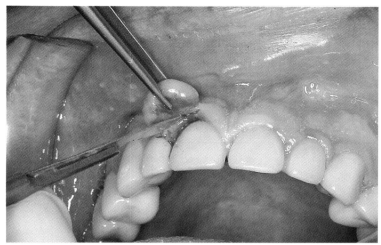

674 Gingival epulis
The immediate clinical impression is one of pedunculated, hyperplastic tissue proliferation that can be deflected without resistance away from the tooth surface.

Left: This 58-year-old man presented with a growth on the marginal gingiva that had slowly increased in size. Clinical inspection revealed a pedunculated, smooth, firm growth emanating from the gingival margin. Radiographic examination did not show any osseous lesions in the area.

(S)

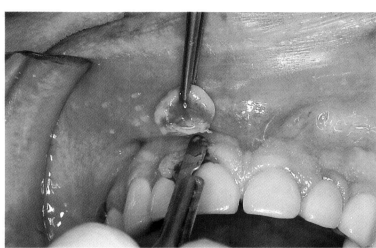

675 Excision
This simple epulis was excised at its base using a scalpel, without altering the gingival morphology in any way.

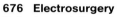

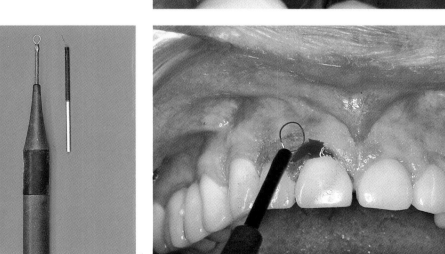

676 Electrosurgery
Delicate modeling at the gingival margin is carried out using an electrosurgical loop.

Left: The operating end of the electrotome allows delicate soft-tissue sculpturing using a loop or a fine, needle-like electrosurgical tip.

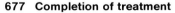

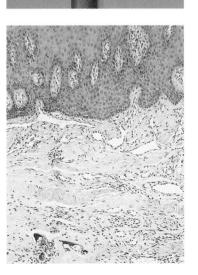

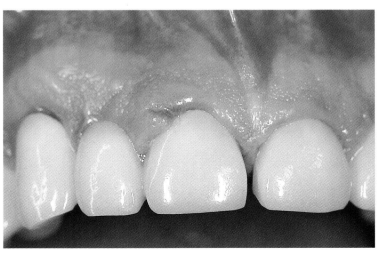

677 Completion of treatment
The follow-up appointment two years postoperatively shows no evidence of recurrence, although there is some minimal scar tissue.

Left: The histopathological examination shows a normal mucosal covering over a fibrous tumor formation without any signs of malignancy: a typical benign gingival epulis (fibroma).

Fibroma of the Cheek

These lesions typically appear as spherical, pedunculated, or broadly based firm growths with an intact, sometimes hyperkeratotic surface. The development of these lesions can often be traced back to earlier trauma. Fibromas of the cheek are usually incidental findings, since they do not cause any clinical symptoms.

Excision is carried out by means of an elliptical incision at the base of the lesion, followed by separation from the substrate using scissors. The resultant wound is closed with interrupted sutures.

Hemangioma of the Lip

A typical hemangioma consists of either an accumulation of vascular elements, or distension of multiple vascular elements. A distinction is made between capillary and cavernous hemangiomas. These lesions can be observed in patients of any age, and in both sexes. The lesions usually protrude beyond the surface. The most commonly affected site is the lip. Hemangiomas that are visible at birth are described as vascular nevi. In these cases, similar manifestations will be observed on the skin at numerous locations on the body. Expansive cavernous hemangiomas can lead to life-threatening

678 Labial hemangioma
This 28-year-old man had bitten his lip many years previously. Since that incident, a firm, bluish, compressible swelling of the internal surface of the lip had developed. The clinical picture corresponded to a small hemangioma. Treatment included total excision of the blood vascular accumulation within the outlined region.

Right: Applying pressure to the lesion caused the color to disappear.

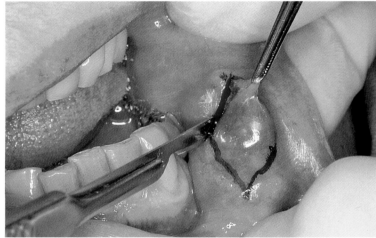
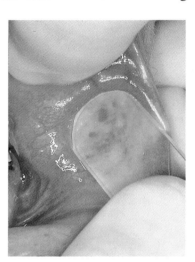

679 Excision
The primary incisions should be made in such a way that the bluish lesion is not encroached on. The dental assistant should grasp and hold the lip with both hands, applying some pressure, which significantly reduces hemorrhage. After an incision through the mucosa, the vascular bundle is freed from its surrounding tissues using blunt scissors.

Right: The wound margins are slightly undermined.

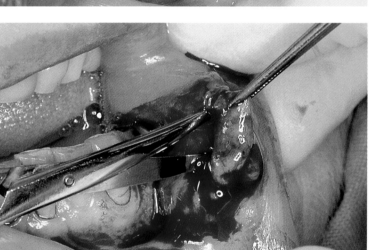
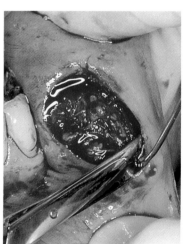

680 Wound treatment
The incision wound runs parallel to the lip, and is closed using interrupted sutures. The tissue that is excised should be sent for histopathological examination. If the lesion is found to consist of multiple thin vessels within loose connective-tissue stroma with an intact mucosal covering, the diagnosis is cavernous hemangioma.

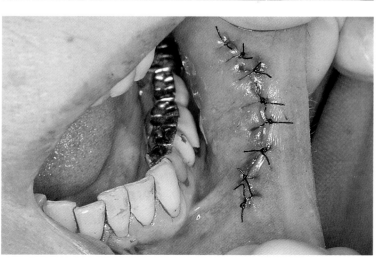

Excision from the Skin of the Face

hemorrhage. Evaluation and treatment should be carried out by a specialist.

Treatment. Small, capillary hemangiomas can be treated by excision, coagulation, or cryotherapy. Cryotherapy is only possible with superficial hemangiomas, since the high degree of vascularization counteracts the cold temperature.

Surgical procedures in the facial area must consider the factors that influence wound healing and scar formation. Primary incisions should correspond to the inherent tension lines of the skin. If an excision is anticipated, the plan should include plastic surgery for esthetic wound closure.

Wound closure is best accomplished with continuous sutures using fine, atraumatic suture material (5–0 to 6–0). Suture removal at 4–8 days. Scar formation is evaluated at the six-week check (Lauer et al. 1995).

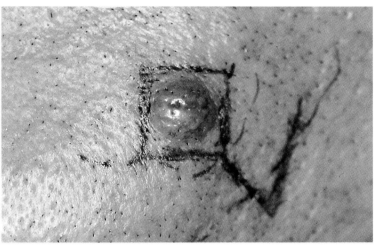

681 Skin excision
Any excisions that are carried out on the external skin surface of the face require appropriate planning to prevent unaesthetic scarring. In this 62-year-old man, the wart-like lesion had been frequently cut during routine daily shaving. The lesion was excised in toto, and the defect was covered with a small rhomboid sliding flap, as shown in this clinical photograph with ink markings.

Ⓐ

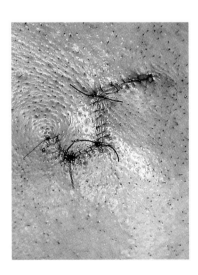

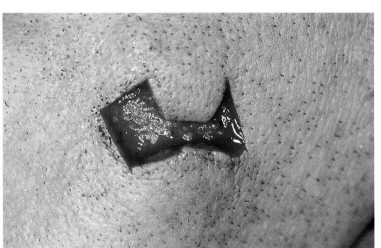

682 Sliding flap
An oblong excision and incisions for mobilizing the small caudal flap allow primary closure of the defect.

Left: The wound was closed using interrupted sutures at the angles and a continuous cosmetic suture along the wound margins, using 5–0 suture material.

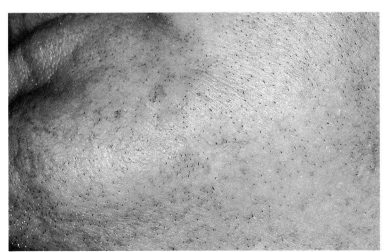

683 Clinical course
At the two-month postoperative check-up, the excision site was practically invisible.

Notes on Biopsy

Soft-Tissue Biopsy

Indelible marks should be made on the tissue surface to indicate the primary incisions, and the excision must follow these marks so that the borders of the biopsy can be continuously monitored during the surgical procedure. The excision should be deep enough to include the adjacent uninvolved tissue layer.

The biopsy is immersed in formalin in preparation for histopathological evaluation. Immunohistological examination can only be carried out on fresh biopsy specimens that are transported to the laboratory in a saline-saturated carrier substance (e.g., wrapped in a saline-soaked gauze square in a Petri dish).

Any special procedures should be discussed in advance with the pathologist.

The proper harvesting of a soft-tissue biopsy demands a certain amount of experience, not least with regard to appropriate plastic surgery to cover the biopsy site. In most cases, the wound can be successfully closed by placing several sutures, and this also serves to stop any bleeding. If the adjacent tissue is spongy and direct suturing might tear the tissue, a Vaseline-coated gauze square can be sutured into place in the "tie-over" technique, with the sutures placed in healthy tissue. Biopsy excisions of gingiva should be oval in shape, and vertical relative to the gingival margin, or they can be wedge-shaped, with the base at the neck of the tooth. This makes it possible to free up completely the adjacent gingival segment unilaterally or bilaterally, using a curtain procedure to cover the defect with secure suturing. If a biopsy is needed in the region of the mental nerve at its exit site from the foramen, it should be taken near to the gingiva whenever possible, to reduce the danger of nerve damage; the same principle applies to biopsies near the orifice of the duct of the parotid gland.

We have found that round dermatological tissue punches are useful for small biopsies of the oral mucosa. The round defect can be easily closed with sutures.

In the case of large excisional biopsies on the palate, where bone is exposed and there is a danger of hemorrhage from the palatine artery, we recommend the use of a surgical stent. An alternative to using a stent is to fix a piece of iodoform–Vaseline gauze, sutured firmly to the adjacent teeth.

Bone Biopsy

The basic surgical principles for harvesting a biopsy from bone are the same as those that apply to soft-tissue biopsy. The biopsy specimen should always include healthy as well as diseased tissue segments. Access to the bone is normally achieved by reflecting a soft-tissue flap, which has to provide adequate visual access as well as allowing wound closure over an intact osseous substrate.

Harvesting of a bone biopsy is usually accomplished using a cylindrical burr. The biopsy specimen must not be subjected to excessive mechanical or thermal forces, to prevent artifacts. It is therefore necessary to provide adequate cooling, and the handpiece must be used at a low speed. The overlying soft tissues are usually not of diagnostic significance, and therefore need not be excised. A specialist should be called in for situations in which bone biopsies have to be harvested in anatomically critical situations (especially in the horizontal ramus of the mandible), or if the dentist is inexperienced in the area of bone pathology. If there is even the slightest radiographic suspicion of a vascular anomaly, osseous biopsy can only be performed in a well-equipped surgical arena. Endosteal hemangioma can lead to extremely severe, even life-threatening hemorrhage, which is extremely difficult to stop.

Evaluation of the Pathology Report

If the findings presented in the pathology report do not appear to match the clinically suspected diagnosis, a discussion between the dentist and pathologist is appropriate. The pathologist may wish to consult a specialist in the particular area of concern. If the pathologist's report does not provide sufficient clarification, a second biopsy may be necessary. If doubt persists, treatment must follow the clinical diagnosis, with careful follow-up.

The differential diagnosis of many fibro-osseous and cemental lesions in the jaw region is complex and difficult.

If the osseous lesion is extensive, it may be advisable to harvest several biopsies to prevent a situation in which the inhomogeneity of the lesion leads the pathologist to an incorrect diagnosis because one tissue component predominates in a single biopsy.

Plastic Surgery Procedures in Soft Tissue and Bone

Definition

Plastic surgery procedures are designed to correct the quantity or quality of tissues, or both. These procedures mainly involve preprosthetic surgery, intended to improve conditions for dental reconstructions, or make these possible.

Functional or aesthetic corrections are also possible. These include procedures intended to allow the insertion of dental implants, involving soft-tissue surgery, osseous surgery, and combinations of the two (Obwegeser 1987).

Corrective Soft-Tissue Procedures

Given the contemporary demand for a good appearance in the facial region, including the oral cavity, there is a strong demand for plastic surgical repair of defects, scar formation, and other disfiguring alterations of the skin and mucosa. Plastic surgeons have developed many new methods for treating these tissue anomalies and abnormalities.

The classical methods of plastic surgery in soft tissues include sliding flaps, rotated flaps, VY-plasty, Z-plasty, and free split-thickness or mucosal transplantation.

There are some very basic anatomical differences between skin and oral mucosa with regard to vascularity, extensibility, and scar formation. The oral mucosa has greater blood circulation and is more extensible than skin, and its tendency for scar formation is less. Keloid formation virtually never occurs on the oral mucosa. On the other hand, in comparison with the functional cheek mucosa, the gingiva and the mucosa of the palate are hardly extensible at all, and are always reflected in connection with the periosteum.

Criteria for Determining the Type of Surgical Procedure

Selecting the method of choice for soft-tissue corrections depends on the following factors:
—The extent of the defect and the distance from usable adjacent tissues.
—The type of tissue required to effect the correction, both functionally and aesthetically.
—Previous therapeutic measures that might influence the course of healing, e.g., radiotherapy.
—Anatomical structures that have to be protected from injury, e.g., nerves and blood vessels.
—Priorities involved in closing a defect, or qualitative correction of soft tissue with regard to function or appearance.

Preprosthetic Surgery

In 1965, Obwegeser published a comprehensive review of the indications for the various surgical procedures for soft-tissue reconstruction in the vestibulum and the floor of the mouth. It is up to the prosthodontist to determine whether surgical procedures can be used to improve the retention for a denture. An indication for surgical corrections in an edentulous arch should be established as early as possible, since relatively minor operations can then achieve better surgical results. It is up to the surgeon to decide which surgical procedure to use to achieve the goal set forth by the prosthodontist. Relatively standardized surgical procedures are used to create a sufficiently deep vestibulum or floor of the mouth. The difficulty lies in creating an immobile epithelial layer for the prosthesis bed. There are three methods for soft-tissue coverage:
—Using mucosa harvested from an adjacent site to cover wound surfaces on the soft tissues or the periosteum.
—Achieving an epithelial covering by allowing the wound surface to heal by secondary epithelialization.
—Covering the wound surface with a free skin transplant.

Healthy vestibular mucosa is qualitatively the best epithelial covering. It is resilient, naturally moist, and thanks to its elasticity it adapts well to the denture base.

Mucosa established after secondary epithelialization is of somewhat poorer quality. It lacks resilience and suppleness. Transplanted skin has the poorest characteristics. It is dry, and does not adapt well to the denture base because it lacks suppleness. Nevertheless, in terms of its load-bearing capacity, transplanted skin is superior to all types of mucosa.

When choosing a surgical procedure, the different mechanisms of denture stabilization in the maxilla (adhesion) and in the mandible (retention) have to be considered. For this reason, a mucosal covering (primary or secondary) is usually the method of choice in the maxilla, while skin transplants may be preferable for the mandible.

The surgical procedures presented in this chapter represent only those procedures for mucosal covering that can be carried out under local anesthesia on an outpatient basis.

Frena

Labial, buccal, and lingual frena usually have to be treated surgically if they are causing functional or esthetic problems. Buccal frena that insert high on the ridge sometimes prevent sufficient extension of the denture border or, in dentulous patients, may aggravate gingival recession. If gingival recession poses a significant clinical problem, a free gingival graft from the palate or a connective-tissue graft can be used to cover the exposed root surface (Schädle and Matter-Grütter 1993, Strub and Kopp 1980).

There are some syndromes involving multiple frenum formation in the oral cavity (e.g., the oral-facial-digital syndrome). The presence and location of frena is genetically determined, but may also occur later in life—for example, in cases of progressive systemic sclerosis (scleroderma).

684 Type of frena
Left: Typical labial frenum radiating into the attached gingiva between the two central incisors, which are separated by a diastema.

Center: This buccal frenum is attached high on the ridge in the edentulous mandible.

Right: Exceptionally short lingual frenum; this is actually a case of lingual ankylosis.

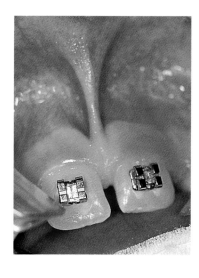
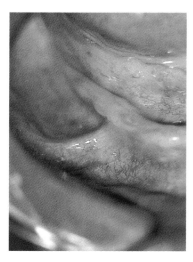
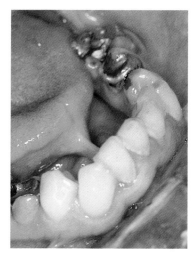

Maxillary Labial Frenum

The midline labial frenum is a genetically determined anatomical structure which varies in appearance from person to person. A thick, firm labial frenum coursing from the facial surface between the central incisors toward the palatal aspect can even cause a diastema.

Indication

If the interdental papilla between the central incisors blanches when the lip is elevated, it is an indication that the frenum should be surgically remodeled.

Complete removal of the labial frenum should be considered if the incisal edges of the central incisors is lateral to the connective tissue fibers. Prophylactic removal of the labial frenum during the deciduous dentition phase is not indicated (Stöckli and Ben Zur 1994), because anatomical changes during the mixed dentition phase in the anterior segment of the maxilla usually takes care of the situation spontaneously.

Documentation

Radiographs can identify other causes of divergent teeth (e.g., a mesiodens or a cyst).

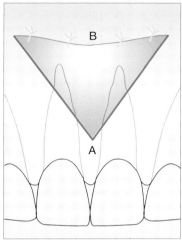
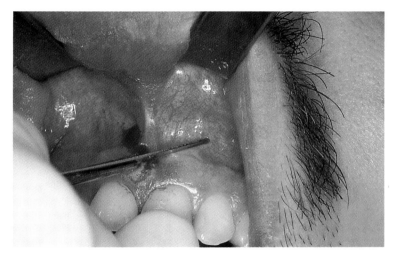

685 Correction of the labial frenum using local vestibuloplasty
The labial frenum in this 22-year-old man is severed broadly at its base in the vestibulum.

Left: The surgical principle: make the incision vertically, and suture laterally. This procedure usually does not lead to complete elimination of the functional disturbance caused by the frenum. The mucosa is released at **A**, and sutured to the periosteum at **B**.

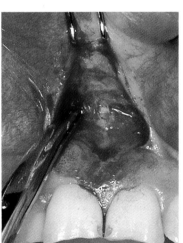
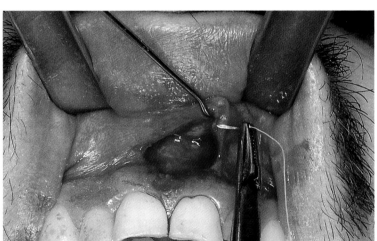

686 Suturing the mucosa
Several resorbable sutures are placed to attach the reflected mucosa to the periosteum.

Left: Blunt scissors can be used to release the mucosa in an apical direction.

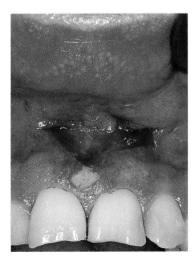
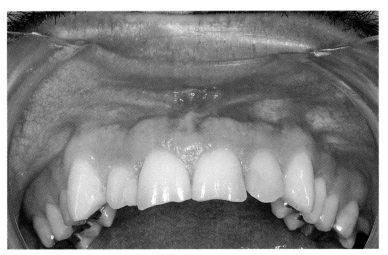

687 Clinical course
The wound surfaces are allowed to heal by secondary epithelialization. A follow-up appointment one year postsurgically reveals a deep, flat vestibulum, with no sign of a residual frenum.

Left: Clinical photograph taken one week postoperatively shows the wound surface covered with a fibrin clot.

Surgical Procedure

If it is found that the labial frenum has to be treated surgically, the goal should be complete excision down to the osseous substrate. The connective-tissue fibers between the anterior teeth must be excised using a wedge procedure from the facial toward the incisive papillae. The firm soft tissues embedded deeply between the teeth must be carefully reflected. During this procedure, the upper lip is reflected cranially. This provides good visualization of the frenum, and scissors or a scalpel can be used in the vestibule to sever the frenum.

Basically, there are two possible methods of correction: *Primary closure.* The rhomboid defect is closed bilaterally and at the vertical extent of the mucosa using interrupted sutures. The small defect that remains can be left to secondary healing.
Secondary epithelialization. Surgical preparation is performed epiperiosteally, as in a vestibuloplasty (p. 292). The exposed surface of the periosteum can be left for secondary epithelialization. This will preclude any shortening or flattening of the vestibulum (p. 257).

688 Diastema
In this 8-year-old girl, the firm, thick labial frenum seems to be maintaining the diastema between the maxillary permanent central incisors, due to its fibrous extent.

Right: The labial frenum is actually pulling the lip itself between the central incisors.

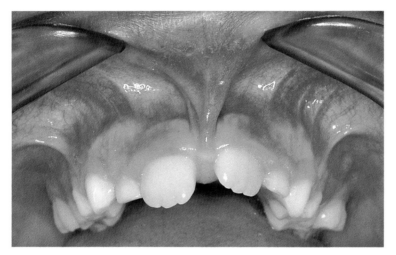
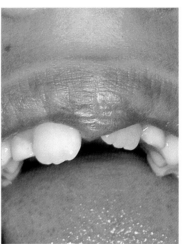

689 Primary incision
A broad-based, V-shaped primary incision of the frenum is made in the vestibulum to free up the frenum.

Right: The firm, fibrous tissue is excised as a wedge.

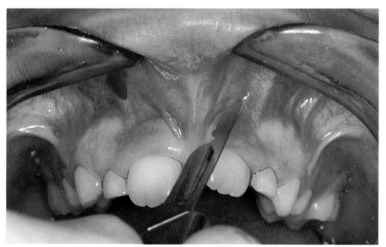
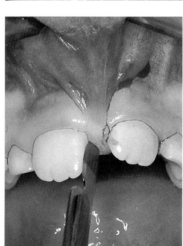

690 Interdental excision
Removal of the fibrous connective tissue between the teeth has to extend far palatally.

Right: Mobilization and excision of the frenum, extending from the vestibule toward the palatal aspect above the periosteum.

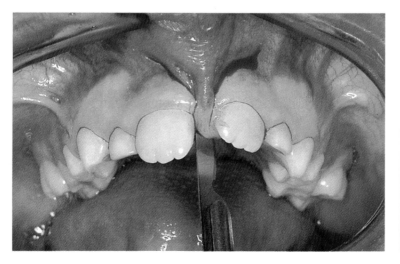
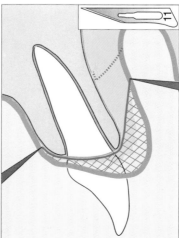

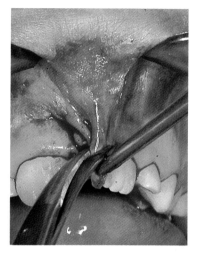
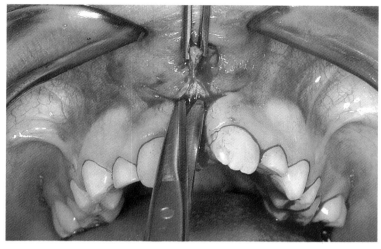

691 Excising the connective-tissue bundle
The epithelial and connective-tissue elements of the frenum are mobilized in an apical direction from the vestibular approach. Blunt scissors are indicated for this procedure.

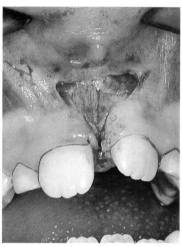
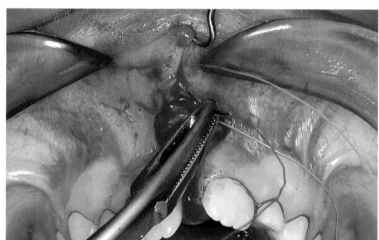

692 Suturing the mucosa
Resorbable sutures are used to attach the flap far apically to the periosteum.

Left: The tension applied to the lip reflects the former labial frenum in an apical direction.

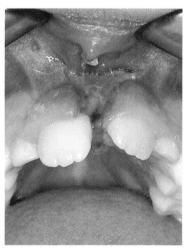
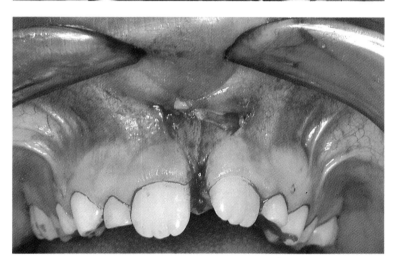

693 Clinical course
The wound surface presents as a triangle. This area is left to secondary reepithelialization.

Left: Clinical picture taken one week postsurgically. The surface of the periosteum is covered with a fibrin clot.

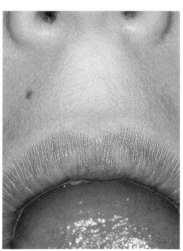
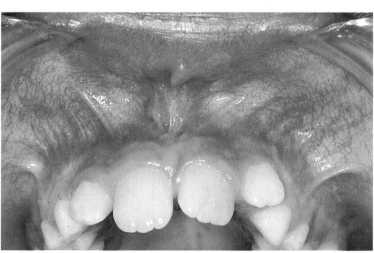

694 Completion of treatment
The clinical check-up one year postsurgically showed spontaneous closure of the diastema between the central incisors.

Left: The patient's lip contour is normal (compare Fig. 688).

Mandibular Labial Frenum

A firm labial frenum in the mandible seldom causes any difficulty. Nevertheless, in adults who have lost marginal gingival tissues due to periodontal disease, the insertion of the frenal connective-tissue fibers near to the gingival margin can serve to accelerate gingival recession. In such cases, surgical correction of the soft-tissue configuration is indicated. The excision is carried out by means of two lateral, slightly arcuate incisions through the mobile mucosa, and subsequent caudal, epiperiosteal preparation.

The narrow band of keratinized gingiva should be preserved. The mobilized mucosal flap is sutured to the periosteum using several resorbable sutures in the vestibulum. The open wound surface is left to secondary epithelialization. A decision must be made as to the possible indication for using a free mucosal transplant from the palate to ensure the desired surgical result (see the section on "Improving Mucosal Quality," p. 268).

695 Mandibular labial frenum
The periodontal pockets in the mandibular anterior segment were treated in this 67-year-old woman. In order to prevent further recession of the gingiva, the dentist suggested removal of the labial frenum.

Right: The surgical principle: epiperiosteal preparation and secondary epithelialization by transposing the mucosa from position **A** to position **B**.

Ⓢ

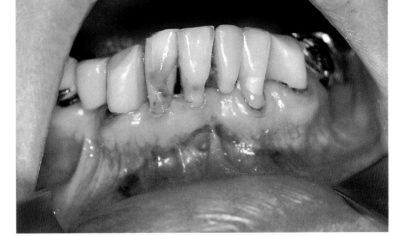
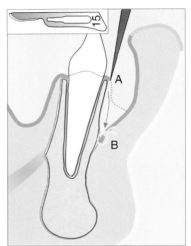

696 Primary incision
The frenum is freed at its base by means of an arcuate incision through the mucosa.

Right: The scalpel blade severs the mucosa, but the periosteum remains intact.

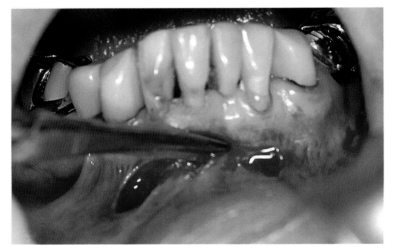
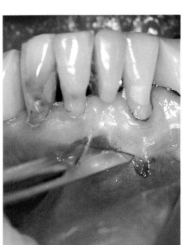

697 Epiperiosteal preparation
Using blunt scissors, the mucosa, with its submucosal tissues and muscle insertions, is separated from the periosteum.

Right: Applying tension to the mucosa using wound hooks simplifies the epiperiosteal preparation.

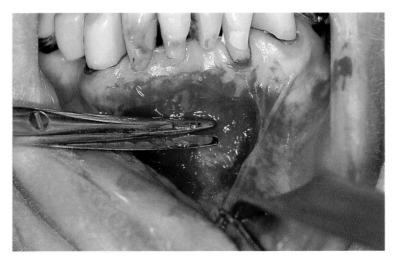
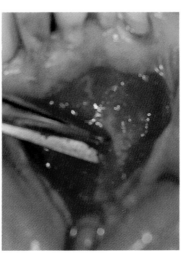

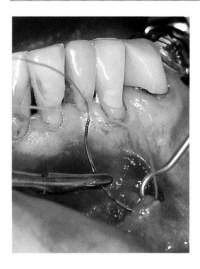

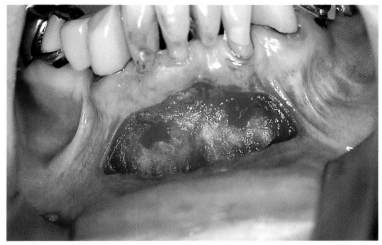

698 Fixation of the mucosa
The tissue retractor is a useful instrument for manipulating mucosa with the least amount of trauma.

Left: The mucosa is sutured to the periosteum apically with interrupted, resorbable sutures.

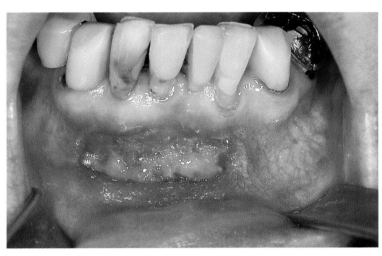

699 Clinical course
The flap must be sutured without tension. The exposed wound surface is allowed to reepithelialize.

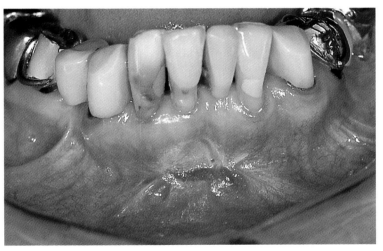

700 Secondary epithelialization
The wound is completely reepithelialized three weeks after the operation.

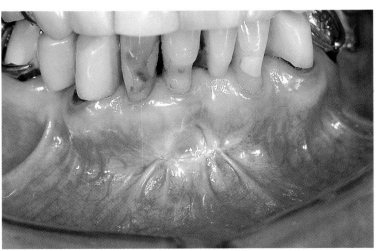

701 Completion of treatment
Six months postsurgically, the clinical situation is stable, and there is no evidence of recurrence. Slight scar formation cannot be avoided. An alternative surgical procedure would involve local epiperiosteal displacement of the mucosa, and coverage with a free gingival graft from the palate. The disadvantage of that approach is that two wounds are created.

Lingual Frenum

Indication

Immobilization of the tongue due to a severely shortened lingual frenum can cause difficulties even in the first weeks of life, by compromising an effective sucking reaction. This type of severe lingual ankylosis is often treated soon after birth simply by severing the frena with scissors. If the mobility of the tongue continues to be compromised by a short, firm lingual frenum, difficulties with speech and possibly even increased susceptibility to caries in the molar region may ensue, as natural self-cleansing in the posterior areas is inhibited. In the connective tissue fibers may protrude between the anterior teeth toward the vestibulum and cause a diastema. Damage to the periodontium on the lingual aspect of the anterior teeth is also possible. The lingual frenum may sometimes form a firm, tendon-like connection to the floor of the mouth, but can also be found as a connective tissue communication with the alveolar process. In patients with scleroderma, progressive shortening of the lingual frenum is seen.

702 Lingual frenum—excision from the tongue
In this 13-year-old girl, mobility of the tongue was limited by the short, firm lingual frenum.

Right: When she was asked to extend the tongue as far as she could, the tip of the tongue only reached the border of the lip.

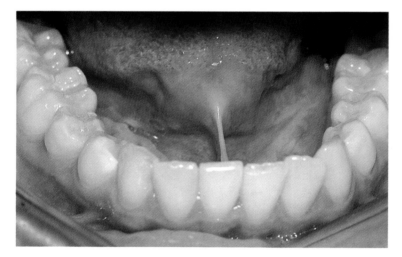
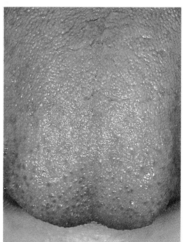

703 Primary incision
Mobility of the tongue is achieved by severing the lingual frenum near its connection to the base of the tongue. A simple scissors cut is sufficient.

Right: The surgical principle: separating the lingual frenum from the base of the tongue.

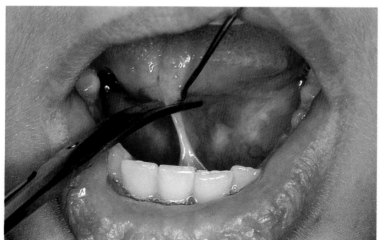
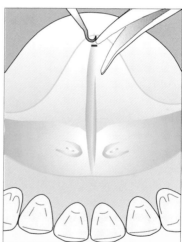

704 Suture placement
The surgical defect has a rhomboid outline.

Right: Interrupted sutures are placed to close the defect longitudinally.

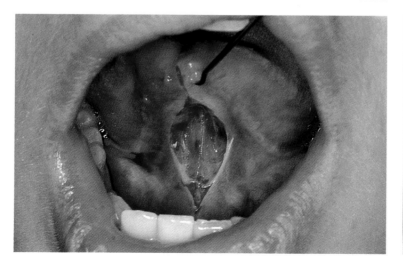
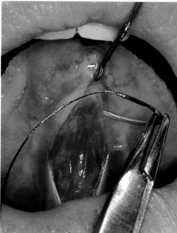

Surgical Procedure

The surgical procedure varies depending on the clinical situation. The simplest method of increasing tongue mobility is to sever the lingual frenum horizontally and place sutures in the midline. This procedure also minimizes the danger of damaging important adjacent structures. The surgical approach is dictated by the configuration and extent of the lingual frenum.

Lingual Frenum Inserting into the Floor of the Mouth

The connective tissue band is severed along the ventral surface of the tongue; suture in the midline.

Frenum Inserting at the Alveolar Process

The frenum is severed transversely at the insertion on the alveolar process and into the soft tissues of the floor of the mouth. Special care must be taken not to damage the orifices of the submandibular duct at the sublingual carunculae. Any injury to these structures can lead to scar tissue formation and stasis of salivary flow. Before placing sutures, the mobility of the tongue should be checked. Wound closure is carried out with interrupted sutures arranged in a vertical line along the wound margins. If any defect persists on the alveolar process, it is left to secondary epithelialization.

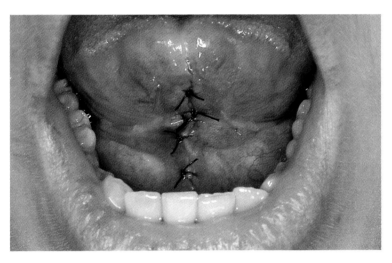

705 Wound closure
The mobility of the tongue is immediately improved.

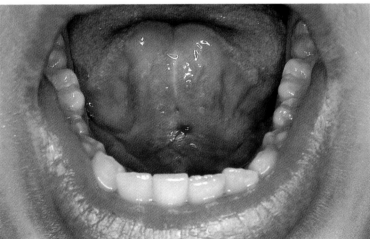

706 Clinical course
The sutures are removed one week after the operation. The patient now has no difficulty in lifting the tongue.

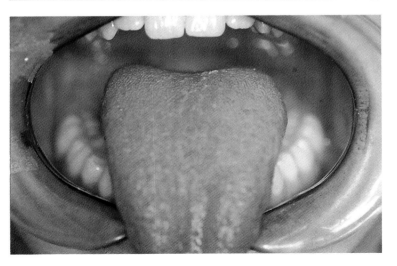

707 Completion of treatment
The follow-up appointment one month postoperatively shows normal tongue mobility.

Free Mucosal Transplant for Gingival Replacement

The quality, stratification, and keratinization of the mucosal surface is largely dependent on the characteristics of the subjacent connective-tissue components. This is an important consideration in choosing mucosa for transplantation. The thickness of the transplant is also important for the success of the procedure; transplanted tissue must not exceed 1 mm in thickness.

Indication

Free gingival grafts are primarily used in periodontal surgery to treat local areas of recession, as well as areas in which attached gingiva is absent. Gingival transplants can also be used to treat undesirable areas of mobile mucosa or buccal frena.

Repairing defects on the gingiva can be readily accomplished using well-keratinized mucosa from the posterior area of the hard palate. The anterior palatal segments are less favorable because of the rugae, which persist after the healing process is complete.

708 Excision at the alveolar process
In this 10-year-old girl, the lingual frenum is attached high on the alveolar process. Lingual mobility is severely limited.

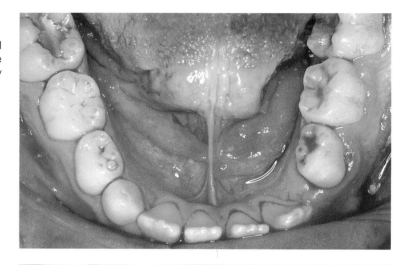

Ⓢ

709 Primary incision
The lingual frenum is severed at the base of the tongue using scissors, and then sutured vertically. A narrow defect may ensue on the alveolar process, but it can be left to secondary healing.

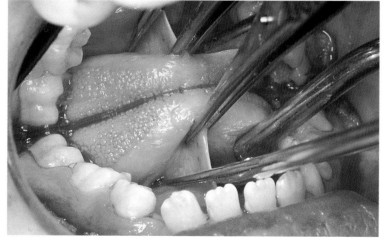
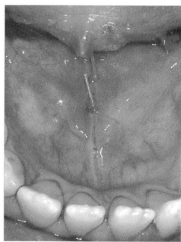

710 Clinical outcome
The follow-up clinical photograph six months postoperatively reveals free mobility of the tongue and normal topography of the anterior floor of the mouth.

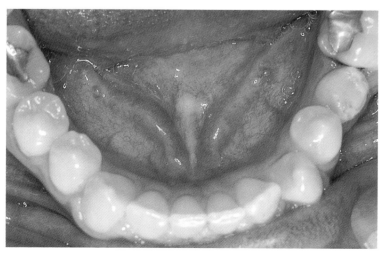

Surgical Procedure

The first step is to administer local anesthesia at the transplant bed. Bed preparation is precisely performed epiperiosteally. The mucosa is secured using resorbable sutures into the newly formed vestibulum. For harvesting the transplant tissue from the palate, anesthetic solution is infiltrated near the palatal foramen, and tissue is removed using a mucotome.

The transplant is applied with pressure to the exposed periosteum, and secured with interrupted sutures (4–0) at the corners. A surgical wound stent will prevent trauma to the surgical site from the tongue or a toothbrush. Oral rinsing with 0.2% chlorhexidine solution is used instead of normal toothbrushing at the surgical site. During the normal course of healing, the epithelial layer of the transplant will become necrotic, even though the subepithelial connective tissue is quickly revascularized. As early as two days after transplantation, the transplanted tissue is revascularized at the new site. Complete healing-in of the transplant can be expected in one week.

Epithelialization of the transplanted tissue develops from the adjacent tissues (Bernimoulin and Lange 1972, Mörmann et al. 1975), and takes approximately two more weeks.

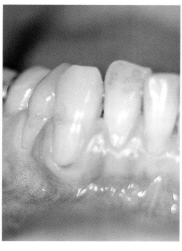
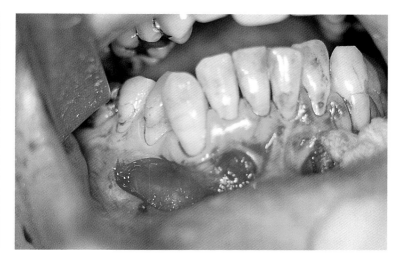

711 Free gingival graft
In this 44-year-old woman, progressive gingival recession was observed on tooth 43. A frenum attachment was located high on the attached gingiva. Because only a small amount of keratinized marginal gingiva remained, the treatment plan included a free gingival graft from the palate to the vestibulum near tooth 43 (*left*).

The mucosa near tooth 43 was reflected, and attached to the periosteum using resorbable sutures (*right*).

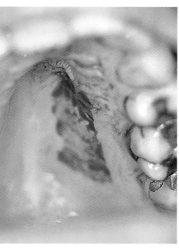
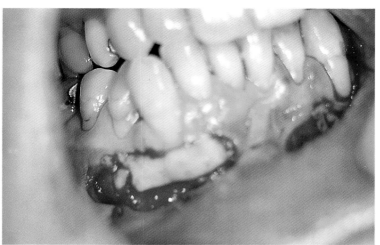

712 Tissue transplant— harvesting and placement
The free gingival graft can be secured by interrupted sutures at its margin or by placing a periodontal dressing (e.g., Peripac). The dressing is removed three days postsurgically and the sutures at one week.

Left: Using a mucotome, a strip of palatal mucosa approximately 0.5 cm thick is harvested for transplantation to the vestibular site near tooth 43, and pressed onto the periosteum.

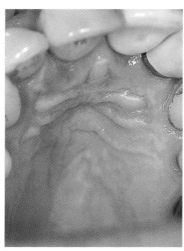
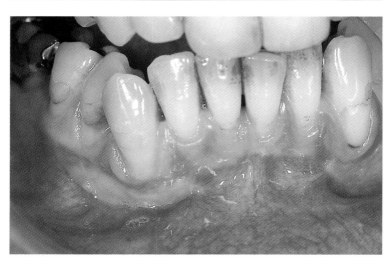

713 Clinical result
The follow-up appointment six months postoperatively shows much better gingival conditions near tooth 43.

Left: The site of transplant harvest on the palate has completely regenerated.

Gingiva–Connective-Tissue Transplant

The free gingival graft is revascularized from the underlying periosteum. It therefore requires a healthy, well-vascularized transplant recipient bed. If a gingival defect is located on or near a poorly vascularized or nonvascularized substrate—for example, over root cementum—other methods for coverage must be sought. One method is to use a sliding flap (curtain procedure). The method illustrated here is an alternative— the connective-tissue sandwich procedure. This method was first described by Langer (1985) for covering exposed root surfaces or gingival margin defects, using a combined gingiva–connective-tissue graft from the palate. This procedure takes advantage of the close contact between the transplanted tissue and the vital tissues of the recipient area.

Indication
In aesthetically critical areas, this method can be used to treat undesirable gingival recession or superficial soft-tissue defects.

714 Gingiva–connective-tissue graft: primary incision
This 33-year-old woman requested coverage of the gingival recession areas on teeth 33 and 34 because of cervical hypersensitivity. The plan involved a combination of gingival and connective-tissue procedures.

Right: The incisions required (*red*). First, an intrasulcal incision is made, beginning at the mesial papilla and extending distally. A separate incision is made in the vestibular mucosa mesial to tooth 33.

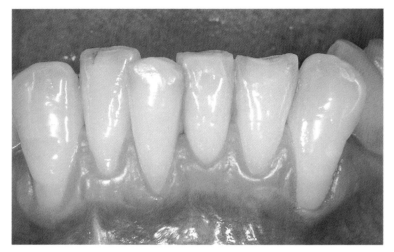
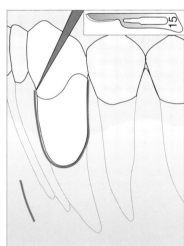

715 Recipient bed
A small elevator or a desmotome is used to free the sulcal gingiva from the tooth and bone surface, creating a "tunnel" contiguous with the vertical incision. The interdental papilla has to be undermined.

Right: Undermining and mobilization of the underlying mucosa.

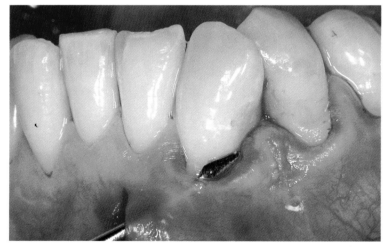
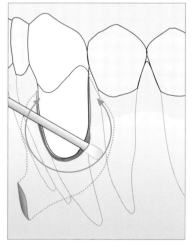

716 Positioning the graft
The width of the connective-tissue graft is adjusted according to the morphology of the sulcus, and the graft is then inserted via the vertical incision to a position subjacent to the oral mucosa. The graft is inserted coronally until the exposed root surface is completely covered by the attached gingiva of the graft.

Right: The epithelial surface of the graft is partially trimmed away.

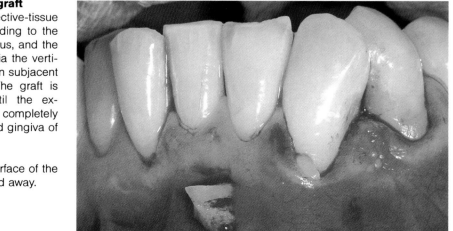
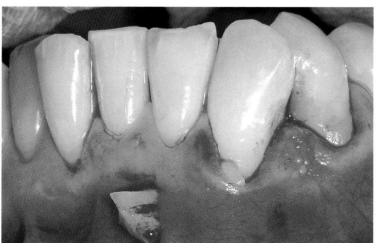

Surgical Procedure

Schädle and Matter-Grütter (1993) proposed a modification of the Langer method that avoids the disadvantage of a vertical incision in the gingiva. To create the connective-tissue graft sandwich, a vertical incision is placed in the mobile mucosa lateral to the defect, and the mucoperiosteum is mobilized by undermining it. Both adjacent gingival papillae are thus preserved, and need only be mobilized as necessary. The connective-tissue transplant is guided coronally through the incision. Fixation of the graft is not necessary. To prevent dehydration, the graft can be covered with a fibrin adhesive (Tissucol) or a tissue adhesive (Histoacryl). The vertical incision is closed with a single suture.

Oral hygiene during the postoperative period is maintained by rinsing with 0.2% chlorhexidine solution.

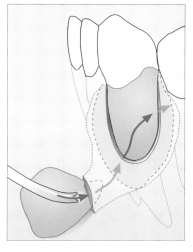

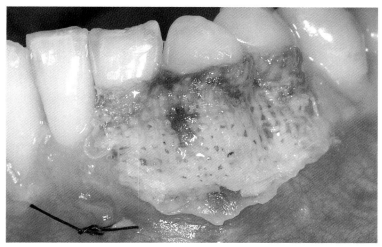

717 Tissue dressing
The grafted tissue is covered with a dressing of iodoform–Vaseline gauze and tissue adhesive (Histoacryl).

Left: Use of an instrument to insert the graft through the vertical incision and manipulate it coronally.

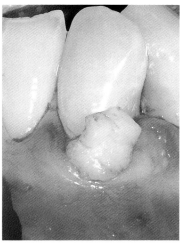

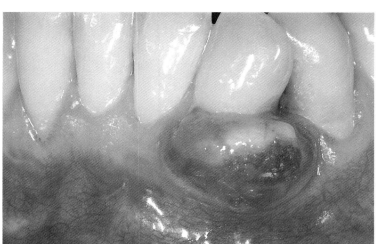

718 Clinical course
The dressing is removed five days postoperatively. After ten days, a vital, well-vascularized graft is present.

Left: Immediate postoperative situation. The graft is slightly over-extended to compensate for the expected shrinkage.

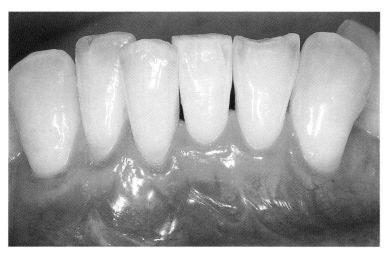

719 Final result
This late postoperative view shows that the areas of recession on teeth 33 and 34, both of which were treated using the procedures described above, have been significantly reduced. The patient can clean the area without difficulty, and the cervical hypersensitivity has disappeared.

Improving Mucosal Quality

Indications
—To eliminate infection-prone areas (candidiasis).
—To improve prosthodontic relationships.
—To increase the area of attached gingiva.
—To improve the appearance of soft tissue.

Surgical Procedure
Qualitative alterations of the oral mucosa can be treated by local modification, or by excision and replacement with new tissue. This goal can be achieved by secondary epithelialization on an intact periosteum over the alveolar process, as well as by submucosal preparation or free grafting (mucosal transplantations). The method selected depends on the extent of the surface to be treated, as well as the ultimate goals of the procedure in terms of soft-tissue quality. Broad papillary alterations, such as hypertrophic candidiasis, are treated with a combination of drug therapy and excision of the diseased mucosa. The electrosurgical loop is well indicated for this purpose. Hyperkeratosis can also be treated cryosurgically.

720 Palatal papillomatosis
This 51-year-old woman, who was a denture wearer, was bothered by the fibrous thickening in the palatal midline. The loose, redundant fibrous tissue had persisted even after correction of the prosthesis.

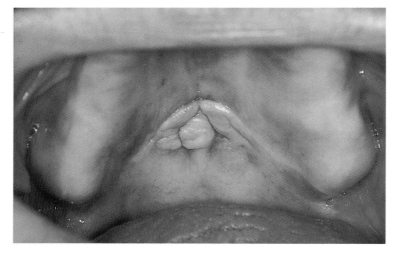

721 Excision using electrosurgery
The electrosurgical loop is used with light, modeling strokes to remove the fibroma. Hardly any bleeding occurs with this procedure. The periosteum remains intact.

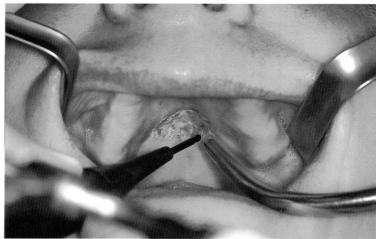

722 Secondary epithelialization
The palatal wound is left to heal by secondary intention. A palatal plate or surgical stent is not necessary.

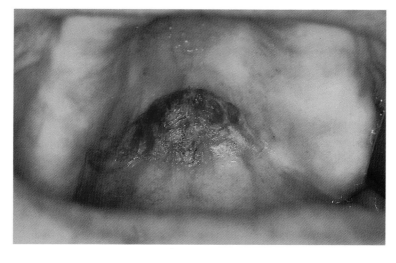

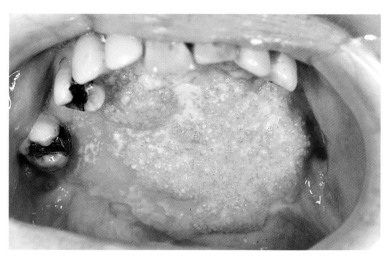

723 Papillomatosis of the palate with candidiasis

In this 60-year-old woman, the bone of the palate had been partially resected ten years previously, and the palatal mucosa had been reconstructed using a skin transplant. For the previous few months, the patient had been suffering from therapy-resistant candidiasis, which eventually led to papillary fibrosis of the entire palatal surface.

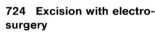

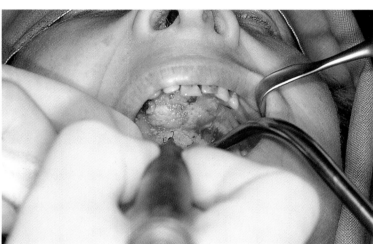

724 Excision with electrosurgery

Various electrosurgical tips are used to remove the papillary lesions layer by layer.

Left: The electrosurgical loop can be used to trim away virtually the entire palatal soft-tissue surface.

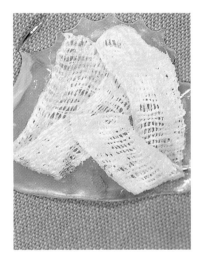
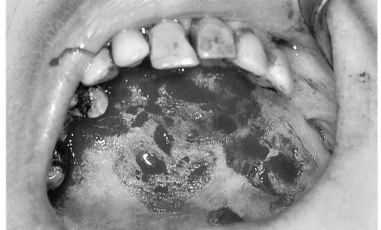

725 Surgical stent

Weeping hemorrhage can be managed by compression applied with iodoform–Vaseline gauze under a transparent surgical stent. The stent also protects the wound surface during meals.

Left: The transparent stent is covered with iodoform–Vaseline gauze; two simple wire clasps hold it in place.

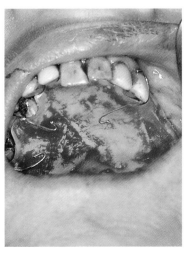
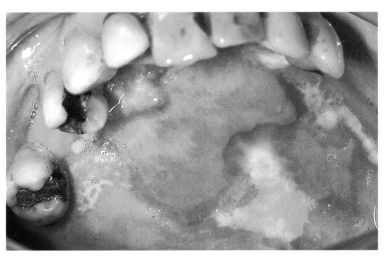

726 Follow-up treatment

The wound is checked and cleaned weekly. Three weeks postsurgically, the regenerative process is underway, and a delicate layer of epithelium is growing in from the margins onto the wound surfaces. Several areas are still showing papillary alterations, which will be dealt with surgically in later procedures.

Left: The transparent stent in situ.

Gingival Procedures Around Implants

Indication

The health of the soft tissue surrounding a dental implant is maintained by a cuff of keratinized gingiva; this can also prevent the formation of osseous defects (Schlegel et al. 1994). Careful oral hygiene can also prevent or minimize peri-implant inflammation (Marinello et al. 1993). In some cases, placement of implant abutments in mobile, nonkeratinized mucosa will be tolerated. Any corrections of the soft tissue required can be carried out subsequently.

Surgical Procedure

A free gingival graft is harvested from the lateral aspect of the hard palate. It should be approximately 10–12 mm wide. It is perforated, and then placed like a collar on the prepared surface of the periosteum around the implants. Buser (1987) proposed a two-phase procedure, in which the soft-tissue situation is improved by vestibuloplasty and coverage with a free gingival graft before placement of the dental implants.

727 Free gingival graft around dental implants
An epiperiosteal bed is prepared by removing the mucosa around the implants, before placing the free gingival graft.

Right: In this 68-year-old woman, two implants had been placed two years previously. The oral mucosa surrounding the implants was mobile. Peri-implantitis developed. A free gingival graft was used to improve the quality of the mucosa around the implants.

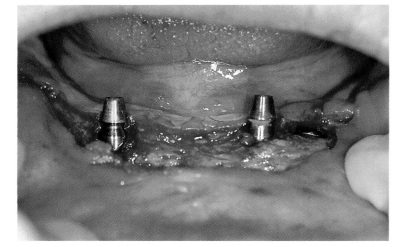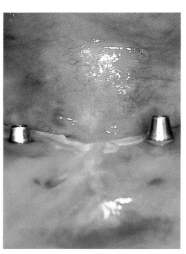

728 Graft placement
Two grafts, approximately 20×10 mm in extent, were harvested from the palate and placed in a collar-like fashion around the two implants.

Right: A mucosal punch was used to perforate the graft so that it could be positioned circumferentially around the implant posts.

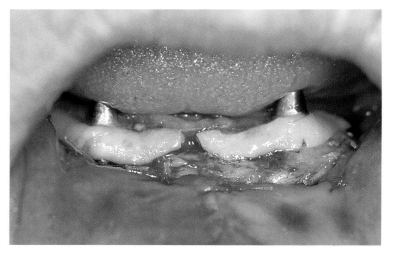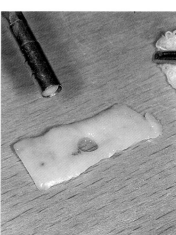

729 Clinical result
The follow-up appointment nine months postsurgically showed that the peri-implant tissue was largely free of irritation.

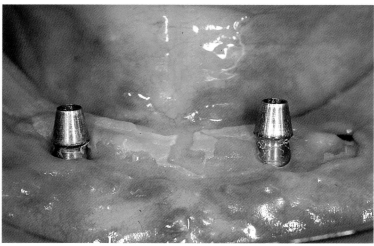

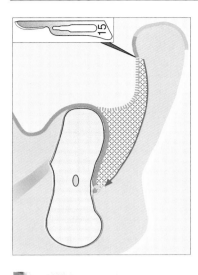

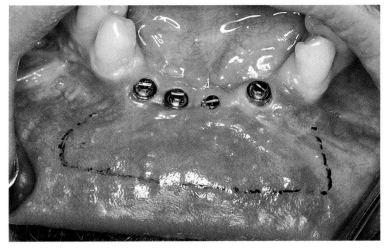

730 The Edlan procedure for mucosal correction

This 22-year-old woman had lost her mandibular anterior teeth in an accident. After osseous reconstruction using autologous bone, and placement of four implants, there was a complete lack of any vestibulum. This made it very difficult to seat a dental reconstruction.

Left: The surgical principle. The mucosa of the internal surface of the lower lip is surgically undermined, and remains attached at the alveolar ridge.

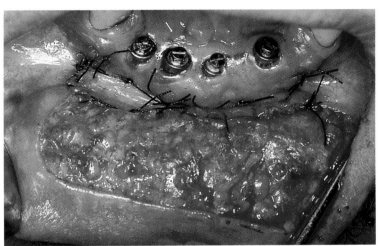

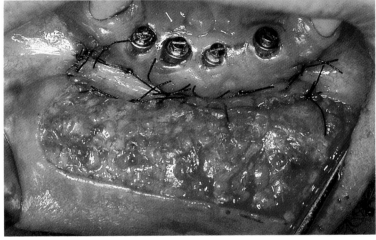

731 Surgical preparation

After a primary incision in the vestibulum, the mucosa is reflected submucosally and epiperiosteally. The submucosal tissue in the vestibulum is excised.

Left: The flap of mucosa, which remains attached at the alveolar ridge, is attached to the periosteum using several mattress sutures.

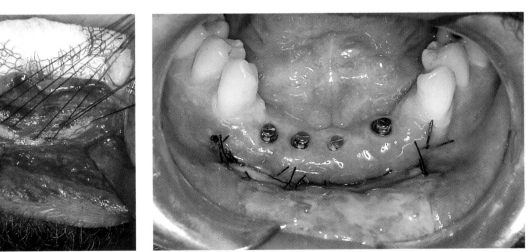

732 Clinical course

After suturing the mucosa down to the periosteum, a broad defect persists on the internal surface of the lip. This is left to spontaneous reepithelialization.

Left: Sutures are attached through the periosteum before the mucosal flap is replaced.

Right: Clinical view ten days postoperatively, before suture removal. The labial surface has healed spontaneously and is covered with a fibrin layer.

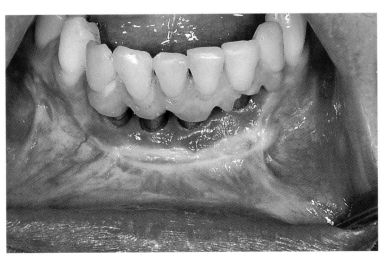

733 Clinical result

Clinical view two months after seating the temporary superstructure. There is a firm, immobile band of keratinized mucosa surrounding the implant.

Z-plasty

Indication

The Z-plasty procedure can be used for purposes such as lengthening a contracted scar, interrupting a straight course of scar tissue, preventing anticipated scar contraction, and lengthening short labial and lingual frena. The elasticity of the skin or mucosa must be taken into account when planning a Z-plasty procedure, and certain mathematical and geometrical requirements have to be observed. The primary incision is made parallel to the scar contracture, and at both ends of the primary incision, oblique secondary incisions are made in opposite directions at an angle of approximately 60° to the primary, forming two triangular flaps, which are undermined, mobilized, and repositioned with regard to each other.

734 Defect coverage using the Z-plasty procedure
This 44-year-old man from Pakistan had extensive hyperkeratosis and fibrosis at the corner of the mouth as a result of intensive betel-nut chewing. The primary and secondary incisions are shown.

Right: The surgical principle. The oval defect resulting after the incisions is covered by repositioning the two flaps (**A** and **B**) as shown (blue arrows).

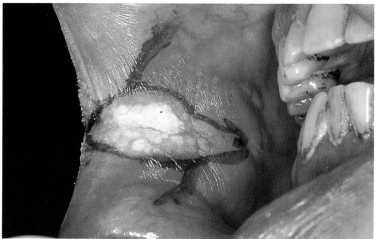

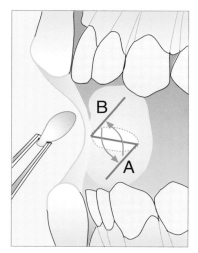

735 Excision
The hyperkeratotic area is excised and freed from the underlying tissues.

Right: The histological section shows the pronounced hyperkeratosis and hyperplasia of the epithelium, with intact layers.

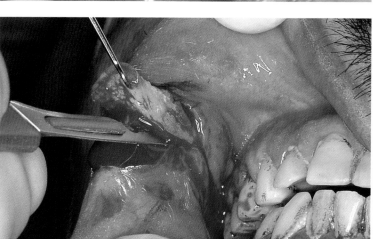

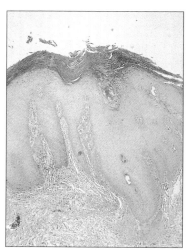

736 Surgical wound
After the excision, an oval wound remains. If the wound margins were simply sutured together, a functional disturbance at the corner of the mouth would result.

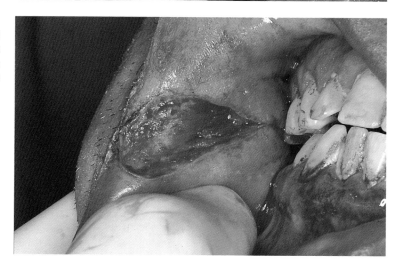

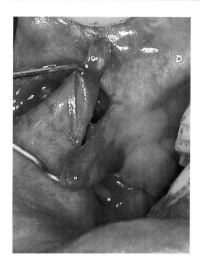
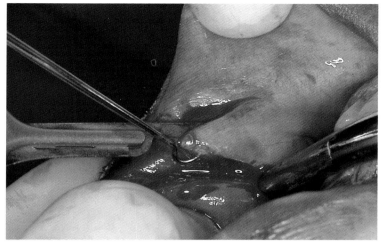

737 Z-plasty

After making the two additional incisions in the mucosa (Fig. 734) and undermining the buccal mucosa, the two triangular flaps are mobilized.

Left: The two triangular flaps are grasped with tissue retractors, repositioned relative to one other, and then positioned within the oval wound.

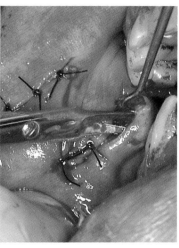
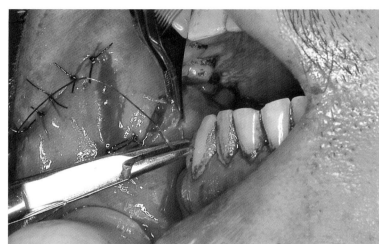

738 Wound closure

The mucosal wound margins are carefully closed using interrupted sutures.

Left: The "dog ears" created by repositioning the flaps are subsequently trimmed away.

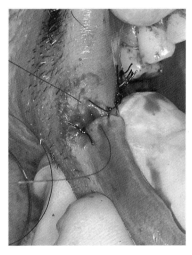
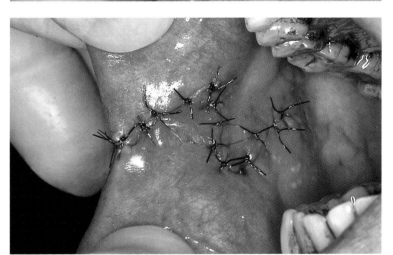

739 Clinical course

When all of the sutures have been placed, the typical Z-shape that gives the procedure its name becomes apparent.

Left: Especially with procedures at the corner of the mouth, extremely careful wound margin adaptation and fine suturing is necessary.

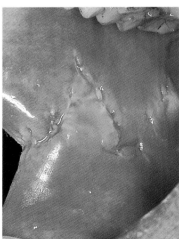
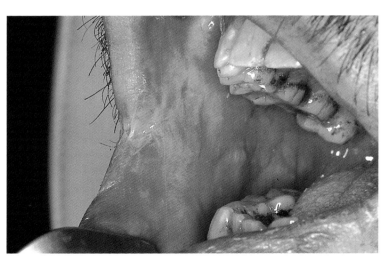

740 Suture removal and final result

The follow-up appointment one year postsurgically shows no recurrence of the condition as well as uninhibited mobility of the mucosa.

Left: The sutures are removed ten days postoperatively.

Excisions on the Tongue

When carrying out excisions on the tongue, it is important to bear in mind that injuries to the lingual nerve can lead to major problems. Excisions should therefore always run parallel to the anticipated course of the nerve. Excisions from the central portion of the tongue are less risky in this respect than those from the lateral border of the tongue, especially those on the lateral undersurface. For treatment of extensive superficial hyperkeratosis, or if a malignancy is suspected, we prefer cryosurgery over excision, since in our experience it leads to less disturbance of sensitivity. Exci-

sions on the tongue may be accompanied by significant hemorrhage from moderately sized arteries; these can be closed using mosquito hemostats, followed by placement of resorbable sutures (e.g., Dexon 3–0 or 4–0). Diffuse hemorrhage from the lingual musculature can be arrested electrosurgically, or by suture closure of the excision site itself. If the excision is very deep into the tongue, we recommend adaptation of the lingual musculature using resorbable sutures. Deep sutures should be placed parallel to the course of the lingual nerve and not pulled too tightly.

741   Excision on the lateral border of the tongue
In this 58-year-old woman, a hyperkeratotic induration was excised from the lateral border of the tongue, including a 0.5-cm band of adjacent healthy-appearing tissue.

Right: The indurated, hyperkeratotic zone on the right lateral border of the tongue is marked by toluidine blue staining.

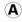

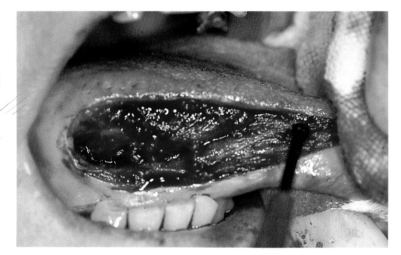
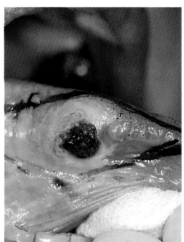

742   Wound treatment
To prevent unilateral elongation of the lingual border, the sutures are placed in such a way that an L-shaped wound closure line is created.

Right: To allow easy orientation for the pathologist, the anterior aspect of the specimen is marked by placing a suture.

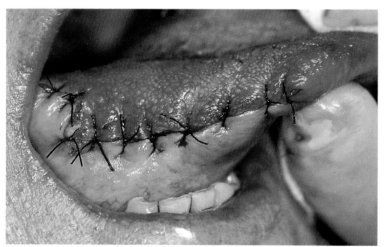
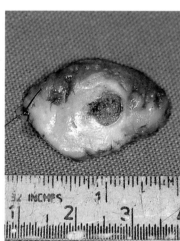

743   Conclusion of treatment
At the check-up six months postoperatively, a completely normal tongue is seen, with unrestricted mobility and normal contours.

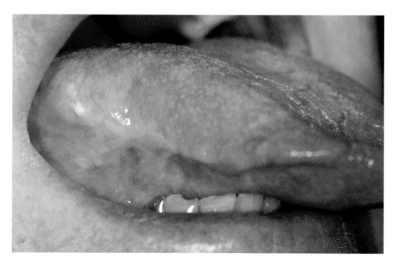

Excision of Pigmentations

Indication
Natural pigmentations of the gingival and oral mucosa are usually genetically determined; due to their size, they can often not be completely removed.

Surgical Procedure
Gingival and mucosal alterations caused by incorporations of amalgam or debris can be treated by excision and coverage. In the area of the alveolar process, the healing of the excision site can be left to secondary epithelialization.

Superficial pigmentation on the external skin surface can be treated by means of dermabrasion using diamond stones, and deeper pigmentation can be eliminated by excision. Dermabrasion should never be performed so deeply as to affect the regenerative, basal skin layers. After dermabrasion, the wound surface heals spontaneously by secondary epithelialization.

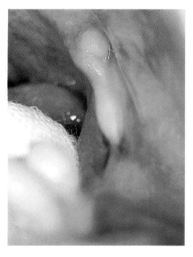
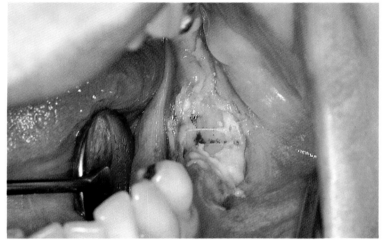

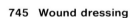

744 Excision and secondary epithelialization
In this 58-year-old man, there was a bluish-gray pigmentation in the edentulous area of tooth 38. The mucosal discoloration extended down to the bone surface, and total excision was planned. In some areas, the defect can be covered with periosteum.

Left: At the previous dental examination, an area of hyperkeratosis had been seen, providing the indication for excision.

Ⓐ

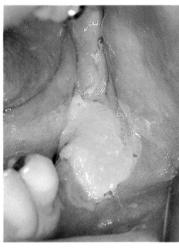
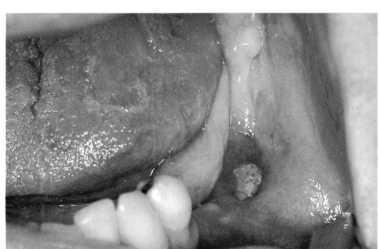

745 Wound dressing
Two weeks postoperatively, the defect is covered with granulation tissue. The histopathological report described foreign-body inclusions, hyperkeratosis, and hyperplasia of the epithelia without dysplasia.

Left: The wound is covered with iodoform–Vaseline gauze, and sealed with acetone adhesive to allow secondary healing.

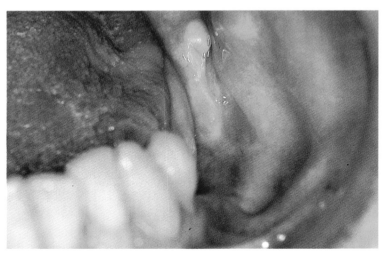

746 Clinical follow-up
The clinical view one year postoperatively shows normal, smooth gingiva in the surgical region.

Cryosurgery

Indication

Necrotization of tissue by the application of cold can be used in cases of superficial, benign lesions of the oral mucosa. The method is described on p. 277. After the epithelium is exfoliated, the wound surface repairs spontaneously by secondary epithelialization. Because the submucosal connective tissue is only partially affected, the new mucosa is qualitatively normal.

Cryotherapy is indicated particularly for well-demarcated, superficial alterations of the mucosa, such as hemangioma, small salivary retention cysts, and areas of hyperkeratosis. An analysis of our cases from the previous three years showed a recurrence rate of only 4% in treatment for hyperkeratosis. However, with lichenoid lesions, a recurrence of 50% can be expected.

In principle, it is possible to harvest a biopsy from the tissue immediately after cryotherapeutic treatment. However, we would recommend that biopsies for histopathological diagnosis should be harvested before applying cryotherapy.

747 Cryosurgery using the liquid nitrogen probe
This 58-year-old man had an extensive, sharply demarcated, partly verrucous, firm, white lesion on the dorsum of the tongue. The condition had been present since early adulthood. A diagnosis of leukoplakia was made after excluding other possibilities and a partial biopsy *(right)*.

Only two days after cryosurgery, the surface of the tongue is coated with fibrin, after blister-like exfoliation of the superficial mucosa *(left)*.

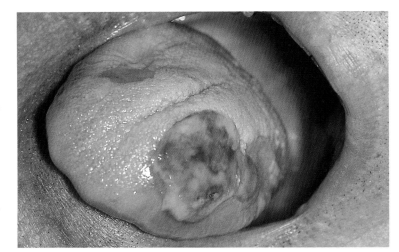

748 Clinical course
This photograph shows the condition eight days after cryosurgery.

Right: The area affected by application of the cryotherapeutic probe can be estimated from the extent of the lateral border of the frozen zone. At −170 °C or −180 °C, a depth of approximately 3 mm into the tissue will be achieved. The cryotherapeutic effect depends on the vascularization and the thickness of the lesion.

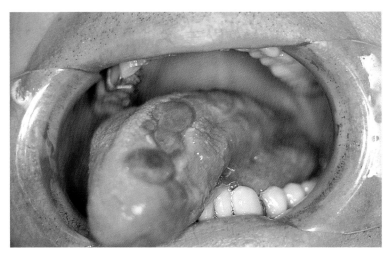

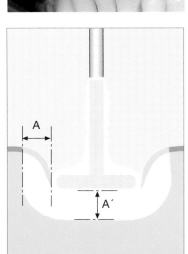

749 Clinical follow-up
A clinical examination one year later revealed small residual areas of leukoplakia on the left lateral border of the tongue. These were again treated with the cryogenic probe *(right)*.

The condition two years later shows a firm, whitish area on the left lateral border of the tongue. Further long-term check-ups are being carried out at one-year intervals *(left)*.

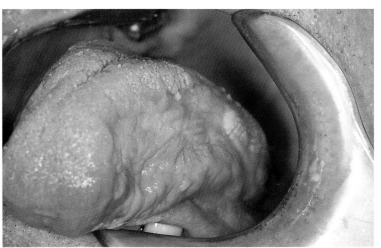

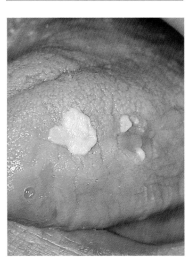

Procedure

The affected area of mucosa is dried using a gauze square. This allows the cold to act directly on the mucosa. Since the cold has an anesthetic effect, it is usually not necessary to administer local anesthesia. The cryogenic probe is applied to the mucosa for 30-second periods, depending on the extent and clinical characteristics of the lesion. The circumference of the iced mucosal surface provides a rough indication of the extent and depth of the effective dose. The procedure is repeated twice at each site. In this way, extensive areas of affected mucosa can be treated at a single appointment.

As soon as the tissue begins to thaw, the patient will experience some pain, which may last for several minutes. Twenty-four hours after cryotherapy, the mucosal surface will have been destroyed, and will be covered with a layer of fibrin.

The clinical characteristics of the lesion will determine the choice of the type of cryotherapy, an N_2O probe ($-80\,°C$) or an N_2O liquid probe ($-180\,°C$). For leukoplakia that is thick and difficult to treat, and in tissue that is well vascularized, we prefer the $-180\,°C$ treatment. Less serious superficial hyperkeratosis or leukoplakia can be effectively treated using the N_2O probe.

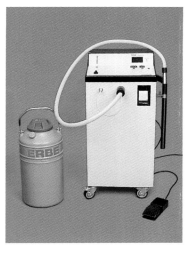
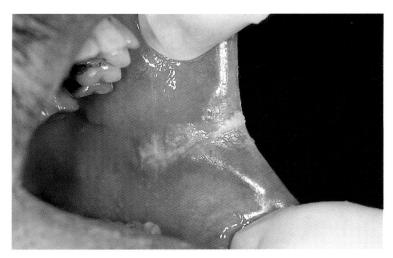

750 Cryosurgery using N_2O
In this 40-year-old man, a firm, white lesion was observed at the left corner of the mouth, radiating into the oral cavity. A biopsy on the right side revealed hyperplasia and epithelial hyperkeratosis without dysplasia. An N_2O probe (at $-75\,°C$) was selected to treat this minor mucosal lesion.

Left: For cryosurgery up to $-180°\,C$, liquid nitrogen is used. The equipment provides automatic temperature regulation and recording.

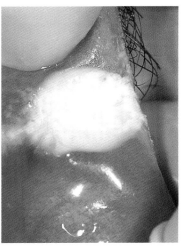
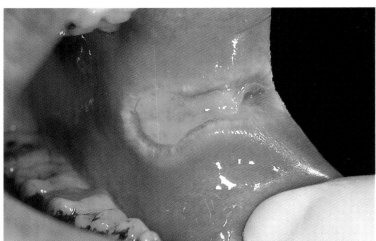

751 Effect of cryosurgery
The clinical view one week later shows a superficial mucosal ulcer.

Left: The cryogenically treated tissue has a bright white appearance immediately after removal of the probe.

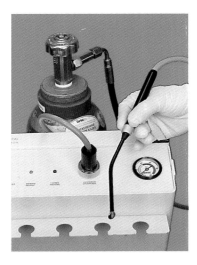
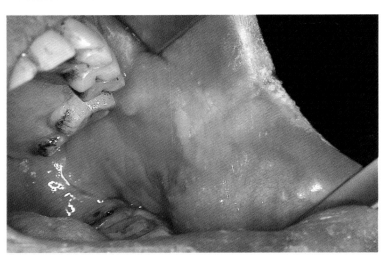

752 Clinical follow-up
One year later, the clinical examination shows normal mucosa at the corner of the mouth and in the oral cavity.

Left: The device is based on the simple Joule–Thomson physical principle. Gas at high pressure is supercooled as it passes through a jet nozzle.

Excisions at the Corner of the Mouth

Indication
In some cases, it is necessary to excise hyperkeratotic lesions situated in the transition zone from the oral mucosa to the external lip surface. The excision of pathological tissue from such areas requires special care. It is important to avoid any unnecessary scar formation and to allow secure lip closure.

Surgical Procedure
The extent of the excision must be carefully marked, to provide sufficient orientation during the procedure. Excision is carried out using the no. 15 scalpel. The oral mucosa is used to cover the wound. With broad undermining, the oral mucosa can be mobilized without tension over the defect. Wound closure is carried out with closely approximated interrupted sutures.

753 Excisions at the vermilion border—excision at the corner of the mouth
Hyperkeratotic lesions are seen at the corner of the mouth in this 40-year-old man, as well as a pronounced hyperkeratotic area with ulceration.

Right: The incision follows the contour of the lip precisely along the marking, to allow complete excision of the leukoplakic segment.

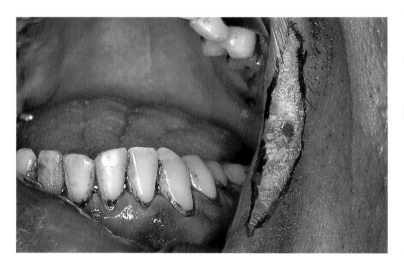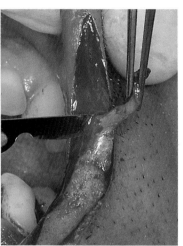

754 Hemostasis
An electrosurgical tip will immediately arrest any hemorrhage at the surgical site.

Right: The wound is long, narrow, and pointed at both ends at the corner of the mouth. This type of wound cannot simply be closed without a risk of aesthetic and functional impairment.

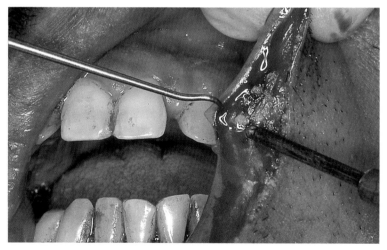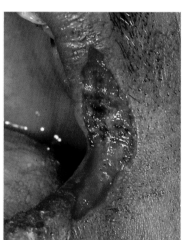

755 Undermining the mucosa
To cover the defect, the oral mucosa is undermined using scissors, and then mobilized.

Right: Pointed scissors are suitable for the delicate initial preparation.

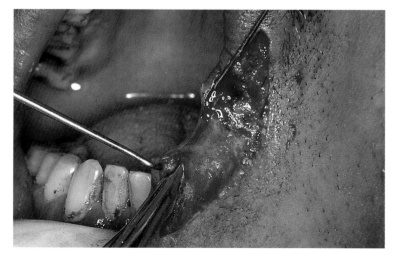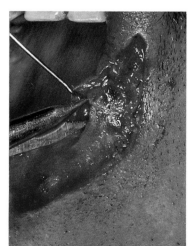

Hair Transplantation

Numerous medications and treatment methods to relieve partial or complete baldness in the head region have been proposed. In addition to the implantation of artificial hair, the use of plugs or larger segments of hair-bearing skin from the head region has been described. Artificial hair implantation is associated with a high rate of complications. This method does not appear to be justified (Künzler and Sailer 1985). On the other hand, in some cases, the transplantation of hair-bearing skin is a valuable method for camouflaging scar tissue.

Indication
This is primarily a cosmetic procedure. It is appropriate for soft-tissue corrections in the hair-bearing facial area (e.g., for cleft lip and palate in men).

Surgical Procedure
Under local anesthesia, a spindle-shaped, full-thickness explant, including hair follicles, is harvested from the retroauricular region or from the back of the head, and transplanted into a recipient bed prepared after removal of scar tissue.

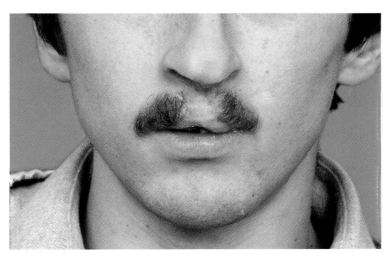

770 Hair transplantation
This 27-year-old man's cleft lip had been surgically repaired. However, he is disturbed by the lack of hair on the midline section of the upper lip, and he also has a "whistling" deformity.

Ⓒ

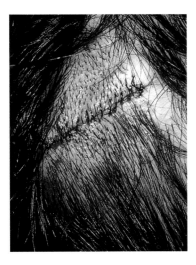
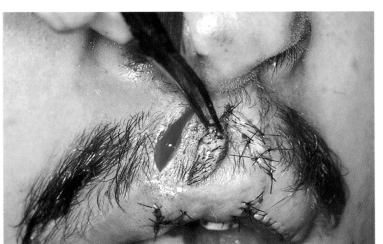

771 Transplantation
Two skin transplants with appropriate hair density are adapted into recipient beds after removal of scar tissue. Interrupted sutures are placed to attach the transplants.

Left: Suture closure of the donor site on the back of the head.

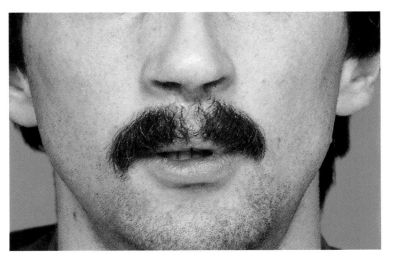

772 Clinical result
This photograph, taken two years postoperatively, shows a significant improvement in the appearance of the patient's mustache. The patient was satisfied with the result and declined additional transplant procedures.

Tuberosity Fibroma and Flap Fibroma of the Alveolar Ridge

Tumor-like fibrous alterations may occur as a result of mechanical irritations. such as chronic pressure from a denture base margin or chronic inflammatory irritation at the gingival margin. Bilaterally symmetrical fibroma of the tuberosities appears to have a hereditary basis. Surgical correction involves a modeling excision designed to restore a functional and physiological situation. Wedge-shaped incisions beneath the gingiva are commonly performed.

Indication
The diagnosis is usually based on the medical history and clinical examination. An indication for plastic surgery correction can only be established in clear cases of reactive fibroma formation. Doubtful cases must be biopsied; such cases belong in the hands of a specialist. Uncomplicated removal of a well-demarcated flap fibroma of the alveolar process as well as "flabby" ridge or buccal fibromas can be carried out on an outpatient basis.

773 Flap fibroma
In denture wearers, the edentulous ridge may be subject to ulceration due to chronic mechanical irritation. Spontaneous "repair" of such ulcerations often results in the formation of redundant, fibrous tissue, which accumulates in the vestibulum in horizontal fibrous flap-like lesions, which are often multilayered.

Right: Fibromas of this type emanate from a base on the alveolar process.

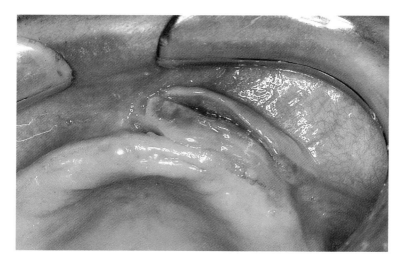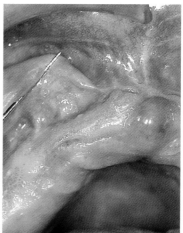

774 "Flabby" ridge
Chronic mechanical loading of the edentulous maxilla, usually in patients with natural teeth in the anterior ridge, often results in an accumulation of fibrous tissue.

Right: A firm, fibrous flabby ridge arises in the anterior maxillary segment.

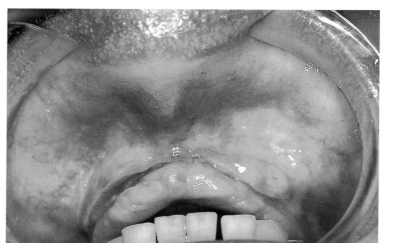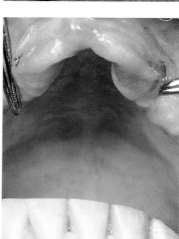

775 Tuberous fibroma
This is a congenital type of fibroma formation that presents as a bilaterally symmetrical accumulation of redundant tissue. The precise etiology is unclear, but periodontal infection seems to accelerate tissue growth. This type of accumulation can lead to functional disturbances, and often makes oral hygiene difficult.

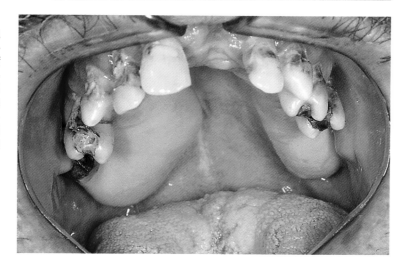

Surgical Procedure

Soft-tissue anesthesia by means of local infiltration in the area is usually sufficient. Local infiltration also inhibits bleeding during the surgery, and simplifies preparation of the soft tissues.

A pedunculated fibroma in the vestibule can be severed at its base, as can local fibromas on the buccal mucosa.

Flat or extensive fibroma formation on the marginal gingiva or the palate must be excised using a wedge procedure in order to avoid leaving tissue defects.

Depending on the extent of the tumor-like lesions, multiple wedge-shaped excisions may be necessary. The goal is to create a morphologically normal situation.

Excision of fibromas in the lingual area is particularly risky (lingual nerve, vasculature, submandibular duct); the surgical approach must be adapted to the anatomical situation, i.e., the tissues must be individually prepared. Only in this way can accidental injury to adjacent structures be avoided.

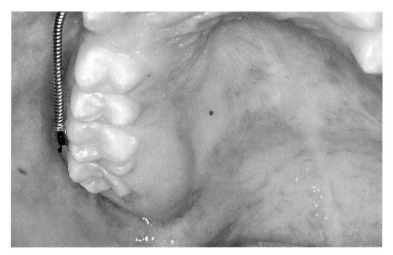

776 Wedge-shaped excision
During the course of his orthodontic treatment, this 18-year-old man developed pronounced fibrous thickening of the palatal gingiva in the maxillary molar region.

Ⓢ

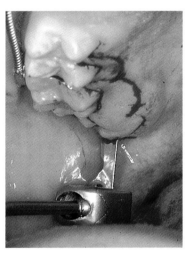
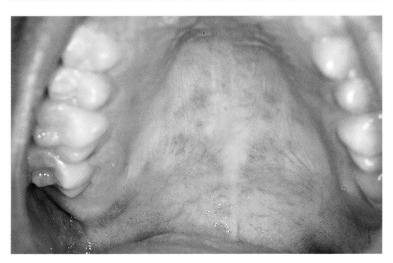

777 Primary incision
Using a scalpel and an angled blade holder, arcuate incisions are made, and the excess tissue is excised to create a situation in which the now thinned gingiva is at its normal location on the teeth.

Left: An angled blade holder is very useful for making precise incisions in the tuberosity region.

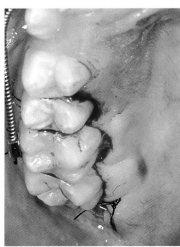

778 Clinical result
A follow-up visit six months post-surgically shows the gingiva with a normal physiological location.

Left: Simple, interrupted, interdental sutures are used to adapt the gingiva to the cervical areas of the posterior teeth.

779 Multiple wedge-shaped incisions from an edentulous area

This 43-year-old-woman required a partial denture after the loss of her maxillary posterior teeth. The clinical examination showed massive undercut fibrotic areas bilaterally in the tuberosity region. The redundant tissue was firm, but mobile.

Right: The surgical principle, involving excision of the fibroma using three wedge-shaped excisions.

 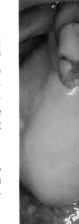

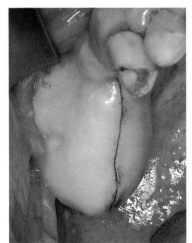

780 Primary incision

Left: The primary incision extends along the length of the edentulous ridge down to the bone.

Center: A surgical forceps is used to hold the fibroma as the second incision is performed.

Right: The second incision courses along the bone surface precisely at the base of the primary incision.

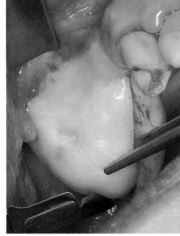 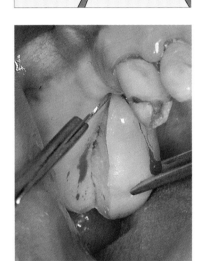

781 Wedge-shaped excisions

Left: Further reduction of the fibrous overgrowth is achieved using another incision subjacent to the mucosa on the palatal aspect.

Center: Removal of the second tissue wedge from the vestibular (buccal) aspect.

Right: The three wedge-shaped excisions.

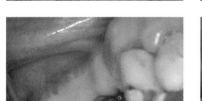 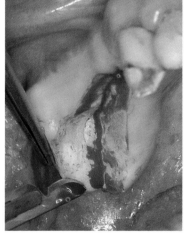 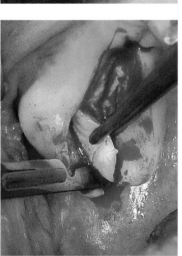 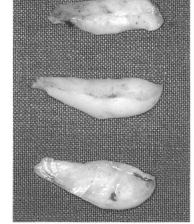

782 Clinical results

Sufficient mucosa must remain just to cover the defect and allow the placement of sutures *(right)*.

The condition two years postoperatively, and after extraction of the remaining teeth, shows the ideal tissue base for a complete denture *(left)*.

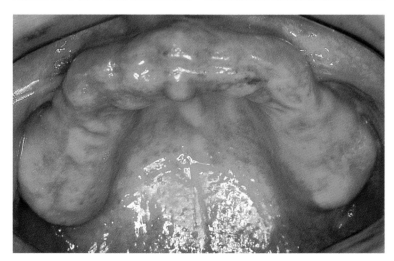 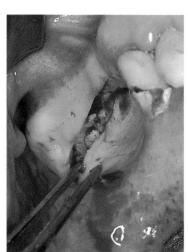

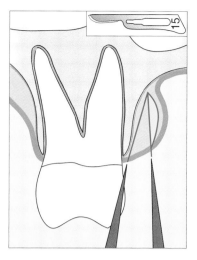

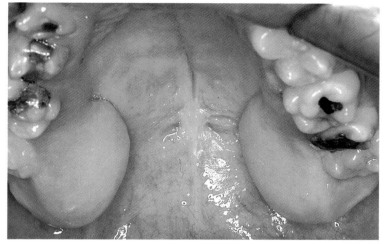

783 Multiple wedge-shaped excisions in a dentulous region

In this 32-year-old man, there was symmetrical fibrotic thickening on the palate, which had a tendency to continue increasing in size. Undercut areas were present on the palatal aspect. The patient found it difficult to maintain good oral hygiene on the palatal surfaces of the maxillary molars.

Left: The surgical principle, involving multiple incisions beneath the mucosa to achieve normal gingival contours.

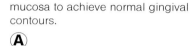

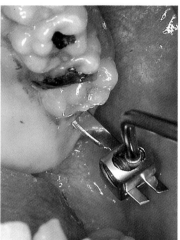

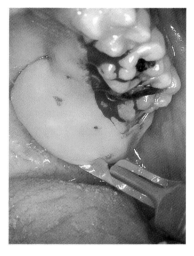

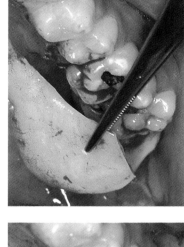

784 Primary incision

Left: A scalloped, inverse bevel incision is made along the palatal segment. At the distal region, an angled blade holder helps to free the fibrous tissue precisely at the sulcus.

Center: A vertical incision oriented distopalatally now follows.

Right: Once it is mobilized, the redundant palatal gingiva blanches because of blood loss. If it were left in situ, it would become necrotic.

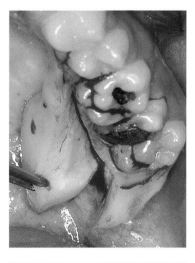

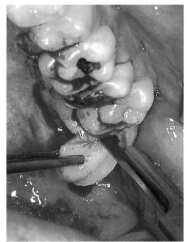

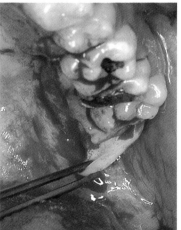

785 Excisions

Left: The palatal portion is excised.

Center: The mucosal flap in the tuberosity region is carefully mobilized using a surgical forceps and a no. 15 scalpel.

Right: The mucosa that remains in the tuberosity region is elevated epiperiosteally.

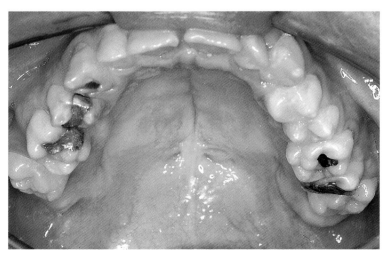

786 Final procedures and clinical result

The gingiva from the tuberosity region is reflected palatally and used to cover the surgical wound *(left)*.

The clinical situation two years later shows normal gingival contours in the molar region, allowing the patient to carry out ordinary dental hygiene *(right)*.

Lingual Flap Fibroma

Indication

Only rarely can simple excision of a flap fibroma near the floor of the mouth achieve any improvement in the denture-bearing area of an edentulous jaw segment. In many cases, the prosthetic situation must be improved by additional surgery, including plasty of the floor of the mouth and skin transplants. If the dental reconstruction treatment plan includes stabilization of the denture by implants, simple excision of redundant mucosal and connective tissue proliferative lesions will suffice.

Surgical Procedure

In the posterior segment of the mandible, care must be taken to avoid injury to the lingual nerve. It is advisable to expose the nerve during the early phase of the surgical procedure; this is the only way to prevent accidental injury to the nerve. The flap fibroma is sectioned so that one portion can be used for soft-tissue closure of the wound, and to avoid flattening the floor of the mouth.

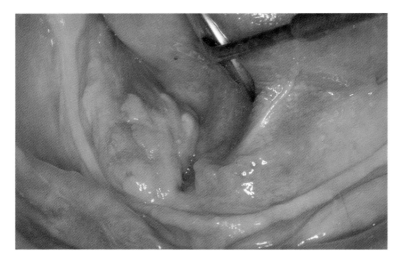
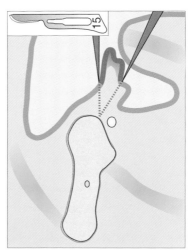

787 Lingual flap fibroma
This 74-year-old woman was suffering constant pain on the right side of the mandible. Clinical inspection revealed a flap fibroma on the lingual surface in the molar area, which was chronically inflamed.

Right: The surgical principle, involving excision of the flap fibroma, with due care being taken to avoid injury to the lingual nerve.

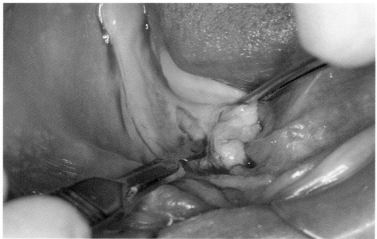
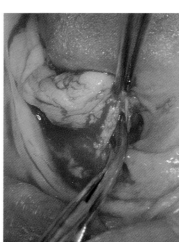

788 Primary incision
The scalpel is guided tangentially to excise the fibrous tissue away from the lingual periosteum, and the scissors are used to help tease out the redundant tissue.

Right: Constant visualization of the course of the lingual nerve to ensure that injury to it is avoided.

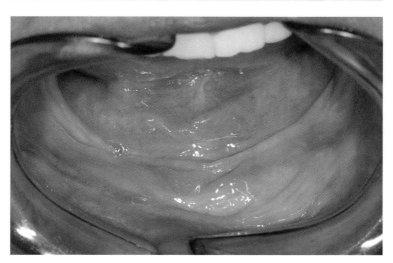
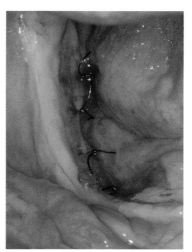

789 Clinical result
The mucosa of the floor of the mouth is closed using superficial interrupted sutures or continuous suturing. Sutures must not be placed so deeply that injury to the lingual nerve might result *(right)*.

One year after the operation and fitting of a prosthesis. There is good healing, and the function of the lingual nerve remains intact *(left)*.

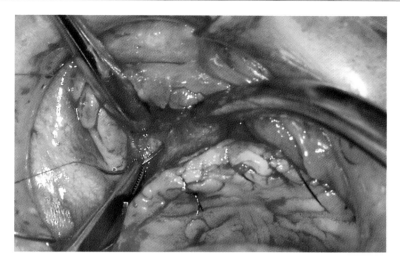

797 Attaching the mucosa
The mobilized mucosa is repositioned apically and attached to the periosteum using resorbable sutures.

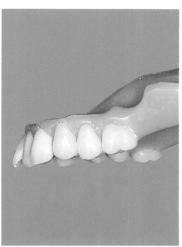

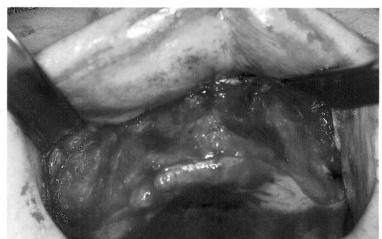

798 Denuded wound surface
The denuded wound surface is not covered by a mucosal flap, but left for secondary reepithelialization.

Left: The patient's denture is completely smoothed off in the area of the surgery, so that absolutely no contact occurs between the denture border and the denuded periosteum.

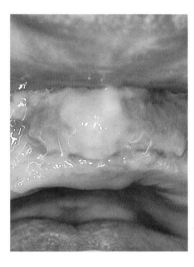

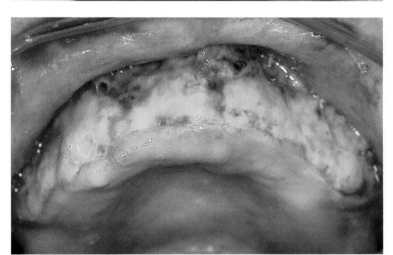

799 Clinical course
Three days after the operation, the clinical view shows the denuded periosteal surface covered by a fibrin clot *(left)*.

The next check-up followed one week later. Any granulation tissue formations are removed with a gauze square, preventing epithelialization of these redundant tissue growths. Otherwise, mobile mucosa would re-form in these areas *(right)*.

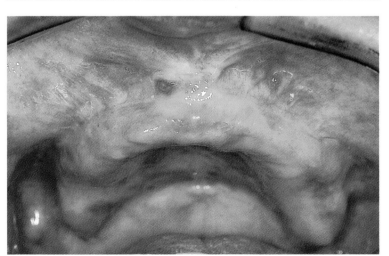

800 Clinical result
The clinical situation one year postoperatively. The vestibulum is capable of supporting dentures, with healthy mucosal conditions, including attached gingiva. Slight scar formation is difficult to avoid.

Excision of Flabby Ridge with Vestibuloplasty

Indication
The surgical criteria are the same as those for simple vestibuloplasty, i.e., after removal of the flabby ridge tissue, there must be an adequate ridge profile for the denture-bearing area.

Anesthesia
In addition to the usual local anesthesia, the fibrous parts of the alveolar ridge mucosa are pumped up with anesthetic solution. This simplifies the surgical preparation and reduces bleeding.

Surgical Procedure
The first step is to excise the flabby ridge tissue using a wedge-shaped excision. On the buccal aspect, enough fibrous tissue should remain to completely cover the epiperiosteal preparation for the vestibuloplasty, with complete coverage of the ridge. The palatal and buccal gingiva are sutured together using firm, continuous sutures. Subsequently, preparation of the vestibular mucosa is carried out (p. 293).

801 Flabby ridge excision—indication
The clinical indication includes situations in which the mucosa is inadequate in quality and quantity, in conjunction with a fibrous alveolar ridge and adequate alveolar crest profile.

In this 52-year-old woman, a flap fibroma and flabby ridge were seen in the maxilla. She had worn a denture for 20 years.

Right: The ridge profile is sufficient for stabilization of a complete denture.

 A

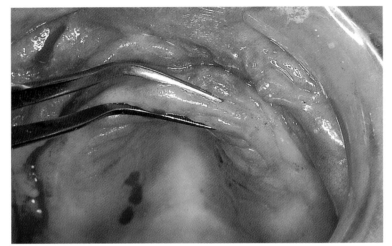
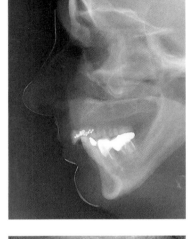

802 Surgical excision
The flabby ridge tissue is expanded by forceful infiltration of local anesthetic solution *(right)*.

The fibrous portion of the ridge is removed using two wedge-shaped incisions *(left)*.

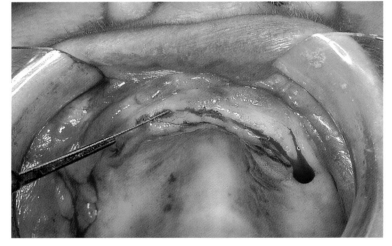
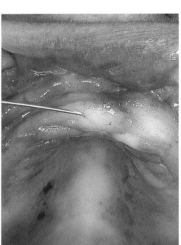

803 Additional procedures
The excised tissue is removed in one piece from its underlying periosteum.

Right: The remaining mucosa should be of sufficient size to cover the surgical wound completely, without tension.

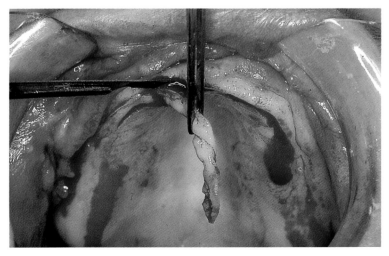
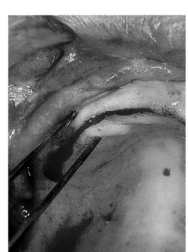

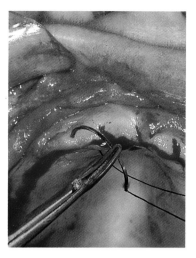 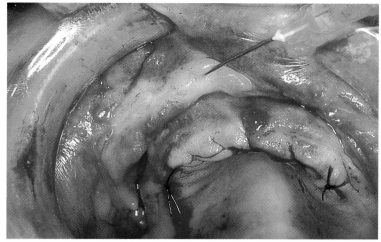

804 Suture closure
The mucosal flaps are repositioned over the ridge and closed with a continuous suture *(left)*.

The flap fibroma in the vestibulum is infiltrated with local anesthetic solution *(right)*.

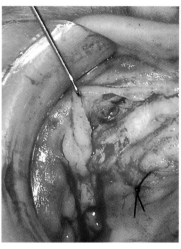 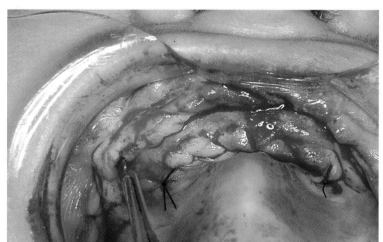

805 Thinning the fibroma
A tissue retractor is used to reflect the pedunculated part of the fibroma, to allow the tissue to be thinned by undermining *(left)*.

The fibroma is severed vertically, and the buccal segment is separated from the underlying periosteum *(right)*.

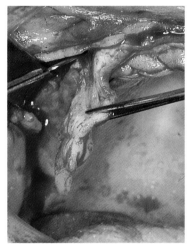 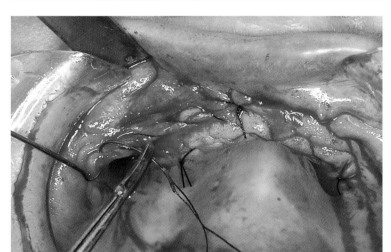

806 Flap closure
The flap fibroma is excised by submucosal and epiperiosteal incisions *(left)*.

After excision of the marginal portion of the fibroma, the vestibular defect is closed with interrupted sutures *(right)*.

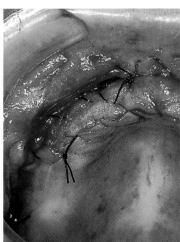 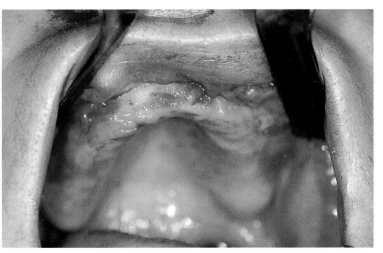

807 Clinical result
Clinical view immediately after the operation *(left)*.

The procedure leaves a shortened vestibulum that is unsatisfactory as a denture base, but the ridge is now covered with firm attached gingiva *(right)*. A vestibuloplasty now has to be carried out using a split-thickness skin graft to deepen the vestibule.

Osseous Surgery

Surgical procedures to correct osseous abnormalities are often necessary in both dentulous and edentulous arch segments. In edentulous jaw segments, it is often necessary to eliminate protrusive bony segments, unresorbed sharp, bony margins, and undercut segments of the ridge that present difficulties for prosthodontic restoration. In addition, there may be pathologic alterations such as exostosis, tori, tumors, and cysts, which may change the shape of the alveolar bone.

Bony Protuberance

Multiple exostoses are a hallmark of Gardner's syndrome. Other exostoses, such as mandibular tori or palatal tori, are often encountered as discrete lesions. Chronic irritation may also cause localized osseous deposition. These conditions can be regarded as benign tumors, and the lesions can be removed surgically by osseous recontouring.

> ### Clinical Tip
> Removal of bone should always be delayed until the final stages of any surgical procedure, in case autologous bone is necessary to fill osseous defects.

Osseous Deficiency

A patient's needs with regard to aesthetic appearance and function often require reconstructive osseous surgery. Mucogingival surgery can achieve relative improvements in vestibular depth. Using mucosal or gingival transplants, local esthetic improvements can be achieved. However, significant improvement with long-term stability can usually only be achieved by primary correction of the osseous substrate. In this connection, prophylactic measures can be applied even during tooth extraction surgery (see p. 62). Residual osseous defects can be treated using various procedures. In every case, the local situation must be fully analyzed in order to select the best possible method of surgical treatment. An abundance of bone in one location may be the cause of an osseous defect at another site. For this reason, bone that has been removed should always be kept in physiological saline solution in case it is needed to fill a defect at later stages of the procedure. An osseous defect can be treated by means of bone apposition or with the sandwich technique, using bone or cartilage from distant sites.

808 Instruments for osseous surgery—hand instruments
The classical instruments for osseous surgery are the mallet and the chisel. The mallet is made of heavy plastic that allows bone work to be carried out with controlled force. The chisel can be of various shapes and sizes, depending on the task concerned.

Right: A heavy lead mallet can be used together with a blunt instrument to arrest hemorrhage from osseous tissue.

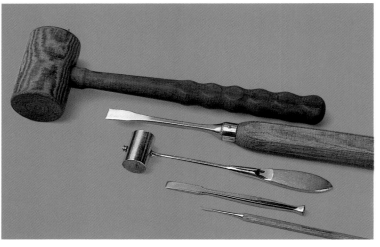

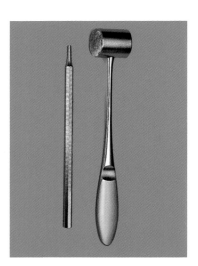

809 Instruments for osseous surgery—powered instruments
Machine-powered drills and bone cutters are suitable for delicate modeling procedures in bone. Certain types of cutter, e.g., the Lindemann bone cutter *(right),* can cause soft-tissue injury, and should therefore only be used when adequate protection of the soft tissues can be achieved.

Hollow cylindrical trephines are used for taking bone biopsies *(left).*

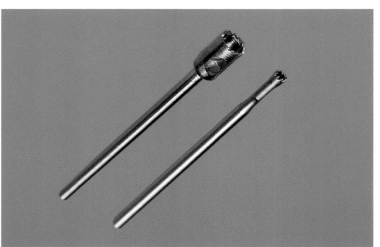

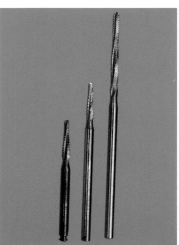

Osseous Surgery

Osseous surgery is carried out using Luer forceps, chisels, files, and bone cutters. The bone is traumatized mechanically or thermally. Using manual instruments leads to superficial necrosis due to compression. Regeneration of such lesions normally proceeds without complications, but may be somewhat delayed. When burrs are used, heat-induced necrosis in deeper osseous layers must be avoided by continuous rinsing with sterile physiological saline solution or Ringer's solution. Intermittent application of the bone cutter also reduces heat.

Mandibular Torus

Indication
If osseous exostoses on the lingual aspect of the mandible are causing speech difficulties or problems with partial dentures, they should be removed.

Surgical Procedure
After block anesthesia, the exostoses are exposed by lingual flap reflection (without releasing incisions). Chisels and burrs are used to remove the bony protuberances. Soft-tissue flaps are repositioned and secured with sutures.

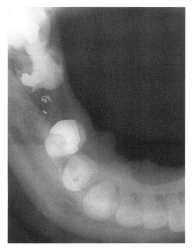
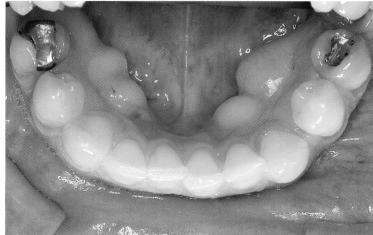

810 Excess bone—mandibular torus
This 32-year-old man presented with typical spherical exostoses on the lingual surface of the mandible in the anterior segment. The exostoses prevented successful placement of a removable partial denture.

Left: The occlusal radiograph clearly shows the isolated osseous extensions.

(A)

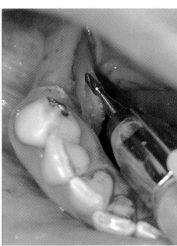
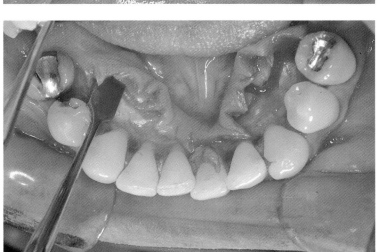

811 Ostectomy
The exostoses are visualized after reflection of a lingual mucoperiosteal flap.

Left: A fissure bur is used to undermine the exostoses, which can then be removed in toto using a chisel.

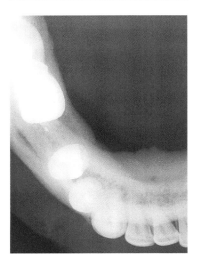
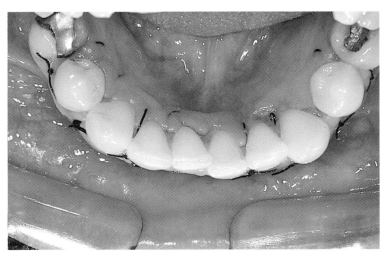

812 Clinical result
Right: An ovoid cutter is used to smooth out any osseous surface irregularities. The soft-tissue flap is repositioned and secured using interdental sutures.

Left: The postoperative radiograph shows normal contours on the lingual mandibular surface after removal of the exostoses.

Palatal Torus

Indication

Exostoses in the midline of the hard palate usually only presents a clinical problem when a maxillary denture needs to be seated and closure of the posterior palatal seal is not possible.

Surgical Procedure

After administration of local anesthesia bilaterally at the palatal foramen, a vertical incision is made from the junction of the soft and hard palates toward the incisal papilla. This incision is followed by two lateral releasing incisions. Any injury to the branches of the palatal artery can lead to hemorrhage, which must be arrested by vascular ligation or cauterization. The exostosis must be completely exposed. A bur is used to create several grooves within the substance of the torus, and the chisel is then used to remove the bony lamella. A large-diameter round bone cutter is then used to smooth the osseous surface. When the wound is closed, any superfluous palatal soft tissue can be excised. Hematoma formation can be precluded by applying pressure, or using a surgical stent.

813 Palatal torus
This 41-year-old woman was bothered by the development of a slowly-growing osseous expansion on the palate. The clinical examination showed a broad-based bony expansion situated symmetrically in the midline of the palate, with an intact mucosal covering.

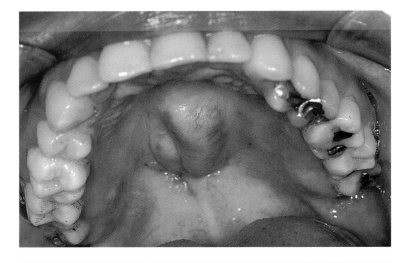

814 Primary incision
The primary incision is made in the midpalatal plane, with lateral releasing incisions both anteriorly and posteriorly.

Right: Sutures are used to reflect the palatal soft tissues and reveal the redundant osseous tissue.

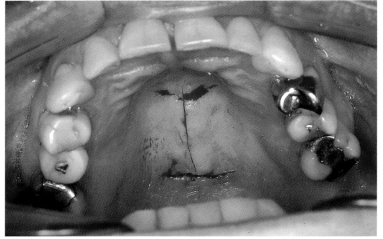
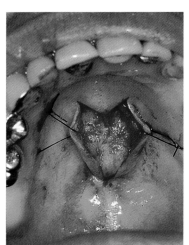

815 Segmenting the torus
A fissure bur is used to create several longitudinal grooves in the exostosis.

Right: Use of a surgical bur to create grooves in the palatal torus.

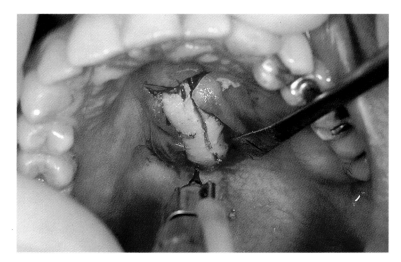
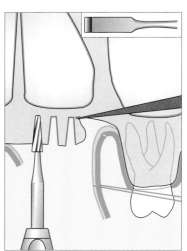

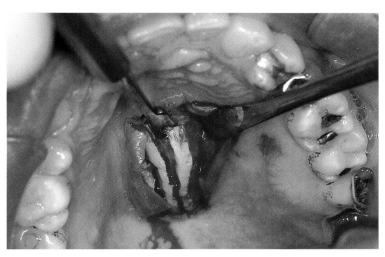

816 Bone removal
The strips of bone are removed using a narrow, flat chisel and a mallet.

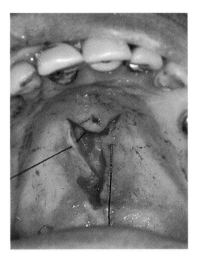

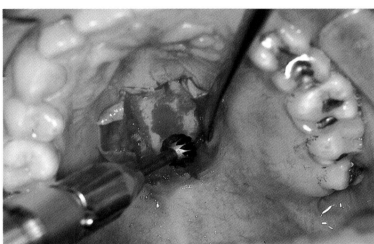

817 Smoothing and suture placement
After smoothing out any osseous surface irregularities, the soft-tissue palatal flaps are repositioned, and trimmed if necessary to avoid any overlapping.

Left: The wound margins are approximated and secured with sutures.

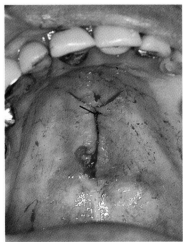

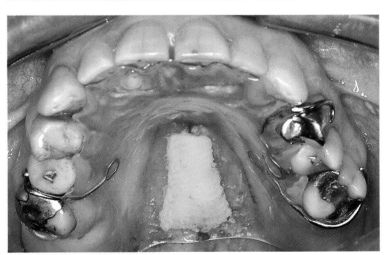

818 Protective stent
The sutures alone will not guarantee that the soft-tissue flaps remain in intimate contact with the surface of the bone *(left)*.
    To preclude hematoma formation or tissue dehiscence, a transparent surgical stent is used to hold the wound dressing in place and to secure the flaps *(right)*.

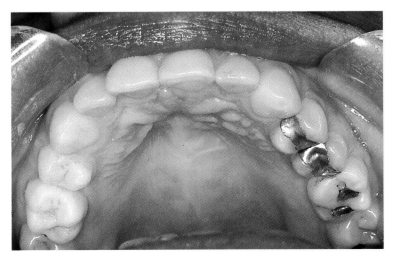

819 Clinical result
The dressing can be removed three days postsurgically, and usually does not have to be replaced. Sutures can be removed five to seven days later. This photograph shows the surgical site two years after the operation.

Osseous Wedge Excisions

Extensive bony protuberances on an edentulous ridge must not be treated by simply grinding away cortical bone, since this would lead to subsequent accelerated resorption of the ridge. The correct procedure is to remove excessive bone from the central portion of the ridge; this can be done by harvesting a wedge of osseous tissue and then collapsing the cortical bone inward. This procedure can also be carried out at the same time as multiple tooth extractions.

820 Vestibular exostosis in the maxilla
A complete denture was planned for the maxilla in this 48-year-old man. There was a broad vestibular exostosis on the left side.

Right: The surgical principle. The buccal cortical plate remains intact after excision of a wedge of bone, and finger pressure is used to collapse the cortical wall into the excision site.

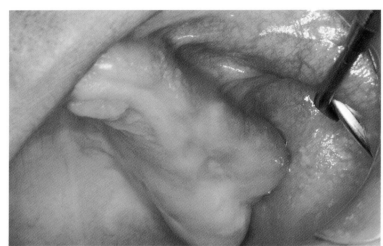 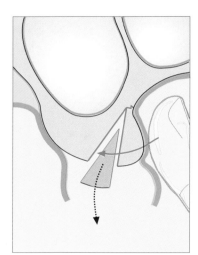

821 Wedge excision
After a primary incision through the soft tissues along the ridge and a vertical releasing incision on the mesial aspect, the soft tissues are reflected to expose the exostosis. The buccal osseous surface should remain covered. A fissure burr is used to create two converging grooves in the bone.

Right: A chisel is used to expand the buccal cortical plate. The wedge of central bone is then removed, and the cortical plate is collapsed inward.

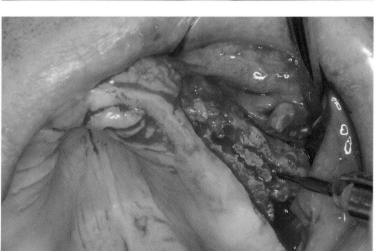 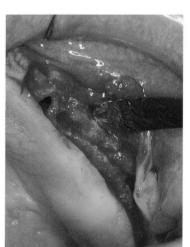

822 Clinical result
Right: Compression of the buccal cortical plate into the defect created by the wedge excision resulted in a satisfactory ridge contour. The soft-tissue flap is repositioned and any excess tissue is excised. Tight wound closure is then achieved using a continuous suture.

Left: The surgical site one year postoperatively, with contours suitable for supporting a prosthesis.

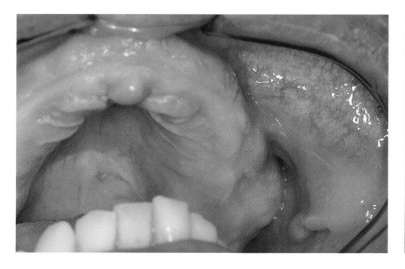 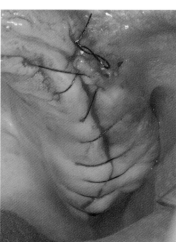

Dean–Köhle–Obwegeser Technique for Treatment of Maxillary Anterior Protrusion

Indication

Dentoalveolar protrusion of the anterior segment of the maxilla may present difficulties during dental reconstruction. One may consider surgical realignment of the alveolar process if the path of insertion for a prosthesis causes displacement of the upper lip. Difficulties in setting prosthetic teeth are an indication for sagittal reduction of the maxillary anterior ridge. A prerequisite for this procedure is that ridge height not be excessively reduced.

If possible, the best time to establish the indication is when the anterior teeth are still in situ. In this situation, the surgical procedure can be combined with tooth extraction. The vertical facial dimension must be taken into consideration, since tipping of the alveolar process may effectively increase the vertical dimension.

If considerable ridge atrophy has already occurred, other methods of surgical correction can be considered (e.g., Le Fort I osteotomy).

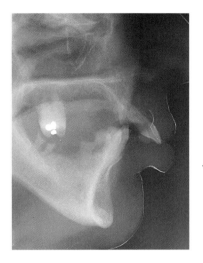 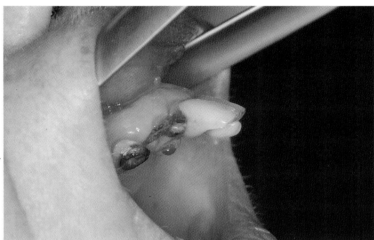

823 Reduction of protrusion in the maxilla
In this 55-year-old woman, the severely protruding anterior teeth, which cannot be preserved, will be replaced by a prosthesis.

Left: The lateral cephalometric radiograph clearly shows pronounced alveolar protrusion in the anterior maxilla.

Contraindications

The Dean–Köhle–Obwegeser procedure for correcting maxillary anterior protrusion is contraindicated if there are any additional skeletal positional abnormalities of the maxilla or of the mandible—for example, skeletal disto-occlusion of the mandible or retromaxilla. From a purely legal standpoint, it is also advisable to consider whether orthodontic surgical procedures might be used to improve conditions before prosthodontic treatment.

Surgical Procedure

After application of local anesthesia, the remaining teeth are extracted, with care being taken to avoid trauma to the surrounding bone. Subsequently, a round burr is used to deepen the alveoli cranially, and to remove any interdental osseous septa, thus creating a deep groove. Next, sufficient pressure is applied from the facial direction to effect breakage of both the palatal and labial bony plates toward the palatal aspect; the fracture line should occur at the base of the groove. Positional fixation to ensure healing is achieved using stiff sutures, and by inserting a stent or prosthesis that has been lined on its buccal aspect and relieved palatally.

824 Surgical procedure—anesthesia and tooth extraction
Local anesthesia is achieved by infiltration bilaterally at the infra-orbital foramina, bilaterally on the palate, and near the anterior nasal spine. The first procedure is tooth extraction, followed by excision of the interdental papilla.

Right: Excision of the interdental papilla.

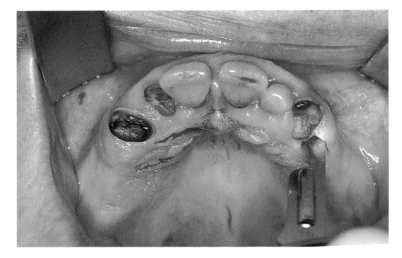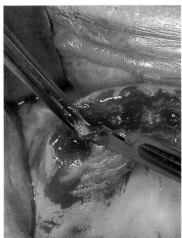

825 Removal of the bony septa
A narrow Luer forceps can be used to remove the interdental bony septa.

Right: A fissure bur is used to carry out horizontal osteotomy and deepening of the alveoli.

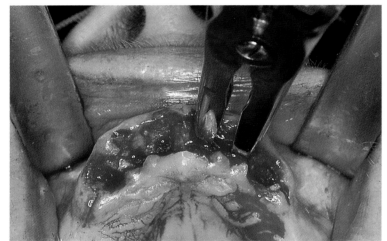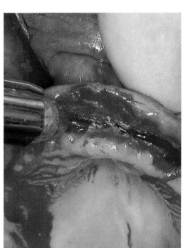

826 Deepening the alveoli
A pear-shaped bur is used to remove additional trabecular bone from the deepened alveoli.

Right: The surgical principle (Dean–Köhle–Obwegeser): deepening of the alveoli in a cranial direction, separation of the buccal and palatal cortical plates, and fracturing and repositioning of the two walls palatally.

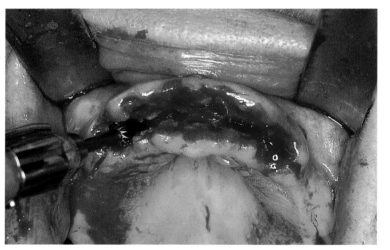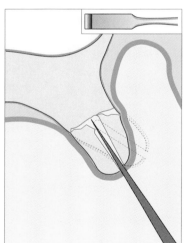

827 Horizontal osteotomy
Targeted fracturing of the labial and palatal bony plates is prepared by carrying out a horizontal osteotomy using fine circular bone cutters.

Right: Circular saw-type burs are available in various sizes to carry out the internal horizontal osteotomy.

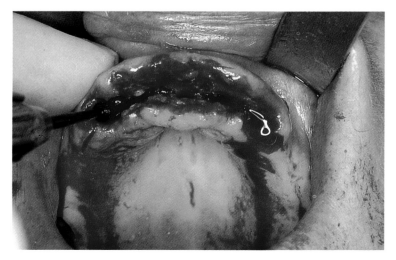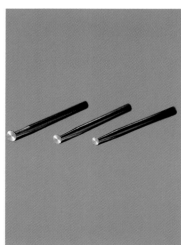

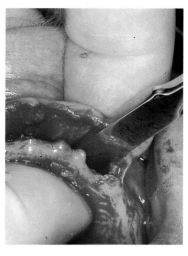
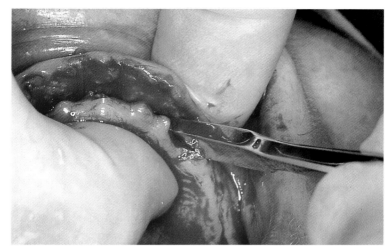

828 Fracturing the cortical bone

Using a wide, flat chisel, the cortical bony walls are fractured by applying buccal and palatal tipping forces.

Left: Fracture of the facial alveolar wall after tipping the chisel buccally.

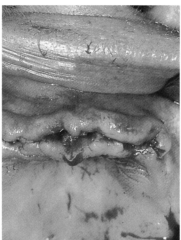
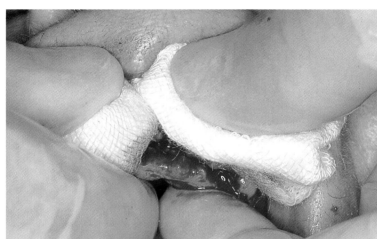

829 Repositioning palatally

Using sterile gauze squares to ensure stability, finger pressure is used to reposition the bony walls in their new, more palatally oriented position.

Left: Situation before suture closure.

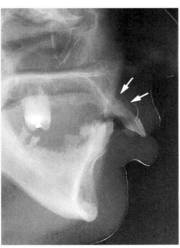
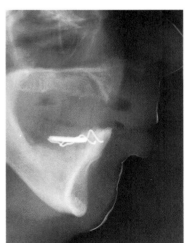

830 Radiographic comparison

The lateral cephalometric films show how the alveolar process has been repositioned palatally (*right*).

Left: Presurgical radiograph.

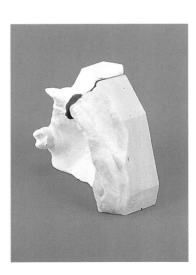
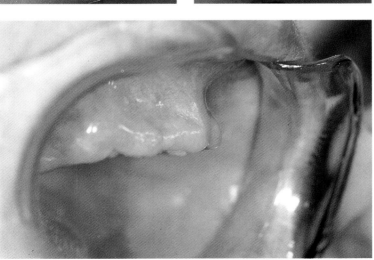

831 Clinical result

This clinical photograph shows an excellent prosthesis bed.

Left: The study model clearly illustrates the geometric configuration. Only the labial and palatal alveolar walls have been tipped palatally. There was no inadvertent bone loss in either the vertical or the sagittal plane.

Relocation (Depression) of the Buccal Bony Plate

Indication

If there is advanced atrophy of the posterior segments of the alveolar process in the maxilla, an extensive zygomaticoalveolar process may prohibit satisfactory extension of the denture base to achieve vertical loading of the posterior denture teeth. If ridge corrections are not required throughout the maxilla, an isolated modification of the posterior segment anatomy may be advantageous.

Surgical Procedure

After anesthesia, the zygomatic process is exposed where it approaches the alveolar ridge, by reflecting a vestibular mucoperiosteal flap. The soft-tissue flap should be wide enough to ensure that the suture line will be on a stable osseous base after osteotomy and opening of the maxillary sinus. A circular saw or an oscillating mini-saw is used to carry out horizontal osteotomy distant from the ridge. Subsequently, vertical osteotomy is performed at 2-mm intervals and extending up to the zygomatic process. Every effort should be made to protect the lining of the maxillary sinus.

832 Correction of the buccal bony plate
A new prosthesis is required due to the loss of the anchoring tooth 21 in this 68-year-old woman. The vestibulum in the left maxilla is shallow, and in the posterior segment it has a horizontal profile. Advanced atrophy of the alveolar process had extended all the way to the zygomaticoalveolar area. The line for the primary incision has been indicated in blue ink.

Right: The circular saw is used to perform horizontal osteotomy distal and cranial to the alveolar ridge.

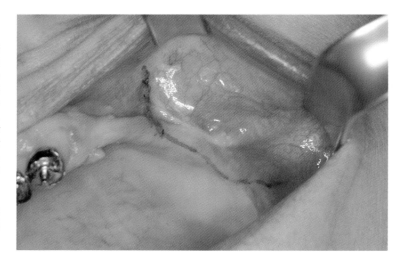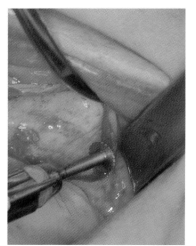

833 Osteotomy
Grooves are prepared vertically along the bony segment of the intact lamella. Using a blunt instrument, the segmented lamella are carefully tipped, step by step, into the maxillary sinus. The mucosal flap is extended by severing the periosteum, allowing complete closure of the wound.

Right: The surgical principle: a cranially directed osteotomy and compression of the osseous lamellae toward and into the maxillary sinus.

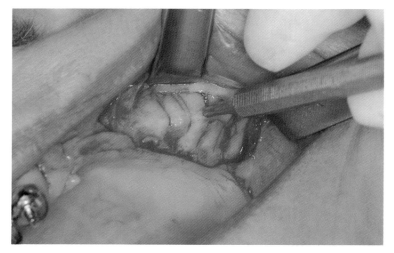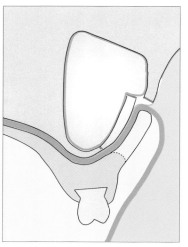

834 Clinical result
To prevent any movement of the bony segments, the margin of the denture is immediately relined using a thermoplastic material.

Right: The results one year postoperatively.

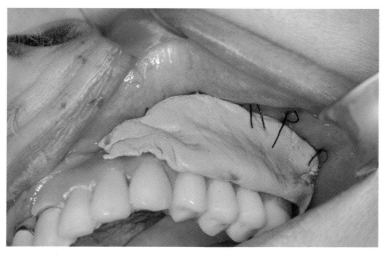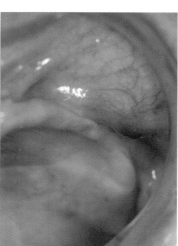

The vertical bony lamellae, which remain attached cranially, are forced carefully into the sinus cavity using a blunt instrument. At this point, the flap can be repositioned. Since the flap now has to cover a larger area of bone, it is necessary to extend the flap by making a periosteal releasing incision. The soft-tissue flap must be positioned without tension into its new position.

Fixation of the flap is accomplished with interrupted sutures. Any oroantral communication must be completely excluded. The patient's denture is now immediately relined using a thermoplastic material in the area of the osteotomy, to ensure that the bony lamellae that were tipped into the sinus will remain in the proper position.

Bone Replacement Materials

Considerations for the Use of Bone Replacement Materials
Since the introduction of hydroxyapatite, tricalcium phosphate, and glass ionomer as bone replacement materials in the late 1960s and 1970s, numerous studies in animals and humans have been carried out to demonstrate the characteristics of these materials. The commercial market for the materials has flourished, and the clinical user often finds it difficult to evaluate individual products effectively. The terms "biomaterials" and "biocompatible," and similar designations, suggest some degree of biological acceptability, or biological and physiological characteristics. In fact, the ideal material for bone replacement is bone from an immediately adjacent area. Bio-inert materials can never achieve this goal. In the best of cases, artificial bone replacement material may be partially osseointegrated, tolerated and (depending on its structure) resorbed and replaced by scar tissue. In the longer term, these bone replacement materials cannot contribute to the adaptation to a physiological remodeling of osseous structures resulting from altered loading. Therefore, although such materials are indeed indicated for use in certain cases, there must be strict adherence to the known contraindications. A reconstructive therapist intent on achieving an ideal therapeutic result should pause to consider the long-term consequences of surgical efforts to modify bone mass or contour, with regard to all of the possible pathological consequences, the aging process, and the future risks that may accompany such procedures.

Contraindications for Nonresorbable Bone Replacement Materials
Absolute:
—Thrombocytopenia
—Recent myocardial infarction
—Pregnancy

Relative:
—Immunosuppression
—Cortisone therapy
—Leukemia
—AIDS
—Rheumatic diseases
—Connective-tissue disorders
—Chemotherapy
—Radiotherapy in the immediate vicinity
—Possible focus of infection

Autologous Bone

In a well-vascularized transplant bed, autologous bone heals in quickly. Bone onlays, however, have a high resorption rate. Physiological loading is necessary to counterbalance the tendency toward resorption. This type of loading is provided by screw-form titanium implants.

Donor Sites for Autologous Bone

In the dentulous jaw, the facial surface of the chin region is a primary site for excision of bone segments up to a size of 1 x 3 cm, and the osseous excision can be performed on both sides of the midline. When bone is being harvested from this area, due consideration must be given to the roots of the anterior teeth, as well as the site of exit of the mental nerve from the mandible. It is also important to ensure that a tunnel-like defect is not created in the lingual direction. Clinical access is achieved via a vestibular flap.

Smaller segments of compact bone can also be harvested from the distal lateral segment of the horizontal mandibular ramus. Care must be taken to avoid injury to the inferior alveolar nerve or roots of the molar.

835 Autologous bone—free transplant from the horizontal ramus
After reflecting a buccal soft-tissue flap, a block of bone is excised from the thick cortical plate near the external oblique line. Care must be taken to avoid the roots of the molars and the location of the mandibular canal. Bone can also be harvested from the retromolar area.

Right: The defects will reossify spontaneously. Relatively small pieces of bone can also be harvested in a similar fashion from the chin region.

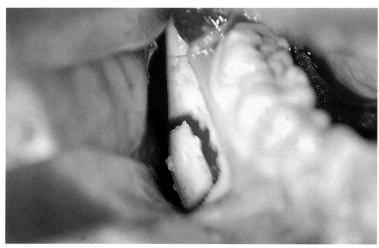
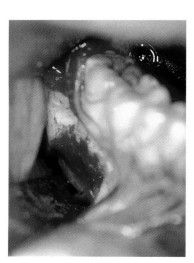

836 Pedicle bone graft—splitting
Minor defects on the alveolar process can be corrected by repositioning a segment of bony lamella, which remains attached in its original location.

Right: The vertical splitting procedure in the alveolar process is a method of correcting sagittal defects, in combination with free osseous transplants, bone bank material, lyophilized cartilage, or foreign substances. The appropriate procedure is largely determined by the comprehensive treatment plan for rehabilitation.

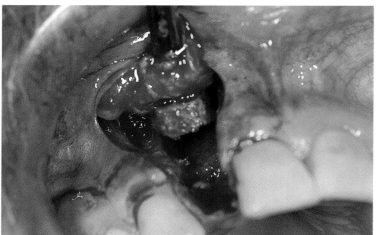
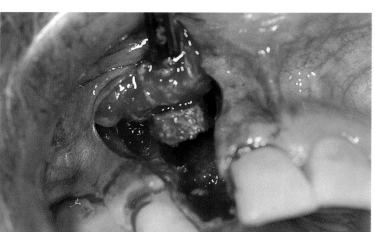
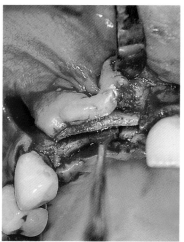

837 Homologous bone—lyophilized bone
Surgical compensation for extensive defects along the alveolar process can be accomplished using appropriately trimmed blocks from a bone bank. Shown here is an onlay of lyophilized material from the sternum, which was placed to compensate for traumatic loss of a segment of the alveolar process.

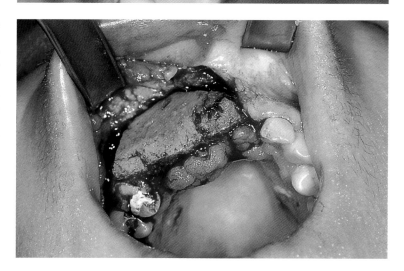

Lyophilized Cartilage or Bone

Sterilized and lyophilized allogenic cartilage or bone is very suitable for use in filling defects in the jaw region, due to the low resorption rate (Sailer 1976, 1983, 1992). Depending on the clinical situation, bone or cartilage pieces can be cut to fit a defect precisely, or cartilage chips can be used to fill the defects. During a phase of calcification, lyophilized cartilage or bone gradually becomes transformed and takes on the histological qualities of the patient's own bone. These materials are also suitable for restoring defects created by harvesting autologous bone.

Lyophilized allogenic cartilage or bone that has been rehydrated in an antibiotic solution is extremely resistant to infection, and can therefore be used even in infected areas.

As it is rehydrated with an appropriate antibiotic, this type of lyophilized material serves as an antibiotic depot at the site.

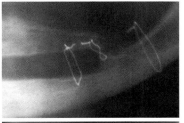
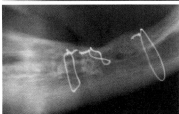
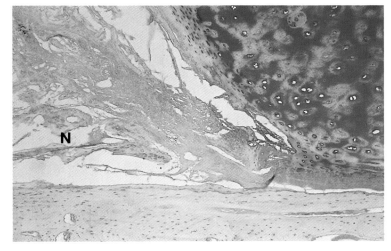

838 Homologous cartilage—lyophilized cartilage
Reossification begins in the empty space at the borders between the periosteum and the section of cartilage. This histological section shows the status 29 days postoperatively (N = newly formed bone).

Top left: A sandwich osteotomy procedure, with incorporation of a section of lyophilized cartilage in the anterior mandible. Ten months after the procedure, calcification and new bone formation are visible.

Bottom left: Six years later, a normal osseous structure is seen.

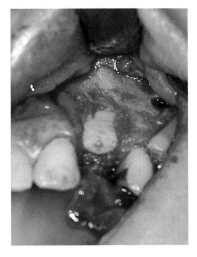
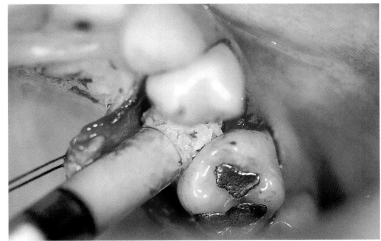

839 Cartilage chips
Periodontal defects can be stimulated to regenerate by applying lyophilized cartilage chips.

Left: Small, superficial osseous defects can be treated by applying a segment of bone as an onlay.

Indication

Lyophilized cartilage, either as individual segments or granulated chips, can be used virtually anywhere, as long as it is possible to achieve tight and secure soft-tissue closure. Due to its antibiotic effect after rehydration in a selected antibiotic solution, this material can also be used in infected areas. As it has only a slight resorption tendency, this material can be used anywhere for superficial augmentation of defective areas.

Free Autologous Bone Transplant

Indication

Autologous bone has a marked tendency to undergo resorption when it is applied to the alveolar ridge. This type of transplantation is therefore suitable for filling cavity-type defects, or in providing an intermediate substance in a sandwich procedure between two vital bony surfaces. As there is a high risk of implant loss in infected regions, autologous bone should not be used in such cases.

Surgical Procedure

In creating the soft-tissue flap, the larger bony area to be covered postoperatively must be borne in mind. The flap must be sufficient to cover the resulting osseous defect completely. Surgical extension of the flap can be achieved as described on p. 37.

A bone cutter is used to create a transplant bed with a clear geometric shape (inlay), so that the transplanted bone will fit precisely. The transplant must fit its bed and remain immobile.

840 Osseous inlay
After traumatic extraction of tooth 44, this 17-year-old boy presented for orthodontic closure of the space. Note the massive defect in the alveolar ridge.

Right: The periapical radiograph shows the osseous situation immediately preoperatively.

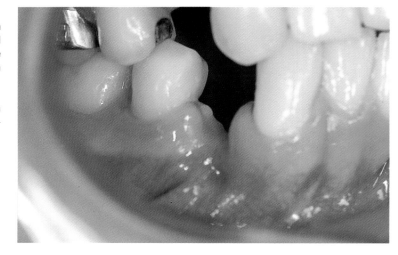
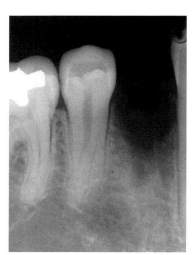

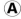

841 Flap reflection
Using a lingual incision and two diverging releasing incisions in the vestibule, a mucoperiosteal flap is created that is large enough to cover the osseous surfaces completely after bony enhancement of the defect. The mental nerve exiting the foramen has been exposed. The distal surface of the root of tooth 43 is largely denuded of bone.

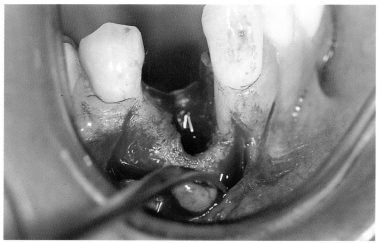

842 Donor site
The donor site is the buccal surface of the chin. An appropriately-sized segment of cortical bone with attached trabecular bone is delineated and removed.

Right: The surgical principle: the free bone transplant takes the form of an inlay to fill the osseous defect.

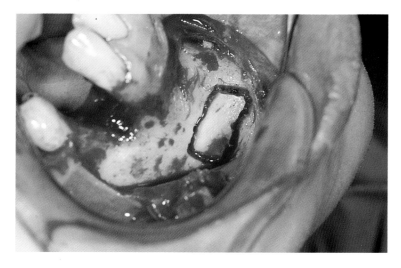
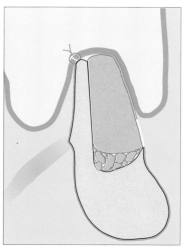

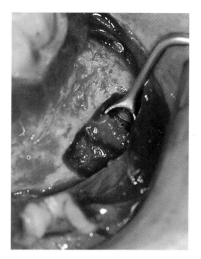

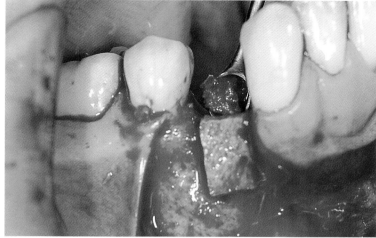

843 Transplantation
The small section of bone is trimmed as precisely as possible to fit the defect. If stable positioning of the transplant is not possible, it may be necessary to use alternative fixation for example, using a mini-implant screw.

Left: Osseous defects can be filled using trabecular bone harvested using a curette.

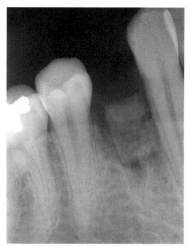

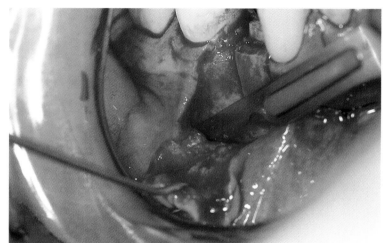

844 Wound closure
It is often necessary to elongate the soft-tissue flap by severing the periosteum. Care must be taken to avoid damage to the mental nerve.
Left: The periapical radiograph taken immediately after the operation.

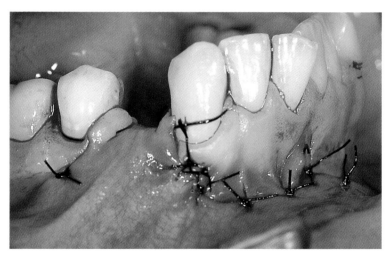

845 Result
After tight suture closure, the improvement in the ridge architecture is clearly visible.

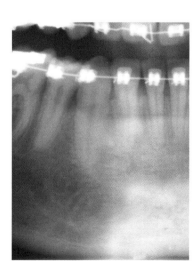

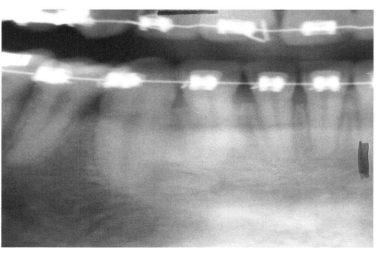

846 Follow-up radiographs
Two months after the operation, orthodontic closure of the space was initiated. The posterior teeth were moved anteriorly. This radiograph shows the osseous architecture on the completion of orthodontic treatment, three years later.

Left: The periapical radiograph does not show any evidence of altered osseous structure in the area of the transplant.

Splitting and Guided Tissue Regeneration (GTR)

Indication

In the case of a localized osseous defect after loss of a single tooth, vertical splitting of the narrow residual ridge is indicated before reconstruction using a dental implant.

Surgical Procedure

First, a mucoperiosteal flap is delineated and reflected vestibularly so that the major part of the vestibular bone remains covered by periosteum. An oscillating saw is used to create two vertical osteotomies, and the buccal cortical bone is gently split using a chisel. A dental implant can now be inserted. This procedure will displace the bony lamella slightly further buccally. Note that the bony wall continues to be covered by the periosteum, with which it is intimately connected. The crevice-like cavity created in this way is covered with a tissue barrier (we prefer resorbable membrane material), and the soft tissue is carefully closed.

847 Splitting and membrane technique
This 26-year-old man lost tooth 11 due to trauma. He had been wearing a removable partial denture for seven years. The comprehensive treatment plan included replacement of the missing incisor using a dental implant. However, the bone quantity was not suitable for implant placement.

Right: The radiograph shows the vertical defect in the area of the missing tooth 11.

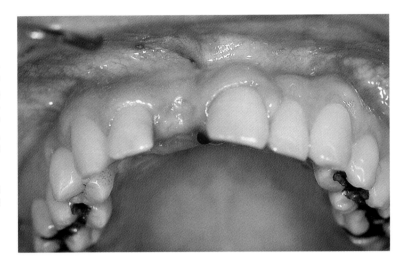 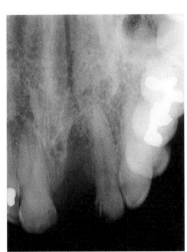

848 Simultaneous implant placement and defect repair
The surgical plan included implant placement with simultaneous osseous augmentation. A buccal mucoperiosteal flap was reflected to reveal the defect. The buccal surface of the bone remains attached to the periosteum (pedicle), and a chisel is used to displace it buccally.

Right: The surgical principle: splitting of the facial alveolar wall, with the breakage site on the buccal aspect.

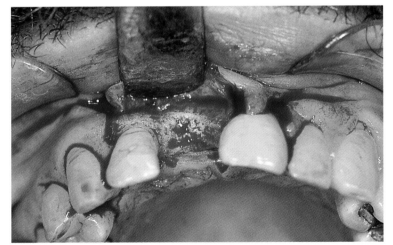 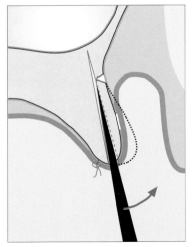

849 Osteotomy
An oscillating saw is used on the buccal alveolar wall to carry out vertical osteotomy.

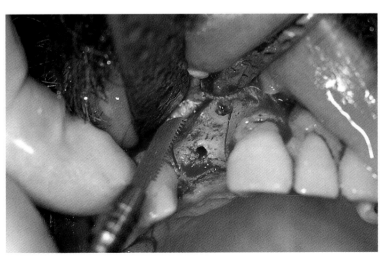

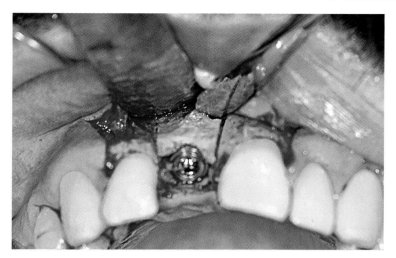

850   Implantation
The process of screwing in the screw-type implant extends the alveolar wall buccally.

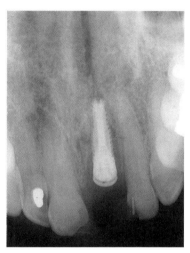
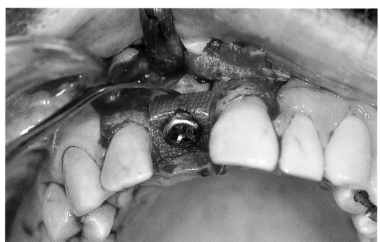

851   Tissue barrier
The resulting defect is covered using a polygalactide membrane. In this case, it was possible to secure the membrane using the healing screw cap of the implant.

Left: This radiograph was taken immediately after the operation.

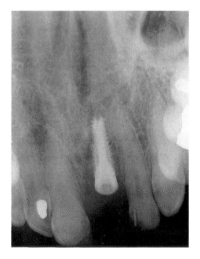
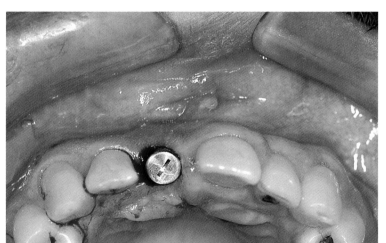

852   Clinical result
The implant was exposed 12 months later, showing irritation-free conditions in the vicinity.

Left: The radiograph shows virtually perfect bony encasement of all of the implant threads.

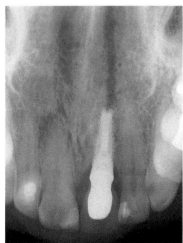
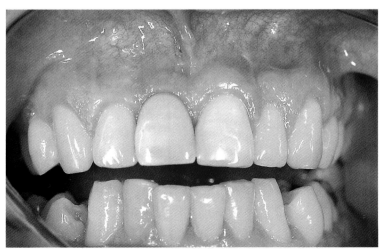

853   Follow-up appointment
The clinical check-up three years later shows that the clinical situation has remained free of irritation.

Left: The radiograph also shows no resorptive processes in the area of the implant.

Defect Closure Using Lyophilized Material and Bone Morphogenetic Protein

Indication

A combination of lyophilized cartilage and bone morphogenetic protein (BMP) leads to significantly faster ossification and restructuring of the transplant. The procedure can be performed anywhere in the jaw region for bone apposition or inlay-type procedures. It is also possible to use lyophilized cartilage in infected regions. For example, a section of lyophilized material can be implanted for ridge augmentation immediately after extraction of a periodontally involved tooth in a compromised jaw segment.

Surgical Procedure

During reflection of the soft-tissue flap, the enlargement of the surgical site must be borne in mind. If the ridge defect is to be treated at the same time as tooth extraction, a preformed implant bed should be created. A section of cartilage is trimmed to fit the defect, but slightly overcontoured and secured in the implant bed using resorbable sutures. Closure of the soft-tissue flap after placement of the cartilage must be secure.

854 Filling a defect with lyophilized cartilage and bone morphogenetic protein
The panoramic radiograph of this 44-year-old man showed a cyst-like defect encompassing the roots of the anterior mandibular teeth, which are hopeless. The medical history included acute infections in this area. Rebuilding the osseous architecture was desirable for prosthetic and esthetic reasons.

Right: The lateral cephalometric radiograph clearly shows the sharply demarcated defect in the anterior segment of the man-
Ⓐ dible.

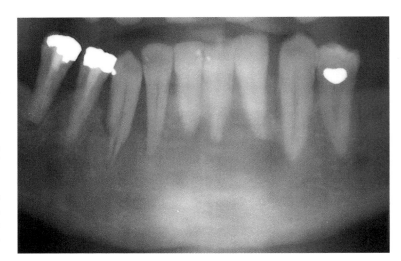
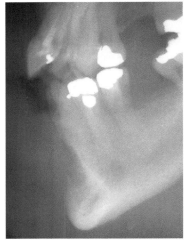

855 Flap reflection
The teeth were extracted, and the labial aspect of the mandible was exposed by reflecting a trapezoid-shaped mucoperiosteal flap.

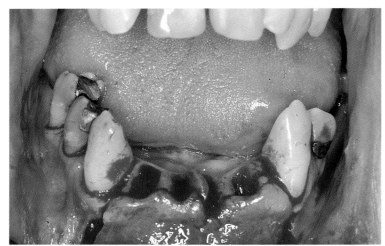

856 Cystectomy
All granulation tissue is carefully removed from the cystic cavity. As in all such cases, tissue should be submitted for histopathological examination in order to substantiate the suspected diagnosis of an infected cyst.

Right: The extensive defect is seen here from an oblique view. A coarse finishing burr can be used to smooth out any sharp bony margins.

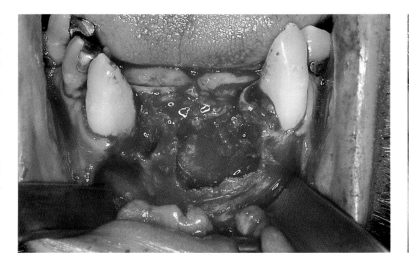
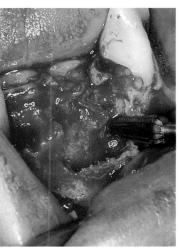

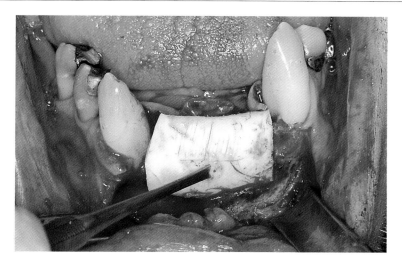

857 Cartilage inlay
To fill the defect, a piece of lyophilized cartilage is trimmed to fit, and then securely sutured into place using resorbable sutures both lingually and caudally. The lyophilized cartilage was rehydrated using an antibiotic solution containing bone morphogenetic protein (BMP).

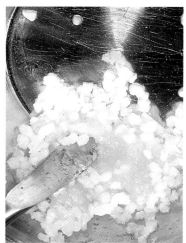
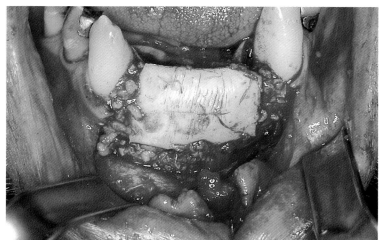

858 BMP paste
Any spaces around the fitted cartilage block are filled using a mixture of lyophilized cartilage chips and bone morphogenetic protein (BMP) paste.

Left: The material is prepared on site in the clinical laboratory. It is easy to apply using a small spatula.

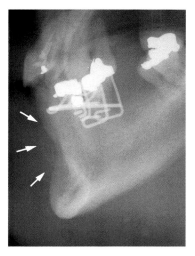
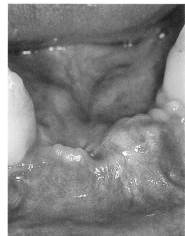
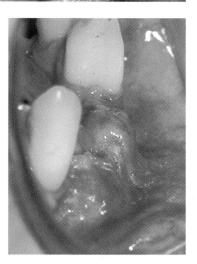

859 Results

Left: After only three months, the radiograph shows islands of calcifying material.

Center: Anterior view.

Right: Lateral view.

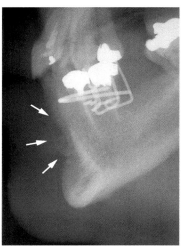
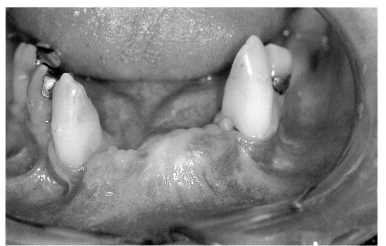

860 Follow-up appointment
Two years after the surgical procedure, the shape and contour of the repaired ridge remains constant.

Left: The cephalometric radiograph shows almost total reossification of the original cystic defect.

Pararadicular Defects

Indications
Osseous defects caused by periodontal pockets, or defects on adjacent teeth after tooth removal (e.g., extraction of third molars that are in intimate contact with the second molars), can be filled using lyophilized cartilage chips to enhance regeneration.

Surgical Procedure
Access to the bony defect is achieved by reflecting a mucoperiosteal flap. The defect is first thoroughly cleared of all inflammatory granulation tissue, to reveal an intact bony surface. A suitable instrument is used to place the rehydrated lyophilized cartilage into the defect; any excess material is removed, and the wound is tightly closed with sutures. Postoperative appointments are made first for suture removal, and then every six months for radiographic documentation of the osseous regeneration. Usually, ossification of the cartilage chips takes more than a year.

861 Correcting a periodontal defect using lyophilized cartilage chips
An interradicular defect between teeth 25 and 26, with a through-and-through pocket palatally, was found in this 12-year-old girl. Both teeth had increased mobility. The defect was accessed by raising a palatal flap; the cavity was curetted and then filled with lyophilized cartilage chips.

Right: Radiographic view preoperatively *(above)* and two months after filling the defect *(below).*

 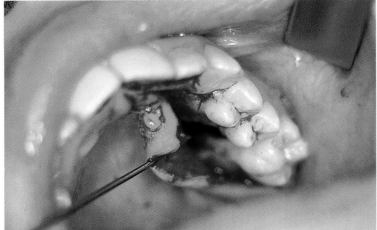 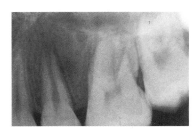 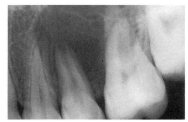

862 Inserting lyophilized cartilage chips
The granular, paste-like preparation is pressed into the defect, and the soft-tissue flap is then closed using interdental sutures.

Right: The radiographs show the course of healing, after one year *(above)* and two years *(below).* Note the normal interradicular trabecular structure and complete regeneration of the periradicular margin.

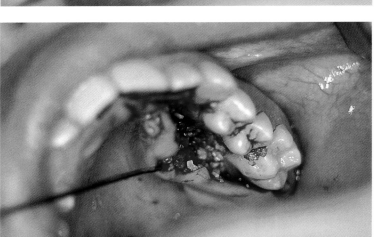 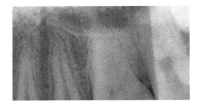 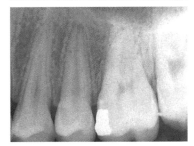

863 Clinical result
One year after surgery, there is a clinically flawless periodontal condition, with normal probing depths. The teeth were still vital.

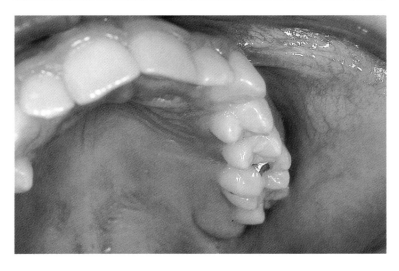

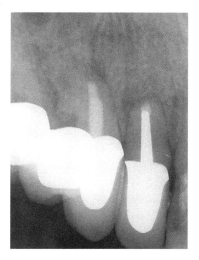
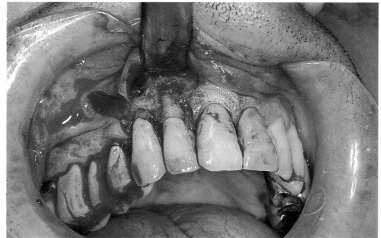

864 Contiguous buccal pockets

In this 57-year-old man, an acute infection developed after a full crown restoration had been seated on tooth 12. During the apicoectomy procedure, a contiguous buccal pocket was detected.

Left: Widening of the periodontal ligament space is clearly visible in the radiograph.

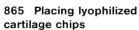

Ⓐ

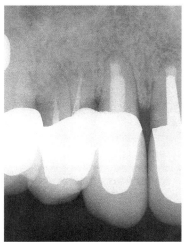
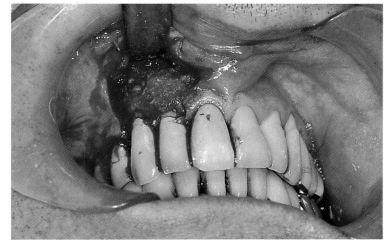

865 Placing lyophilized cartilage chips

After minimal resection of the root tip and curettage of the pocket walls, the defect is filled with lyophilized cartilage chips; the root surface is also covered. Uncomplicated healing followed in this case. The periodontal pockets can no longer be probed clinically.

Left: The radiograph one year after the operation shows the osseous situation. The periodontal ligament space has normalized. There is no evidence of bone resorption.

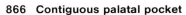

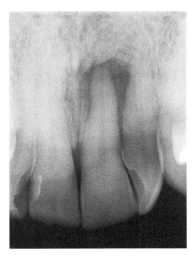
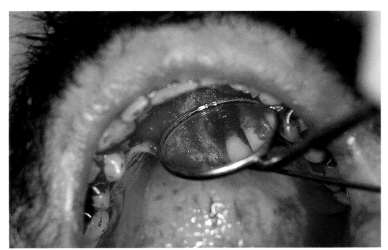

866 Contiguous palatal pocket

In this 33-year-old man, there was a contiguous osseous defect on the palatal aspect of the root of tooth 21. The defect is clearly visible after reflection of a palatal flap. The tooth was vital.

Left: The radiograph clearly shows the area of osteolysis in the periapical region of tooth 21.

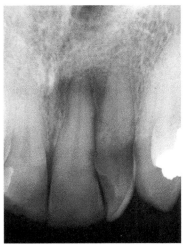
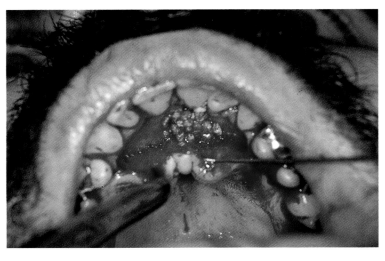

867 Clinical result

From a palatal approach, the defect is thoroughly curetted to remove granulation tissue, and then filled with lyophilized cartilage chips. The soft-tissue flap is repositioned and tightly sutured. The course of healing was without complication, and the one-year postoperative visit showed healthy conditions.

Left: The radiograph clearly shows increasing osseous restructuring in the former bony defect.

Sailer Lyophilization Technique

Rib bone, rib cartilage, or sternum is excised from a cadaver donor (under 30 years of age, with no infectious diseases), and all fatty tissue is removed (chloroform/methanol 1:1, 48 hours at room temperature). Lyophilization can then be carried out (freeze-drying for 72 hours at 25 °C and negative pressure of 10^{-2} bar), followed by gas sterilization (ethylene oxide, four hours at 37 °C; gas clearing for 48 hours at 37 °C).

The material can be stored indefinitely without any problem. Before use, the material is rehydrated for 24 hours in an antibiotic solution of choice (usually penicillin or streptomycin). Lyophilized cartilage chips can be used directly, even without rehydration. They are simply rehydrated in antibiotic solution immediately before being placed in the osseous defect.

Bone Morphogenetic Protein

New bone formation can be accelerated using BMP (Sailer and Wolf 1994a, b). This phenomenon can be exploited during surgical attempts to correct osseous defects. A combination of lyophilized cartilage or lyophilized bone with BMP for the repair of osseous defects leads to much faster calcification of the transplanted material.

Hydroxyapatite

Since the basic building material of bone is hydroxyapatite, it is reasonable to suppose that this material could also be used as a bone replacement. It is important to bear in mind, however, that although this material is well accepted by host bone, resorption of the transplanted material can be expected to a greater or lesser degree, depending on the characteristics of the implanted hydroxyapatite (particle size, pore size). Depending on the method employed, the particles may become surrounded by a scar-like encapsulation, or may be partially penetrated by newly formed bone. Implanted hydroxyapatite basically continues to behave like foreign body within the bone. As such, it must be regarded as a site of lessened resistance. Over the long term, therefore, potential complications, such as infections, can be expected. The risk is higher if the implanted material cannot be rendered immobile at the implantation site. A particularly feared risk is possible migration near the mental nerve, which can cause neuralgiform symptoms.

Guided Tissue Regeneration (GTR) and Guided Bone Regeneration (GBR)

Guided tissue regeneration using barrier techniques (membrane, foil) is based on the principle of inhibiting connective-tissue regeneration within osseous defects. To accomplish this, the bony wound is separated from the overlying connective tissue by means of a barrier. By forming a tent-like cavity with the membrane, a certain degree of osseous augmentation of the alveolar ridge can be achieved. Since the process involves new formation of autologous bone, corresponding resorption can be expected if there is no loading. By contrast, in arch segments subject to loading from dental implants, the method appears to be successful in the longer term.

Use of Connective Tissue to Improve Contours

Indication
Treatment of osseous defects on the alveolar process using connective tissue is only possible for aesthetic corrections. The long-term prognosis for success with soft-tissue defect closure is still an open question, since follow-up studies have not yet been published. An alveolar ridge that has been augmented with a connective-tissue transplant should not be loaded prosthetically. Free connective-tissue transplants from the palate can be used to increase the volume of the alveolar process. The quality of the mucosa usually requires a subsequent free gingival graft. Combined surgical procedures have been described, but in our experience, these cannot be regarded as routine procedures.

Traumatology

Definition

Trauma is defined as the destruction of tissue integrity, with causes including:

—Mechanical trauma
—Chemical trauma
—Thermal trauma
—Radiation trauma

An "accident" is defined as an unintentional, sudden, damaging effect of an abnormal external factor or force on the human body.

Basic Principles

Severe or life-threatening injuries to the mouth, jaws, and facial regions must be treated in hospital. Isolated mild trauma, in which any life-threatening injury can be excluded with certainty, can be treated on an outpatient basis.

The need for immediate treatment depends on the severity of the injury.

Clinical Tip
Trauma cases should be handled as emergencies that require attention without delay.

If injuries to the facial skeleton are apparent, additional injury to other parts of the body should be excluded either on the basis of the medical history or by requesting further clinical examination. Due consideration must be given to the possible effects of alcohol or other drugs on the patient's current general condition, particularly when diagnosing neurological disturbances.

Medical History

The medical history should include inquiries concerning the place and time at which the trauma took place, as well as the surrounding circumstances. It is important to ascertain whether the patient can provide precise information about the accident. If the patient's memory is cloudy, and examination by a physician is indicated (possible concussion), information provided by third parties is often helpful in reconstructing the circumstances surrounding the incident. The need for a tetanus booster should be clarified.

If there are injuries to the teeth, it is important to ascertain the exact length of time that has elapsed between the accident and the start of initial treatment. If teeth have been completely luxated, the length of time during which they have been outside the mouth and the transport medium are important aspects of the prognosis for attempts to re-implant the teeth, and therefore also play an important role in treatment planning. The patient's responses to questions concerning the temporal aspects should be entered in the chart. The rest of the medical and dental history is obtained as described in the section on patient examination (p. 6).

Data Collection

Extraoral Examination

A complete and thorough examination should be carried out, with special attention being given to tissue contours, sensitivity, occlusion, tooth mobility, and step formation. Left–right comparisons should be made throughout the examination in order to correctly interpret apparent deviations. The surface of the face and skull should be carefully examined for indentations, pressure-sensitive areas, abrasions, and hematoma formation.

Any apparent inconsistencies between clinical observations and the description of the trauma should be noted. It is also important to note whether observed injuries correspond to the time of occurrence of the accident. Clinical signs of previous trauma or surgery (scars) should be noted.

868 Inspection after trauma
Special attention should be given to penetrating soft-tissue wounds of the lip. If teeth have been fractured, it is likely that there are small dental fragments in the wound. Other foreign bodies may also be encountered in fresh wounds that are not swollen. The extraoral examination is carried out systematically following the diagrams on page 10.

Right: The same wound from the facial view.

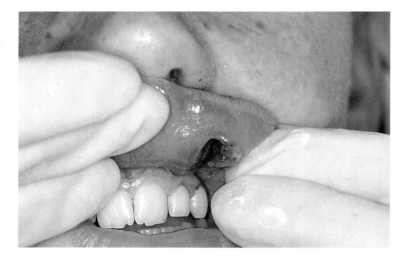 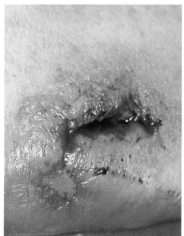

869 Oral examination
A systematic inspection of occlusion, assessment of tooth mobility, elongation, premature contacts and tooth fractures should be carried out. Soft-tissue reddening and elongation of teeth are signs of luxation or tooth fracture, as seen here in tooth 21.

Right: A radiograph of tooth 21 reveals a transverse fracture of the root.

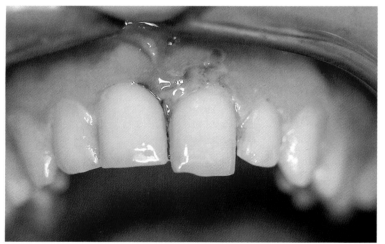 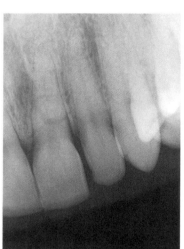

870 Counting the teeth
After carefully cleansing the area, clinical inspection of these multiple injuries to the alveolar process can begin. First, the teeth are counted; this often provides evidence of tooth loss. Due to crown fractures and displaced jaw segments, there is not always a space where a tooth has been luxated.

Right: In cases such as this, the radiograph is an absolute necessity.

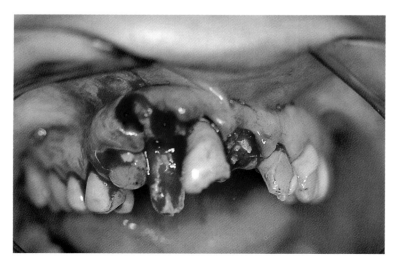 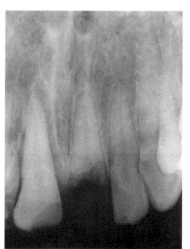

Intraoral Examination

In patients who are dentulous, observing the inter-cuspation of the teeth provides a very precise finding that helps to identify dislocations. It is imperative to take impressions of the jaws and to create a wax bite to record the existing occlusal relationship. Plaster models of the jaws are an important means of documentation in trauma cases. In edentulous jaws, the patient's prosthesis can also provide information about dislocation in the bones of the jaw. Dentures that have been fractured during the trauma incident should be available during the intraoral examination.

Clinical Tip
If there is suspicion of a jaw fracture, or apparently disturbed tooth contact, study models to check the occlusion must be prepared.

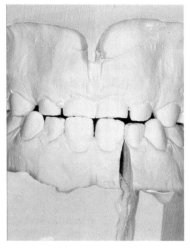
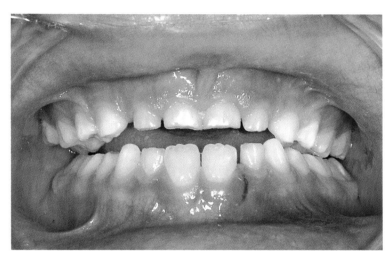

871 Occlusal disturbance
Occlusal disturbances are not easy to detect in cases of trauma, as the patient may position the jaw so as to avoid pain. Study models are absolutely necessary to evaluate the occlusion. The clinical view reveals step formation and false mobility of tooth 31 and deciduous tooth 72, with a premature tooth contact on the left side.

Left: In patients with occlusal steps, the model is duplicated, and then sawed apart in the fracture area. This allows the correct occlusion to be identified and re-established on the study models.

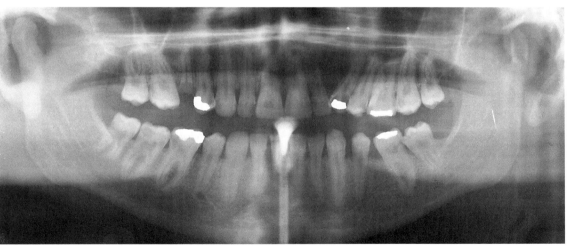

872 Panoramic radiograph
The panoramic film is the best way of obtaining an overview of the masticatory apparatus. Interruptions of the continuity of osseous structures can be detected, as well as displacements of the anatomical axes, as seen here in the bilateral fracture of the heads of the mandibular condyles at the temporomandibular joint.

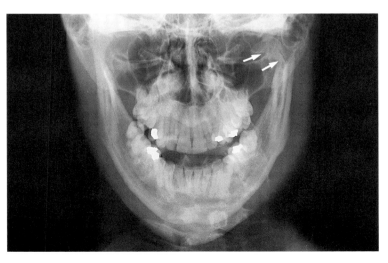

873 Posteroanterior skull radiograph
The second plane for depicting osseous injury to the mandible is provided by a posteroanterior mandibular radiograph, taken with the mouth maximally opened. Here, the dislocation of the left condyle in a median direction is easily seen (arrows).

Radiographic Examination

Although injury to bone often elicits clinical symptoms, only radiographs can provide direct confirmation. The anatomy of the skull has several typical predilection sites for fracture lines. The dentist or surgeon must have detailed knowledge of the osseous radiographic anatomy of the skull so as to be able to diagnose fractures using conventional radiographic methods.

Several basic principles must be followed without fail:
—Radiographs of a suspected skull injury must be taken in at least two planes.

—Selective radiographs should be made, depending on the suspected diagnosis (Machtens and Heuser 1991, Düker 1991).
—Computed tomography (CT) provides excellent information in all three planes; it can replace all other skull projections. The sections should be oriented axially (with the patient in the supine position) and, if possible, also coronally (with the patient positioned in the prone position). Sagittal sections are required for complete imaging of the temporomandibular joints.

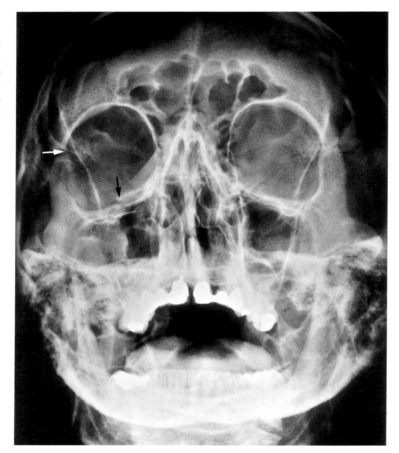

874 Injury to the midface—posteroanterior skull film
A posteroanterior skull radiograph is indicated in cases of facial fracture. Using this film, the trained eye can accurately observe the contours of the midface. Depicted here (arrow) is a fracture of the right zygomatic bone.

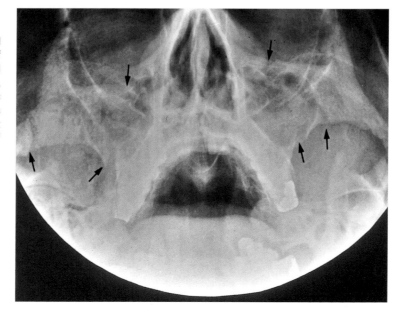

875 Fracture of the midface—semi-axial maxillary radiograph
This projection is especially useful for depicting injuries in the area of the midfacial skeleton, the lateral borders of the maxillary sinuses, the zygomatic bone, zygomatic arch, and the borders of the orbits (arrows). In this case, the patient had suffered a complex fracture of the midface.

Standard Radiographic Projections

Panoramic radiograph: An overview film that is useful for the horizontal ramus of the mandible and the zygomatic complex. The chin, temporomandibular joints, and midfacial region are difficult to evaluate.

Semiaxial skull projection: Excellent for the alveolar process, lateral walls of the maxillary sinuses, and the lateral and ventral regions of the orbit.

Axial skull projections: Favorable for evaluating the zygomatic bone, especially the zygomatic arch.

Lateral skull projection: provides good imaging of the frontal region, orbital complex, and alveolar processes. Fractures are not always well visualized.

Posteroanterior overview of the mandible with maximal mouth opening: Good for visualizing fracture lines and dislocations in the angle of the mandible, in the ascending ramus and the joint process, as well as the muscular process.

Laterally separated mandibular projection: For imaging the angle and ramus of the mandible.

Occlusal projections of maxilla and mandible: Good for detecting fracture lines in the chin region and canine area, as well as the canine fossa region.

Intraoral periapical films: for imaging dental injury, root fractures, and fractures of the alveolar process.

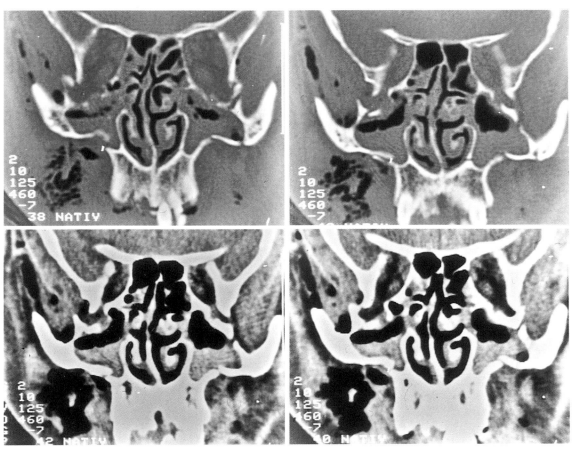

876 Computed tomogram (CT)
By changing the projection parameters, special views of bone and soft tissues can be achieved. The coronal section shows a massive impression in the midface in the so-called "bone window."

Below: Soft-tissue window. The same CT projection, this time showing the soft tissues, shows extensive emphysema in the soft tissues of the cheek on the left side.

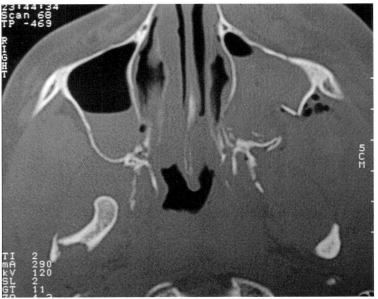

877 Computed tomogram (CT)
In cases of complex multiple injuries, only a CT can provide definitive information. For example, this axial projection shows destruction of the rear wall of the left sinus, fractures in the region of the pterygoid process bilaterally, bilateral sinus hemorrhage, and massive dislocation of the right temporomandibular joint process.

Injuries

Soft-Tissue Injuries

Depending on the causative agent, the following types of soft-tissue injury can be distinguished:
—Tear or crush wounds
—Laceration wounds
—Incision wounds
—Caustic burns (e.g., from acid contact)
—Burns
—Radiation injury
Depending on the type of tissue destruction, the following types of injury can be distinguished:
—Tissue loss defect
—Penetration from the oral cavity
—Penetration into bone
—Injury to vessels
—Injury to nerves (facial nerve)
—Injury to salivary ducts (e.g., the secretory ducts of the parotid gland and the submandibular gland)
—Foreign-body incorporation

Determining and defining the type of injury is very important for recognizing the etiology. A discrepancy between the type of injury and the patient's description of the accident may be of legal significance.

Dental Injuries

Injuries to the teeth are only described here in broad terms.

The teeth are often injured during trauma to the jaw region. Depending on the severity of the trauma, teeth may be directly affected, especially in the anterior region, or indirectly if the jaws are forced together. Damage to enamel and dentin may occur, as well as damage to the tooth root that is not clinically apparent, or combinations of the two. The initial examination should determine whether the pulp chamber is still covered by hard tissue. If the pulp has been opened, an infection can progress into the alveolar bone by way of the pulp canal. In addition to alleviating the patient's pain in such situations, immediate dental treatment should be carried out. An examination of a traumatized jaw must therefore also include an assessment of the condition of the individual teeth. This is done by checking the occlusion, palpating the individual teeth, checking for abnormal mobility, using the probe to detect defects of the tooth crowns, and finally by vitality testing. Doubtful teeth must be further assessed using intraoral radiographs to check for root fractures or the presence of root canal fillings.

Injuries to Bone

Direct and Indirect Injuries to Bone
Damage to underlying osseous structures usually does not occur without some sign of injury to the overlying soft tissues. However, in certain sites, osseous fracture can occur without direct impact.

A distinction is therefore made between direct and indirect injuries to bone. An example of indirect bone injury is temporomandibular joint fracture, where the force exerted usually impacts on the chin, and is transferred through the mandible to the joint processes, where the trauma actually occurs.

Dislocations
With injuries to bone, dislocation of the fragments usually occurs to a greater or lesser extent. In addition to the direct forces of the trauma, the muscle insertions on the individual areas of the bones may have a major role. Depending on the effect of the muscles, a distinction can be made between a favorable or unfavorable direction of the fracture line. When the fracture line is favorable, the muscles tend to hold the fragments in their normal position, and when it is unfavorable, the muscular effects tend to dislocate the sections of bone. Fracture of a bone without any dislocation and without severing of the periosteum is known as "greenstick fracture." The type and extent of dislocation have a critical role in the selection of the appropriate treatment.

Open and Closed Fractures
An open fracture is one in which the soft-tissue injury is such that bone is exposed to the environment. Open fractures involve increased susceptibility to infection, and appropriate antibiotic coverage is therefore indicated. Injury to oral tissues with penetration to the site of fracture, e.g., via the periodontal ligament space, is also referred to as open fracture.

Injury to Bone in Dentulous or Edentulous Jaw Segments
Injuries to bone in the jaw region are also classified in relation to the type and degree of dentulousness. Whether interarch occlusion is present or not is an important factor in selecting treatment. It is important to include the patient's removable prostheses in the overall assessment. Prostheses can usually be used for repositioning and stabilizing jaw fractures.

Temporomandibular Joint Fracture

Temporomandibular joint fractures usually occur as a result of secondary forces, i.e., a blow to the chin with forces transferred to the condylar heads. The degree of dentulousness and the position of the mandible when the trauma occurs affect the direction of force transmission: edentia and an open mouth allow forces to be transmitted directly to the temporomandibular joint structures. However, if the mouth is closed and teeth are present, a more likely sequela is injury to the teeth themselves.

Clinical and Radiographic Findings
Clinical:
—Tear or crush wounds in the chin region
—Pressure sensitivity, with possible swelling of the affected temporomandibular joint
—Condyle not palpable, or without movement during mandibular excursions, including protrusion
—Deviation of the mandible toward the affected side during opening
—Lack of occlusal contact on the healthy side
—Displacement of the midline toward the affected side

Radiographic:
—Axis deviation on the affected side
—Dislocation of the condyle
—Fracture lines in the mandible
—Axis deviation of the articular process

In cases of bilateral fracture of the condyle, mouth opening and mandibular excursions are often symmetrically inhibited with temporomandibular joint pain. The occlusion usually shows a retruded position of the mandible with an anterior open bite.

When fractures in the temporomandibular joint region occur, injury to the external auditory canal may also occur. Trauma to, or perforation of, the very thin condylar fossa is also possible. Any signs or symptoms of injuries that are difficult to diagnose require the participation of an appropriate specialist during the clinical evaluation.

Caution
Temporomandibular joint fractures in children are often symptom-free. Mouth opening may not be inhibited.

TMJ Luxation

A spring-like fixation of part of the temporomandibular joint in an abnormal position is referred to as luxation. Temporomandibular joint luxation may be unilateral, bilateral, habitual, or traumatic.

Clinical Tip
Radiography can never provide definitive information about temporomandibular joint luxation. The clinical findings are decisive.

Disk Luxation

There may be lateral, anterior, medial, or posterior dislocation of the articular disk. The function of the temporomandibular joint will be correspondingly inhibited. This condition is usually unilateral, with the disk dislocated anteriorly or sometimes posteriorly.

After extended dental treatment with the patient's mouth maximally opened, pressure damage to the articular disk can occur, with resultant inhibition of the functional translation movement within the temporomandibular joint. Normal mandibular function will only return when the dislocated disk is repositioned, and this can also happen spontaneously. If this occurs repeatedly, there may be excessive distension of the ligaments, and temporary stabilization of the temporomandibular joint may be necessary.

Anterior luxation: Limitation of jaw opening (often in the morning, especially in patients with nocturnal bruxism and clenching parafunctions); this can be painful. There will be deviation of the mandible toward the affected side during jaw opening and attempts at mandibular translation.

Posterior luxation: Jaw closure may be painful or even impossible, and there may be a slight open bite in the posterior segments. Some difficulty with mouth opening may be observed.

Diagnostic measures may include radiography (arthrography) and CT or magnetic resonance imaging (MRI).

Radiation Injury

Radiotherapy is still a treatment of choice for malignant tumors in the orofacial region. The adverse effects of radiotherapy depend on the radiation dose affecting the local tissues. Long-lasting and irreversible injury to teeth, soft tissue and bone can be expected.

Injury to Bone
Ionizing radiation causes damage especially to the intima layer of blood vessels, and this leads to circulatory disturbances. In the bones of the jaw regions, this often leads to necrosis (osteoradionecrosis). Natural reparative processes are either completely lacking or delayed, and the host defense mechanisms are impaired. Irreversible damage to bone must be expected at doses higher than 50 Gy.

Injury to Soft Tissues
Soft tissues are also injured by ionizing radiation. This leads to a reduction in saliva flow (due to atrophy of the acini) and to inflammatory atrophy of the oral mucosa, sometimes even with ulceration (radiation stomatitis). Caries activity increases significantly. For all these reasons, it is necessary to eliminate any potential or obvious sources of infection (foci) before radiotherapy in the head and neck region is carried out.

As the time between the diagnosis of a tumor and the initiation of radiotherapy is often short, dental treatment in the affected jaw segments cannot always be performed.

Our clinical criteria for detecting foci of infection before radiotherapy are given on pages 20 and 55. Planned treatment measures should be discussed in advance with the radiotherapist. Once the radiotherapist has planned the procedure, the precise zones that will fall within the field of irradiation can be identified. Modern radiotherapy techniques allow precise delineation of the radiation field and prediction of the expected dose in the area affected.

It is advisable to establish the procedure firmly before, during, and after radiation treatment in each individual case. Long-term care of such patients (recall) must be ensured, despite the fact that some patients show insufficient cooperation. It is the task of the dental therapist to provide knowledge and understanding as well as a feeling of empathy for the patients concerned, who are likely to have priorities other than their dental treatment.

Preparations for Reimplantation

Local anesthesia should be administered, followed by careful cleaning of the alveolus, including removal of the coagulum and any bone fragments or foreign bodies.

Careful cleaning of the tooth using only physiological saline solution. Do not use disinfecting agents, as they have necrotizing effects on the remaining periodontal tissues.

Repositioning the tooth: depending on the occlusal situation, the tooth is manually repositioned into its alveolus.

Fixation: the stabilization must allow physiological mobility of the reimplanted tooth. Rigid fixation carries a risk of root resorption and ankylosis. Fixation is maintained for two weeks, followed by stepwise detachment at the individual sites, and complete splint removal after four weeks.

Systemic antibiotic coverage is indicated (p. 331).

Follow-up: the clinical and radiographic signs and symptoms determine the need for additional measures.

Endodontic Therapy

When a tooth is reimplanted, a root canal filling should never be carried out immediately, as this reduces the chances of pulpal regeneration and maintenance of the periapical periodontal tissues. Endodontic therapy is only indicated after the first signs of pulpal necrosis. If root growth is complete, the first stage of endodontic therapy involves placing calcium hydroxide treatment paste. The calcium hydroxide acts as a mild chemical irritant, inducing regenerative processes within the pulpal and periodontal tissues. Information about the condition of the pulp can be obtained from clinical findings such as sensitivity to percussion or heat, and radiographically by the appearance of widening of the apical periodontal ligament space, or osteolysis indicating an inflammatory process or an infection. Small areas of root resorption can be identified radiographically after three or four weeks. If the condition is noninflammatory, any incipient resorption can be reversed by immediate therapy, including slight movement of the tooth and loosening of its fixation.

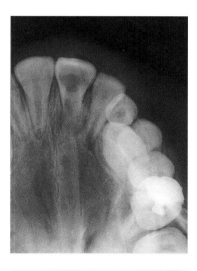
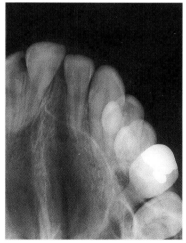
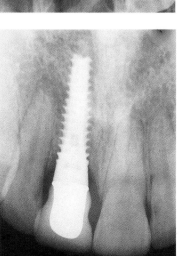
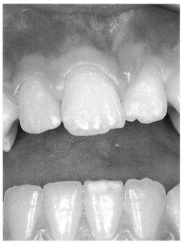
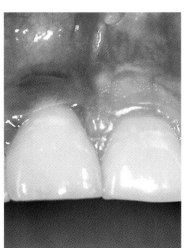
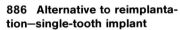

885 Alternative to reimplantation—space closure
To avoid the need for a conventional fixed bridge, the alternative solutions of closing the space by orthodontic movement of the adjacent teeth and aesthetic crown recontouring, or an aesthetic build-up, can be considered. This approach requires a precise and comprehensive orthodontic consultation.

Left: Resorption of the reimplanted tooth 21.

Center: Radiographic appearance.

Right: Clinical view.

886 Alternative to reimplantation—single-tooth implant
This type of treatment requires a comprehensive, full-mouth treatment plan.

Left: Radiographic view one year after the loss of tooth 11, showing osseous regeneration.

Center: Periapical radiograph two years after placement of a dental implant.

Right: Clinical view two years after implant placement.

Insurance Matters

General

Not all oral surgery procedures are covered by a patient's medical insurance policies or government-provided benefits (e.g., Medicare-Medicaid). Industry and government regulations concerning payments for oral surgery procedures vary widely within the insurance industry, from state to state, and from country to country internationally. In the broadest sense, the holder of an "accident insurance policy" can expect the insurer to pay for oral surgery services rendered if the "preponderance of the evidence" demonstrates that these services were, in fact, necessary because of an accident. When payment is requested from an insurer, the request must therefore be accompanied by a plausible and convincing description of the accident.

Injuries During Mastication

The teeth are routinely exposed to numerous mechanical, chemical, and thermal influences. These influences cannot be regarded as falling into the category of "uncommon" in most insurers' definition of an accident. Fractures of the teeth that occur during mastication cannot therefore always be classified as accidents. The actions of the teeth during the chewing of foodstuffs are intentional, and therefore not uncommon. It is quite normal for people to use the teeth for chewing food, for gnawing on bones or to separate fruit from pits, but not to attempt to actually chew on bones or fruit pits or seeds. Unintentional biting on a hard substance within a foodstuff may be defined as "uncommon," and can therefore be categorized as an accident. On the other hand, insurers may differentiate between injuries resulting from biting on substances that are naturally part of foodstuffs, on the one hand, and biting on unexpected or uncommon substances on the other (Heusser 1987). In layman's terms, this means that all substances usually found within or on common foodstuffs do not qualify as uncommon factors in the sense of causative agents in an accident.

Additional Questions

What about situations in which an injury to a patient's health can only *partly* be attributed to an accident? What if an accident merely worsens a preexisting condition? Should medical and accident insurance pay the entire cost of treatment in such cases? The answer to this question will vary considerably from insurer to insurer, and certainly also from country to country.

What about questions concerning remuneration for pain, suffering, reduced quality of life, or the reduced ability to enjoy life? The financial responsibility of insurers may vary, depending on the severity of the extraneous consequences of an injury. With regard to dental injuries, remuneration for pain, suffering, etc., may only be forthcoming if the consequences are considerable and of long duration. Here again, the decision to pay or not to pay, as well as the scale of coverage, can vary considerably, and any preexisting condition may play an important role. Severe dental defects and posttraumatic jaw deformities that can be treated unsatisfactorily or not at all may serve as valid reasons for increased levels of payment. The same may apply to any accident-related reduction in chewing capacity or aesthetic impairment resulting from dental defects (Wüthrich 1987).

In summary: before providing treatment—except in acute circumstances—it is advisable for oral surgeon to clarify whether or not treatment falls into the applicable private or public insurance coverage system.

Antibiotics and Root Resorptions

After the reimplantation of luxated teeth, one factor that can lead to failure is progressive root resorption. If the surgeon is successful in preventing such resorption, healing of the periodontium can occur. In addition to maintaining the periodontal soft tissues on the root surface before reimplantation, the use of systemic antibiotics also appears to inhibit root resorption (Hammarström et al. 1986). However, if root resorption has already begun, antibiotic therapy will not serve to stop it.

Andreasen (1993) recommended the simultaneous use of systemic and topical doxycycline in tooth reimplantation. No data or precise information concerning the optimum choice of antibiotics, the dosage, or the duration of such treatment are available. In any case, however, it is reasonable to provide antibiotic coverage in cases of attempted tooth reimplantation.

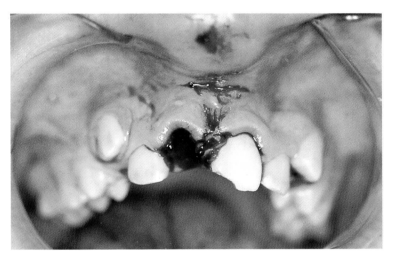

887 Total luxation of tooth 11
This 14-year-old boy had fallen while ice-skating, causing the total luxation of tooth 11 and subluxation of tooth 21, with fracture of the incisal edge. The boy was treated more than an hour after the accident; he brought tooth 11 wrapped in a moist cloth. Apart from a crush injury to the upper lip, there were no other injuries discernible.

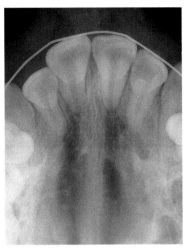

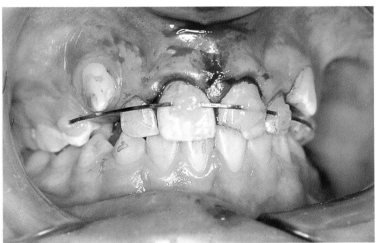

888 Preparing for reimplantation
After administration of local anesthesia, both the tooth and the alveolus were carefully cleaned. Using only finger pressure, teeth 11 and 21 were repositioned in such a way that proper centric occlusion was achieved. An arch bar was formed using a square stock, and attached using cement on teeth 14 through 24.

Left: Radiograph taken immediately after splint application. Note that apical root growth is not yet complete.

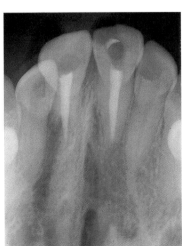

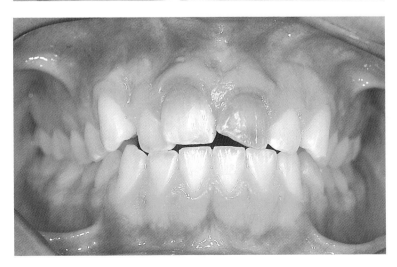

889 Clinical course
Ten days after the accident, the pulps of teeth 11 and 21 were opened, and calcium hydroxide treatments were applied. Permanent root canal fillings for both teeth were carried out four months later. The clinical picture shows severe darkening of both teeth, which can be referred to as "natural temporaries."

Left: The radiograph shows advanced resorption of the tooth roots. It was possible to retain the teeth until the patient was 20 years old, when definitive treatment was planned.

Fixation Splints

The fixation of luxated and reimplanted teeth must allow for a certain degree of physiological mobility. For this purpose, a cemented external arch wire or a custom acrylic splint can be used if the occlusal situation permits (sufficient space on the palatal aspect).

Caution
Manipulations on deciduous teeth can cause subsequent damage to the permanent teeth. Whenever a deciduous tooth suffers trauma, periodic examination should be carried out until the time of eruption of the permanent teeth in order to assess any possible consequences of the trauma.

Clinical Tip
An external arch secured with wire ligatures is not indicated for fixation of reimplanted teeth, since the ligatures pull the arch marginally, and if the wire ligature is reinforced with acrylic, it produces rigid fixation. An external arch of this type should only be used for fixation in cases of fracture of the alveolar process.

890   Instruments and material for preparing a cemented splint
Acid gel for enamel cauterization, light-hardening composite material, quadratic arch wire, cement spatula, pointed pliers, side-cutter, and plugger.

Right: The clinical photographs show that teeth 21 and 22 have been luxated.

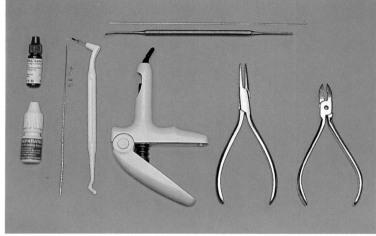
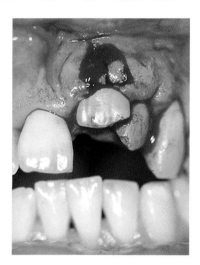

891   Clinical procedure
The arch wire is adapted free of tension to the buccal tooth surfaces, which are then prepared to receive the splint by cauterization of the cleaned and dried enamel surfaces. The areas of attachment on the teeth and splint are painted with composite resin. Polymerization of the acrylic to attach the splint is started on the healthy teeth.

Right: The luxated teeth are repositioned using finger pressure, and then attached to the splint.

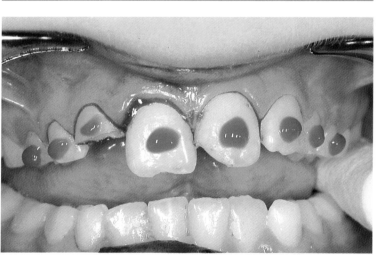
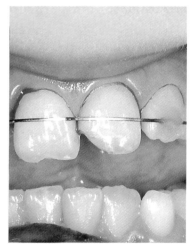

892   Removal of the splint
After about three weeks, the side-cutter can be used to release the mounds of acrylic from the wire, and a rotating abrasive disk can then be used to remove any remaining acrylic from the tooth surfaces.

Right: The tooth surfaces must also be carefully polished.

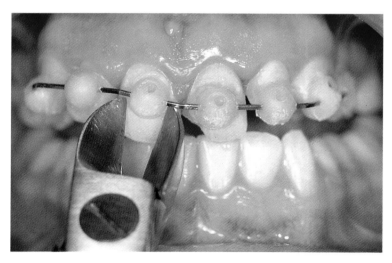
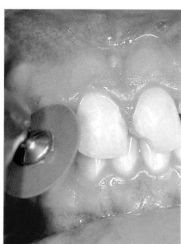

Treatment of Bone Fractures

The treatment of complex fractures of the maxilla and mandible, including Le Fort I, II, III, and multiple fractures should be carried out by a maxillofacial surgeon. Contemporary treatment approaches today involve primary treatment with reconstruction of the facial skeleton in all three dimensions (Rowe and Williams 1985, Sailer and Grätz 1991, Schuchardt 1966). Treatment of this type should never be rendered on an outpatient basis in a private practice.

Maxillary Fractures

Maxillary fractures are classified according to the facial region affected:

—Central midface fracture: Le Fort I, II, III
—Lateral midface fractures: zygoma, zygomatic arch,
                                                 and combinations

Midface fractures are often complex fractures. The diagnosis must be precise and comprehensive.

Clinical Tip
Fractures of the maxilla are usually complex, and should be treated only by specialists.

Fractures of the Alveolar Process

Even in adults, luxated teeth should be retained as long as possible until the fracture line has healed. Reimplantation of teeth makes it easier to reposition the bone fragments and to fix them in the original position. In the case of isolated fractures of the alveolar process, intermaxillary fixation is not necessary. For immobilization of alveolar process fractures, an external arch bar attached using cement or wire ligatures is indicated. In individual cases, it may be necessary to carry out open fracture reduction, with fixation using miniplates or microplates.

The ability to chew will be restricted, and a soft diet is indicated for a three-week period. The patient should receive weekly check-up appointments so that any infection of the remaining teeth can be identified and treated.

Mandibular Fractures

Location
Mandibular fractures are classified according to the typical locations of the fracture line, as shown in Figure 893.

1 Fracture in the anterior segment. The genioglossus muscle tends to dislocate the fractured segment dorsally.

2 Fracture in the canine region (long root).

3 Fracture of the horizontal ramus. The mylohyoid muscle tends to dislocate the fractured segment medially.

4 Fracture at the angle of the mandible. Dislocation may be caused by the masseter muscle, the temporal muscle, or the medial pterygoid muscle (Fig. 896).

5 Fracture of the ascending ramus between the angle of the mandible and the semilunar suture. Dislocations will occur due to pulling from the masseter muscle, the medial pterygoid, and the temporal muscle.

6 Fracture of the articular process. The lateral pterygoid muscle will dislocate medially.

7 Fracture of the coronoid process. Dislocation by the temporal muscle.

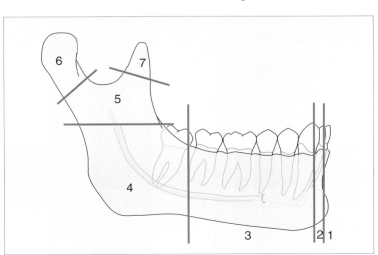

893 Classification of mandibular fractures—location

1 Anterior region
2 Canine region
3 Horizontal ramus
4 Angle of the mandible
5 Ascending ramus
6 Articular process
7 Coronoid process

Type of Fracture

The type of the fracture involved is also classified. It depends on the type and direction of the impact force applied (blunt, hard, rapid, slow).

F1 Simple fracture with or without dislocation. Usually easy to reposition manually.

F2 Multiple fractures. Depending on the type of dislocation, simple manual repositioning may suffice, or open surgical repositioning of the fragments may be necessary.

F3 Comminuted fracture, with numerous fracture lines and isolated osseous fragments. This type of fracture has to be treated surgically for repositioning and fixation.

F4 Multiple fracture lines with loss of substance and lack of continuity. These are complex fractures that require comprehensive reconstruction.

Additional Criteria

Occlusion:
0 = No occlusal disturbance.
1 = Maxillary/mandibular tooth contacts are disturbed.
2 = Edentulous mandible.

Soft tissues:
1 = Mucosal tear up to the fracture site.
2 = Tear or crush wound externally up to the fracture site.
3 = Combination of 1 and 2.
4 = Soft-tissue defect up to the bone; primary closure not possible.

894 Types of dislocation and fragments

F1 Simple fracture
F2 Compound fracture

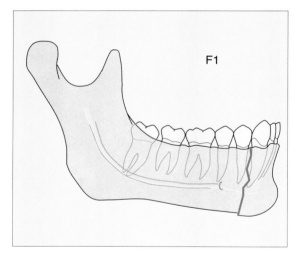
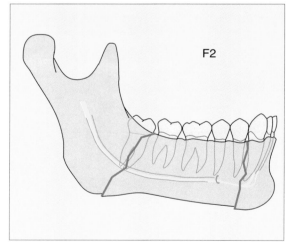

895 Types of dislocation and fragments

F3 Compound, comminuted fracture
F4 Fracture with defect

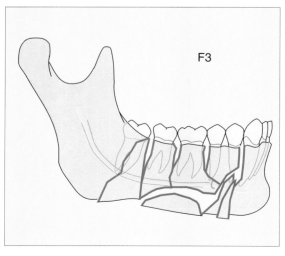
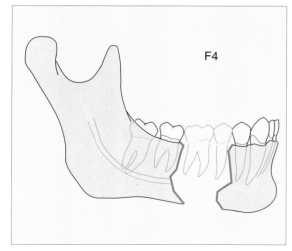

Surgical (Open) Fracture Treatment with Osteosynthesis

Consideration should always be given to the surgical repositioning and fixation of osseous fragments using screws and plates (Hardt 1986, Schmoker et al. 1983). The treatment is performed on an in-patient basis, but postoperative intermaxillary fixation is often not necessary.

Conservative Treatment of Fracture

This usually involves manual repositioning, with stabilization using intermaxillary fixation. At least half of the maxillary arch must be intact, since it serves as the basis for stabilization of the mandible. If the maxilla is mobile, immobilization can also be achieved using interskeletal fixation around the intact zygomatic arch or other intact osseous structures of the facial skeleton. However, these procedures usually require general anesthesia.

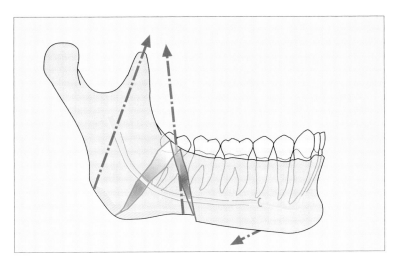

896 Fracture at the angle of the mandible—muscle pulling
Depending on the location of the fracture line, the bone fragments will either be dislocated or repositioned by tension from the masseter muscle and the medial pterygoid muscle, as well as the temporal muscle and the muscles of the floor of the mouth.
Red: Favorable fracture lines.
Blue: Unfavorable fracture lines.

Criteria for Evaluating Potential Treatments

It is not possible to establish absolute treatment guidelines for selecting either surgical or conservative methods. The advantages and disadvantages should be considered in each individual case.

	Conservative	Osteo-synthesis		Conservative	Osteo-synthesis
Dentulous	X		Open fractures	X	X
Edentulous		X			
Stable occlusion	X		Closed fractures	X	
Disturbed occlusion, step formation	X	X	Tooth in fracture line	X	X
Simple dislocation, manually repositionable	X		Tooth bud in fracture area	X	
Fragment formation, defects		X	Fractures within the dental arch	X	
Favorable fracture line	X		Fractures outside the dental arch	X	X
Unfavorable fracture line		X			

Intermaxillary Stabilization
(Conservative Treatment)

Using models as a guide, manual repositioning and intermaxillary fixation provide almost rigid stabilization of the bone fragments in dentulous patients. Fracture healing takes three or four weeks.

With intermaxillary fixation in place, adequate oral hygiene is difficult. Nevertheless, intensive hygiene measures should be observed (p. 343).

Clinical Tip
Emergency dental treatment measures (e.g., endodontic treatment, treatment for tooth fractures) must be carried out before splint therapy. The patient must be informed about the potential methods of conservative treatment as well as surgical treatment for the fracture.

Even though intermaxillary fixation over extended periods of time is not necessary for osteosynthesis, in simple fracture situations the more conservative treatment should be considered. It can be regarded as the treatment of choice.

Clinical Tip
Patients who are treated with complete intermaxillary fixation should be advised to remain at home (off work) for the entire duration.

Nutrition During Intermaxillary Fixation

An important problem for patients with intermaxillary fixation is their nutrition (Perko 1966, Spiessl 1975). Associated problems include the lack of hygiene with oral wounds and the ingestion of qualitatively and quantitatively appropriate nutrition. In patients with a complete dentition, taking sufficient food is especially difficult during the period of intermaxillary fixation. Special cups and straws used lateral to the dental arches allow liquid diets to be taken.

Nevertheless, only a limited amount of nutrition per meal can be taken in, and additional between-meal eating is therefore needed.

The patient must be informed about the necessary shift to a liquid diet, and also must be given information about a balanced diet.

If surgical wounds are exposed in the oral cavity, a diet of only pure liquids should be taken on the first postoperative day: tea, coffee, mineral water, fruit juices and bouillon.

Viscous substances, such as bread, potatoes, pasta, rice, salad, creamed vegetables, or milk and egg dishes are inappropriate.

If there are no open wounds, or in any case on the second postoperative day, the following regimen is appropriate: five or six meals per day in the form of soups, milk shakes, or blended liquids. These can be prepared and seasoned according to individual taste. Appropriate foods include meat, poultry, and vegetable soups, vegetable puree, mashed potatoes, baby food, fruit puree, fruit cocktail (vitamin C), milk shakes, chocolate drinks, and yogurt.

All meals can have butter, margarine, cream, sugar and honey added to enhance the energy content.

Supplementary vitamins and trace elements are needed if intermaxillary fixation continues for more than three or four weeks.

Splints

Splints that are used in outpatient surgery on the teeth must be atraumatic, gentle on the periodontal tissues, hygienic, sufficiently stable, and easy to apply (Obwegeser 1952). We have found the following types of splints useful for conservative treatment of fractures.

Wire loop splint: useful for fractures of the jaw, for fixation of intermaxillary elastic or wire ligatures; in complete dentition, partial edentia with stable occlusion, or individually missing teeth.

Acrylic splints: useful for alveolar process fractures, tooth luxation without intermaxillary fixation (for isolated intramaxillary fixation).

External arch bar: this can be attached with ligatures or reinforced with acrylic resin, or both; applicable in partial edentia, with intermaxillary fixation, rubber bands or wire.

Prosthesis splint: useful for fractures of the alveolar process and simple jaw fractures; it must be attached to the remaining dentition or using perimandibular wires.

Cast cap splint: useful for bilateral temporomandibular joint fractures with massive eccentric movements and a tendency toward open bite; it can be left in situ for several months.

Caution
When a splint is being placed or removed, injury to the teeth, periodontal structures, or restorations can occur. Patients must be informed about this, and any apparent risks should be documented.

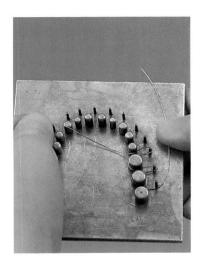
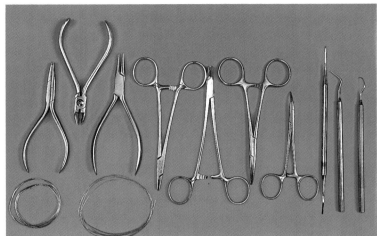

897 Instruments for making a wire loop splint
Pointed pliers, side-cutter, flat pliers with groove, wire clamp, wire loop pliers, curved clamp (large and small), plugger, blunt probe, scaler, soft steel wire (0.5 mm).

Left: The 0.5-mm wire is pre-stressed and arranged with appropriate bends. A metal template with pegs for the appropriate tooth sizes is helpful for preparing the wire.

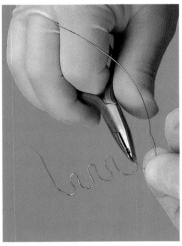
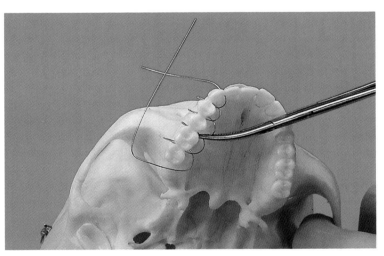

898 Creating the eyes
Flat pliers are used to compress the loops that were created on the template, and tip them vertically *(left)*.

A large, curved clamp is used to insert the eyes through the interdental spaces *(right)*. The distal end of the wire is passed around to the buccal aspect and through the various eyes. The two ends of the wire are then temporarily and loosely twisted together.

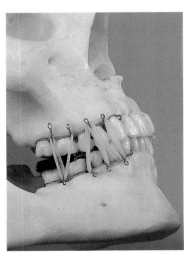
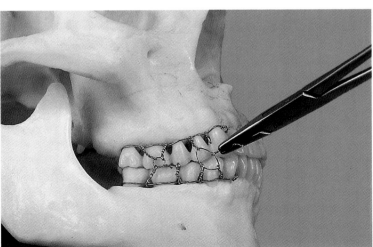

899 Completing the fixation
Under constant tension from the clamp, the eye is grasped and twisted definitively. Kinking must be avoided when the wires are being manipulated in this way.

Left: The eyes can also serve as retentive elements for intermaxillary fixation using elastic.

Further Treatment after Intermaxillary Fixation

Three to four weeks later, after healing has been checked radiographically, the intermaxillary fixation is gradually released. Mandibular function is reinstituted over a period of one or two weeks.

In the absence of any complications, the splint is definitively removed a week later. Professional tooth cleaning for prophylactic purposes should be carried out immediately after the splint is removed. As soon as the mouth can be opened sufficiently (30 mm), definitive dental treatment can be initiated.

For the first two weeks after splint removal, nutrition should be limited to soft foods. Stable and centric occlusion, and increasing normalization of mandibular function, should be documented at weekly appointments.

If limited ability to open the mouth persists, the ensuing two-week period should include energetic exercise by the patient using mouth-opening instruments (Heister) or wooden tongue blades, and the results should be documented daily. If no definitive progress is made, the patient should be referred to a specialist.

Clinical and radiographic check-ups should be made at six and 12 months.

900 Conservative fracture treatment
The diagram shows a fully dentulous mandible with multiple fractures and dislocated fragments. Note in particular the fracture lines between the teeth in the arch.

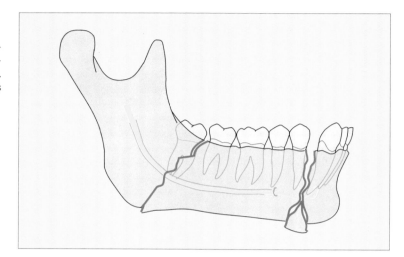

901 Repositioning using elastic
After seating a twisted wire splint in both the maxilla and mandible, rubber bands are placed to reposition the bony segments. It is often necessary to apply manual pressure to reposition the fractured segments and achieve proper occlusal relationships.

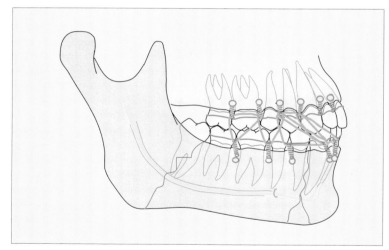

902 Intermaxillary fixation
After one or two days, the repositioning achieved by the rubber bands should be complete. The wire loops are then tipped occlusally, and wire ligatures are used to establish secure intermaxillary fixation. Three of the wire eyes are connected with a single wire ligature (0.5 mm). At weekly intervals, clinical check-ups are carried out for any loosening of the fixation, and the patient's oral hygiene is checked during the course of the healing process.

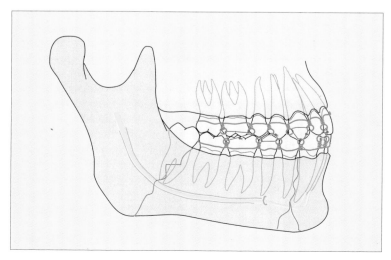

Treatment of Fractures in Deciduous and Mixed Dentition

The diagnosis and treatment of fractures occurring during jaw growth have a special place in oral surgery (Hardt and Von Arx 1989a). Special consideration has to be given to the stage of the dentition and the presence of dental primordia. In most cases, conservative methods of treating the fracture are preferable to open osteosynthesis.

In small children, conservative methods involving perimandibular ligatures for fixation of an acrylic splint can still be used to stabilize mandibular fractures.

There has been renewed interest in osteosynthesis procedures using miniplates and microplates screwed onto the cortical bone in children, because these methods seldom cause damage to tooth buds.

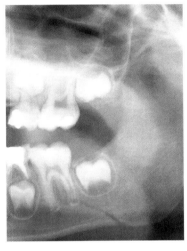
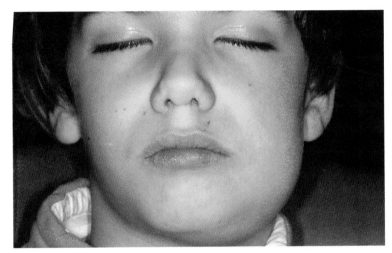

903 Fracture during the mixed dentition stage
This eight-year-old boy experienced trauma during judo training. He presented with swelling of the left side of the mandible.

Left: This detail of a panoramic radiograph shows a fracture at the angle of the mandible, but no dislocation.

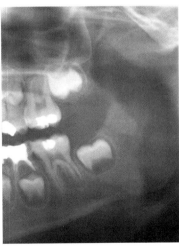
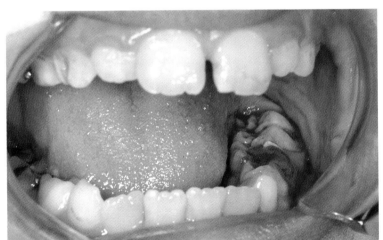

904 Intraoral findings
The patient experienced difficulty in opening the mouth, and there was deviation to the right. It was possible to achieve centric occlusion when the jaws were closed.

Left: This detail of a panoramic radiograph shows progressive healing of the fracture only three weeks after the start of treatment.

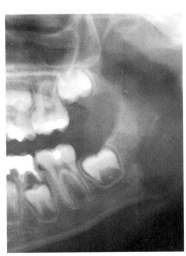
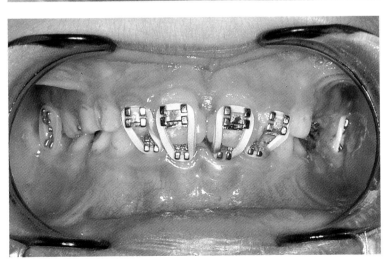

905 Fixation using elastic
For a three-week period, intermaxillary fixation with rubber bands ensured immobilization of the fracture. Retentive brackets were cemented to the incisors and the first permanent molars to receive the rubber bands. Three weeks later, the fixation devices were removed, and it was possible to check the fracture clinically.

Left: This radiograph was taken six months later. The fracture line can no longer be identified.

Treatment of Teeth in the Fracture Line

Controversy continues over whether or not a tooth located in a fracture line can be left in place (Shetty and Freymiller 1989). In 1970, Killey proposed a differentiated procedure. He suggested that only those teeth that had been rendered nonvital by the fracture should be removed. In 1974, Converse favored the removal of impacted teeth located in fracture lines before repositioning and fixation. If teeth have no apparent periodontal or apical infection, leaving them in place within a fracture line does not appear to influence the frequency of subsequent infection (Kamboozia et al.

1993, Marker et al. 1994, Neal et al. 1978).

Teeth with evident pathological involvement (periodontal pockets, periodontitis, apical osteitis, or cysts) represent an infection risk and must be removed. However, if removing this type of tooth would involve additional problems—such as making it impossible to reposition and fix the bone fragments, or a risk of additional dislocation, nerve damage, etc.—the tooth may be temporarily left in place. Systemic antibiotic coverage is absolutely required.

906 Fracture in the permanent dentition
This panoramic radiograph shows a fracture line coursing vertically in the region of tooth 45 in this 39-year-old man who had fallen on his chin. Mandibular continuity is not disrupted, and there is no dislocation of the fragments. However, note the fracture of the condylar process on the left side, with dislocation of the peripheral fragment axially and caudally.

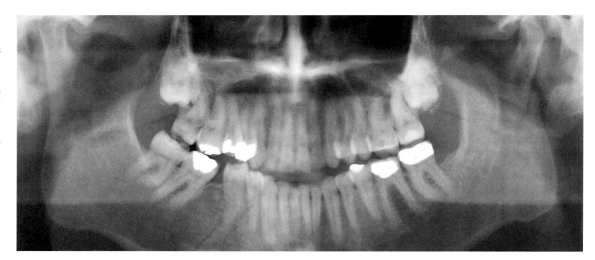

907 Intermaxillary fixation
Repositioning was achieved manually, and the teeth were kept in occlusion using intermaxillary fixation for four weeks.

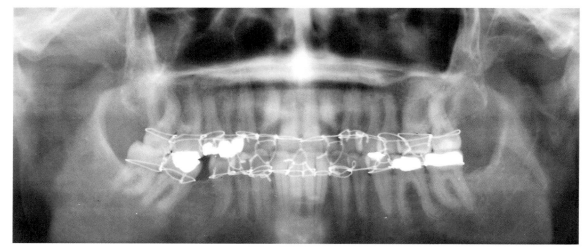

908 Clinical course
This panoramic radiograph shows the situation six months later. Complete osseous restructuring near tooth 45 has occurred, and normal vitality of all teeth was maintained. Osseous restructuring occurred in the condylar region on the left side, and the movement of the mandible was normal.

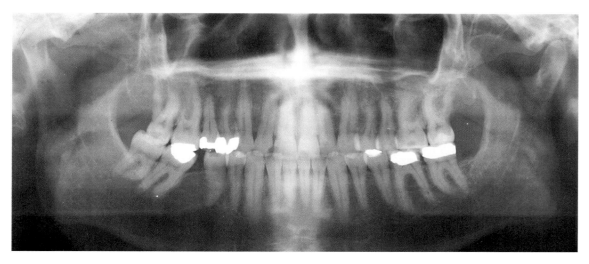

Treatment of Fractures in the temporomandibular joint Region

Conservative treatment by securing the occlusion and providing stabilization, with subsequent functional therapy, is associated with the fewest complications. If treatment is properly carried out in the individual case, late sequelae such as arthrosis or ankylosis are rare (Schmidt and Luhr 1976, Takenoshita et al. 1990, Kristen and Singer 1976, Zou et al. 1987).

There has been a recent trend toward surgical treatment of temporomandibular joint fractures. Since it is very difficult to achieve precise repositioning of the fragments, and because the blood supply to the area may be compromised by surgical exposure of the fragments, subsequent disturbances of joint function due to necrosis of the fragments cannot be excluded.

Unilateral intracapsular fractures:
—Stabilization for up to two weeks
—Avoid even minor additional trauma
—Possible use of muscle relaxants or analgesics
—Functional therapy after releasing the fixations

Unilateral extracapsular fractures:
—48-hr distraction of the joint with a hypomochlion
—Stabilization of the jaws for three weeks

—Maintenance of the vertical dimension
—Ensure and maintain occlusion
—Exercise therapy after releasing the fixations

Fracture of the condylar head in young patients: this situation requires long-term follow-up to check for appropriate development of the affected side.
Temporomandibular joint fractures in children: up to eight years of age, patients often require only functional treatment (monoblock), since during the mixed dentition stage, it is often impossible to secure the occlusal relationship. In addition, rapid healing processes usually obviate the need for stabilization.

Treatment of Bilateral Fracture of the Condylar Head

These fractures are associated with a tendency toward caudal malpositioning of the mandible, and therefore often require additional measures for repositioning, as well as appropriate follow-up observations.

Caution
Bilateral fractures of this type are associated with a special set of problems. They should be treated only by specialists.

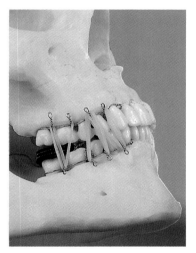
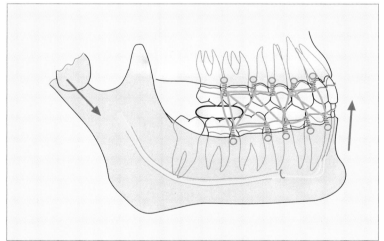

909 Temporomandibular joint fracture with distraction of the condyle
Rubber bands and an interocclusal rubber hypomochlion are used to achieve distraction within the right temporomandibular joint. This compensates for the shortening of the joint support on the right side.

Left: This skull preparation shows the wire splint with rubber bands and the hypomochlion in place. Rubber bands are placed more densely in the anterior area to increase the pulling force on the mandible.

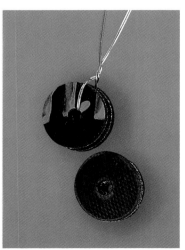
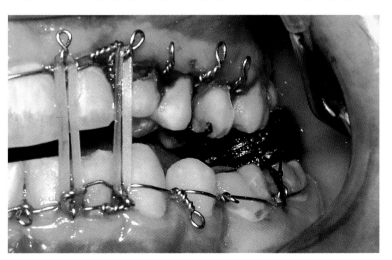

910 Hypomochlion
In this 36-year-old woman, splinting and rubber bands were used, with a rubber ring (hypomochlion) shown in place.

Left: The hypomochlion consists of hard rubber, and should always be attached in the mouth using a wire ligature to prevent swallowing or aspiration.

Treatment for temporomandibular joint Luxation

Repositioning

Repositioning is carried out manually. If this simple procedure fails to achieve proper positioning, mechanical repositioning can be attempted by placing a hypomochlion in the molar region and applying elastics in the anterior segment to counteract the forces exerted by muscles. Repositioning of the condyle usually has to be carried out within a few hours of the luxation. In difficult cases, manual repositioning may have to be carried out under general anesthesia, with muscle relaxants.

Fixation

After repositioning, intermaxillary fixation for one to two weeks will prevent recurrence and provide stabilization of the overstretched tissues.

In uncomplicated cases, fixation using rubber bands for one or two days is usually sufficient, followed by replacement using wire fixation as soon as the occlusion can be properly aligned. Elastics should not be left in place for more than a week in patients with healthy periodontal conditions, because otherwise the constant forces might actually supererupt the teeth.

911 Condylar fracture
This 44-year-old man had suffered a blow to the chin, fracturing the condylar head on the right side. The panoramic radiograph shows the situation immediately before splinting. Treatment consisted of repositioning and reestablishing the occlusion using rubber bands and a hypomochlion, with subsequent intermaxillary wire fixation for stabilization over a two-week period.

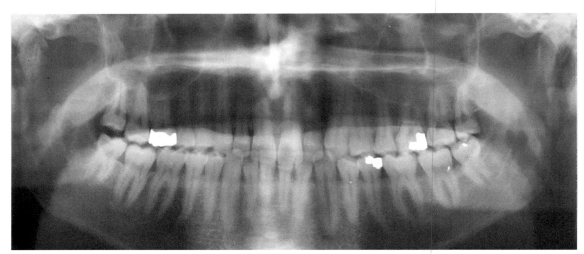

912 Functional physiotherapy after splint removal
Energetic exercises should be carried out to retrain the patient for mandibular movements. The patient can gradually extend the ability to open the mouth by biting on successively larger numbers of tongue blades *(right)*. The patient should keep a record of the extent of mouth-opening ability both morning and evening.

If self-training does not lead to reestablishment of satisfactory mouth opening after a few days, Heister's spring-loaded mouth-opening device *(left)* may be useful.

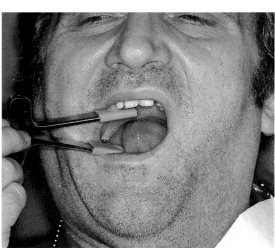 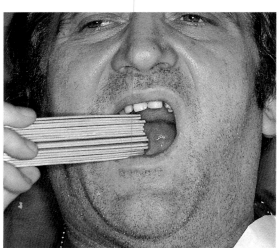

913 Clinical course
This panoramic radiograph shows the situation immediately after splint removal. The condylar process has returned to its normal position. The goal of the treatment was ultimately to achieve normal mandibular movement. In contrast to other fractures, no effort is made to reposition the bone fragments to enhance osseous consolidation.

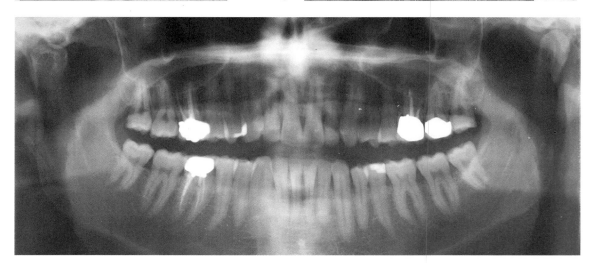

Oral Hygiene When the Jaws Are Wired Shut

In these cases, access to the teeth for oral hygiene (with a toothbrush) is severely restricted, and the patient is normally ingesting a calorie-rich, cariogenic diet. It is therefore necessary to initiate special measures for plaque control. Failing this, there is a risk of dental caries and gingival inflammation.

Oral Hygiene Measures

Patients should be advised to brush the buccal surfaces of the teeth three times daily using a small toothbrush (e.g., a children's toothbrush) and dentifrice. After each meal, patients should rinse with a commercially available chlorhexidine solution.

After removal of the splint, or if the splints are left in place for more than four weeks, professional tooth cleaning (dental hygienist) should be performed.

Rinsing the mouth with salt-water solutions may also be recommended, especially in cases of soft-tissue injury or if trauma occurs due to the splinting.

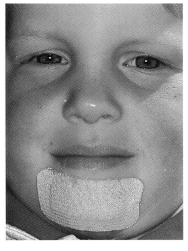
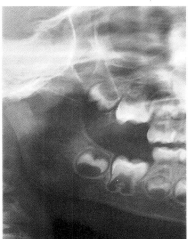
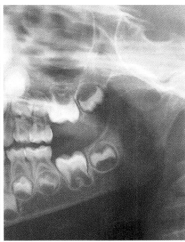

914 Temporomandibular joint fracture in a child
This four-year-old boy had fallen on his chin during a bicycle accident. He suffered a fracture of the right mandibular condyle, which led to the typical functional disturbances and immobilization of the mandible *(left)*.

The panoramic radiograph shows anterior tipping of the temporomandibular joint process *(right)*.

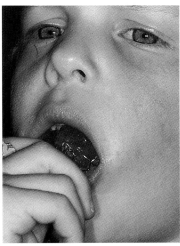
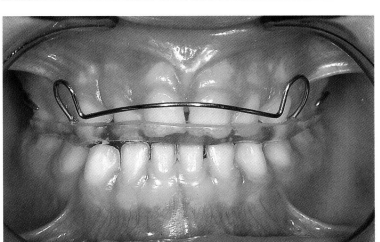

915 Treatment
The therapy consists of inserting a monoblock to reestablish occlusion, with simultaneous functional treatment for mouth opening.

Left: The child was very cooperative, and was able to insert and remove the training device himself.

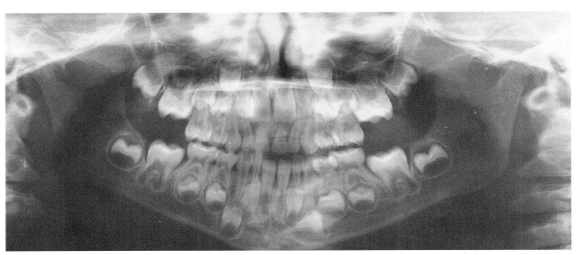

916 Clinical course
This panoramic radiograph, taken ten months after reconstruction of the fracture site, shows correct location of the head of the condyle. Additional follow-up visits are necessary to ensure proper growth of the mandible. In very young patients, trauma in the temporomandibular joint region can lead to disturbances of subsequent joint development.

Treatment for Radiation Injury

During Radiotherapy

It is important to protect the remaining dentition. Trays should be made for topical application of a fluoride gel.

Professional dental prophylaxis and treatment of any existing periodontal pathology should be carried out before and during radiotherapy.

The patient should be carefully instructed in oral hygiene techniques, including chlorhexidine rinsing. In most cases, recall appointments should be scheduled at weekly intervals.

If the patient develops stomatitis during radiation therapy, oral rinses with fluoride-containing solutions should be prescribed. If mucositis occurs, patients may be instructed to use artificial saliva. Daily home care for the oral mucosa during the period of radiotherapy may include glycerin-containing saline solutions or bicarbonate solutions. Salves for the oral mucosa can also be used, incorporating anesthetic agents if necessary.

Prescription for Artificial Saliva

Any artificial saliva solution should have a neutral pH to prevent decalcification of the remaining teeth. Ideally, such solutions should serve to remineralize enamel surfaces, as well as providing a lubricating function during the ingestion of foodstuffs.

Gel 7 B+ (pH: 8)

Ammonium fluoride:	0.25 %
Ammonium phosphate:	1.00 %
Sodium cyclamate:	0.075% (can be varied)
Sodium saccharine:	0.125% (can be varied)
Lycasine:	0.125% (can be varied)
Sodium benzoate:	0.10 %
Natrosal HR250:	0.50 % (can be varied)
Viscosity, H_2O:	Up to 100%

(This solution has been recommended by the Preventive Dental Medicine Clinic, Dept. of Periodontology and Cariology, University of Zurich, Switzerland; Chairman, Professor Felix Lutz).

Treatment Measures after Irradiation

Continuation of professional hygiene measures at intervals of three or four weeks.

Treatment for mucositis and continued use of artificial saliva.

Prosthodontic measures can be performed after the radiotherapy course, but these must be followed by short-interval recall appointments to deal with any prosthesis-related mucosal injury. It is critical to avoid any mucosal ulcerations resulting from pressure spots, because the mucosal tissues cannot heal on a radionecrotic bony substrate. In such cases, even slightly traumatized soft tissue ulcers may be the causative factor in the loss of entire segments of irradiated bone.

If surgical procedures are considered to be absolutely necessary, they must be carried out with antibiotic coverage and with primary soft tissue closure of any defects. In such cases, referral to a specialist is indicated.

Treatment for Burns and Caustic Burns in Soft Tissues
(Cf. p. 324)

Superficial chemical or thermal damage often leads to necrosis.

Treatment consists of local wound care by cleaning with a 3% H_2O_2 solution and topical application of physiological saline to the demarcation zone between healthy and necrotic mucosa. The wound surface can also be covered with an adhesive intraoral paste. Small areas of ulceration (ca. 2 cm^2) can be left to secondary reepithelialization, while larger defects have to be covered surgically. During the surgical procedure to carry out this coverage, care must be taken to anticipate scar formation. Cases such as this should be treated by specialists.

Laser Surgery

Definition

LASER is an acronym that stands for "Light Amplification by Stimulated Emission of Radiation." "Laser light" is created by applying energy into a medium so that electrons change their orbits and therefore emit light rays. Through appropriate reflection within the resonance chamber, these light rays can be targeted as a very precise, bundled energy source. Laser light is monochromatic, coherent, parallel and very energy rich.

There are four main categories of media that can be stimulated to emit laser light:
−gases: CO_2, argon
−solids: neodymium YAG (yttrium-aluminum-gallium), erbium YAG, holmium YAG
−fluids: dyes or chromatic lasers
−diodes: diode light in the red and infrared spectra

The therapeutic spectrum for medical lasers ranges from ultraviolet (e.g., eximer laser), through the visible range (e.g., ruby laser), and to the near infrared (e.g., neodymium YAG), middle infrared (e.g., erbium YAG) to the far infrared (e.g., CO_2 laser).

The mode of application can be continuous, pulsed, and super-pulsed. In the pulsed mode, especially high energy can be achieved for short time periods (0.1–0.8 ms). In super-pulsed (or Q-switched) mode the energy level is correspondingly higher (> 100 mJ) with a pulse duration of 1-10 ns.

Laser Application in Oral Surgery

In contrast to medical applications, the use of lasers in dentistry is a relatively young science. At the present time, there are three systems used routinely in oral surgery:

1. Erbium YAG laser (2,940 nm): For removal of superficial skin and mucosal lesions and of dental hard tissue.

2. CO_2 laser (10,600 nm): Universal use for soft-tissue surgery in the oral cavity. Flexible hollow wave guide with a nuclear diameter from 0.4 to 1 mm are indicated for very precise manipulations. Systems with super-pulsed laser rays (50–1,300 µs) and pulse energy from 15 to 50 mJ reduce the zone of thermal injury to several µm.

3. Neodymium YAG laser (1,064 nm): For disinfection of root canals, removal of smear layers, and for sealing of dentinal tubules, as well an interstitial therapy for circumscript oral and perioral hemangiomas.

CO_2 Laser

Indication: Universally useful for treatment of skin and mucosal lesions, hyperkeratosis, scars, gingival lesions, skin wrinkles.

Application: Superficial application via flexible hollow wave guide of 1 mm diameter.
Intermittent application: pulse 0.01 s, pause 0.1 s.
Energy level: 5–7 W.

Treatment on the Gingiva

In contrast to other possible modalities of treatment, such as cryosurgery or electrosurgery, the CO_2 laser is especially well indicated for treatments on the marginal gingiva. Damage to tooth hard structure does not occur, nor does post-treatment hypersensitivity.

> **Caution**
> The patient as well as the treatment team members can be injured by laser light. Protective measures (eyewear, signs or placards) must be strictly adhered to.

917 Indication for CO_2 laser
Therapy-resistant leukoplakia. Using a sweeping motion, the handpiece is moved parallel to the tissue surface and in three directions, without touching the tissue.

Right: protective measures. Appropriate eyewear for patient and treatment personnel. The treatment room must be designated by a placard outside, to prevent entrance by unauthorized persons.

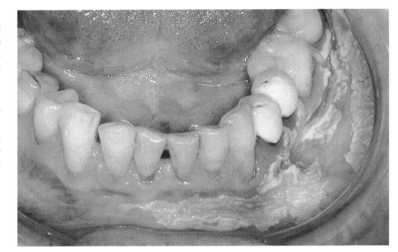
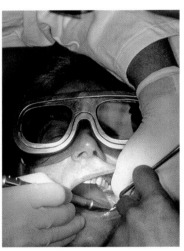

Ⓐ

918 Laser apparatus
Modern laser devices have a clear visual display and provide for desired adjustments. A warning system is built in to announce any operational problems.

Right: anesthesia. To insure a painless procedure, topical anesthesia is generally employed, e.g., xylocaine spray.

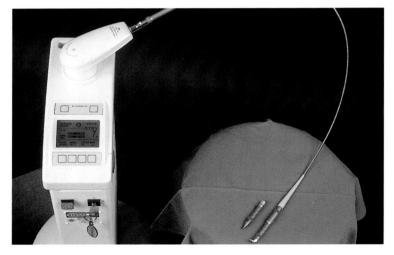
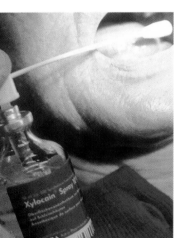

919 Clinical course
Ten months after the laser application, there was no recurrence of the leukoplakia. The mucosa appears free of irritation or scar tissue.

Right: treatment of the gingiva. The laser probe tip can be very precisely guided along the margins of dental restorations.

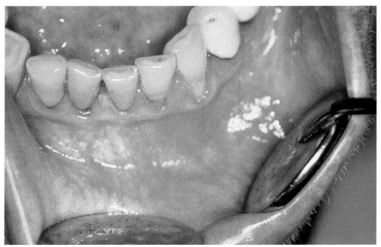
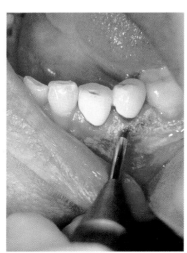

Laser-tissue interaction

The adequate laser source must be evaluated according to the coloration of the tissue. The depth of penetration and effectiveness of the laser is dependent upon the wave length and the spectrum of absorption of the tissue. As an example, hemoglobin exhibits two absorption peaks, at 488 and 514 nm wavelength.

With specific regard to dental hard tissues, the morphologic crystal structure (hydroxyapatite) and the course or the dentinal tubules also play important roles. Finally, the interaction between laser energy and tissue will be determined by laser power (W = Watt), and energy (J = Joule) as well as the power density (W/cm^2) and energy density (J/cm^2).

Clinical Tip
It is absolutely necessary to submit mucosal tissues excised by means of laser technology for histopathologic evaluation. If this is not practical, the laser surgery should be preceded by a conventional biopsy.

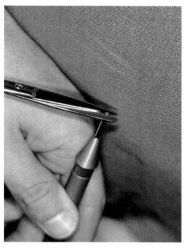
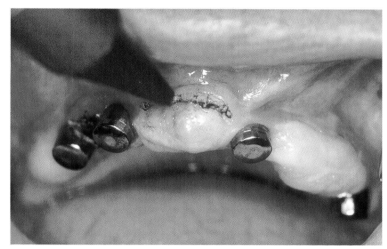

920 Indication
Undesirable fibrous tissue has developed between the implants. Tissue removal is accomplished by excision, using a fine hollow fiber.

Left: intra-operative. The end of the fiber must be freshly cut. The display on the laser apparatus will signal if the fiber is not suitable.

Ⓢ

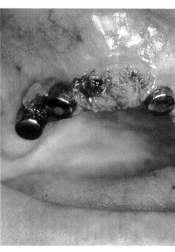
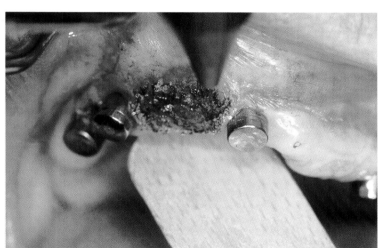

921 Protective measures
A wooden spatula is used to provide protection from inadvertent laser effects on adjacent tissues.

Left: wound surface. Following laser ablation of a lesion, the wound appears raw, however, hemorrhage seldom occurs. No wound dressing is needed.

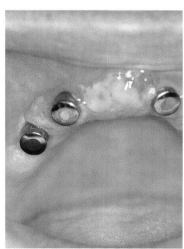
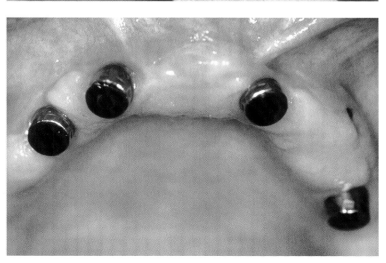

922 Late clinical view
Six months postoperatively, there is no evidence of recurrence in the anterior region of the maxilla.

Left: clinical course. One week following laser surgery, the wound surface exhibits a fibrin coating that is free of irritation. Postoperative pain is not a common problem.

Neodym YAG Laser

Indications: Blood-rich lesions such as localized hemangiomas or vascular malformations. Can also be applied in cases of dental hard structure or osseous preparations.

The tissue interaction and specific wave length (near infrared) and the energy density of the fiber optic handpiece permits simultaneous cutting and coagulation.

Application: Superficial and interstitial treatment of blood-rich tissues.

Pulsed laser with transmission through quartz fiber, targeted light application with helium-neon laser.

Power: 25 W

Pulse duration: 200 µs, 25 Hz

Interval duration: 20 s

Cooling: Surrounding tissues must be cooled with 5–7 °C saline solution.

923 Indication

Esthetically objectionable bluish malformation on the lower lip. Well demarcated, observed for many years, and unchanged over that time.

Right: interstitial treatment. By means of interstitial necrotization, a scar-free and esthetically acceptable removal of the vascular anomaly could be achieved.

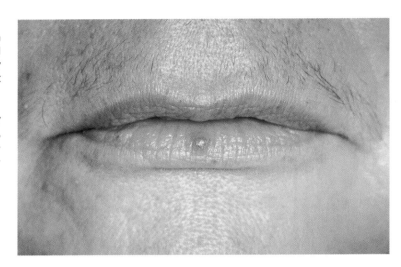
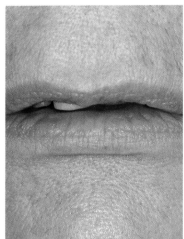

924 Indication

Esthetically objectionable blue-black lesion in the vestibular region near tooth 33.

Right: interstitial treatment. Using a quartz probe, the internal structure of the malformation is necrotized.

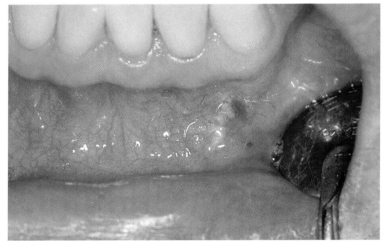
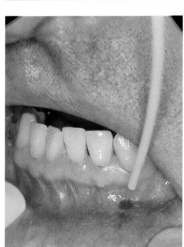

925 Postoperative result

Immediately following the laser surgery, the persistent lesion is no longer visible.

Right: later clinical result. One month following the interstitial laser treatment, the lesion can scarcely be detected clinically.

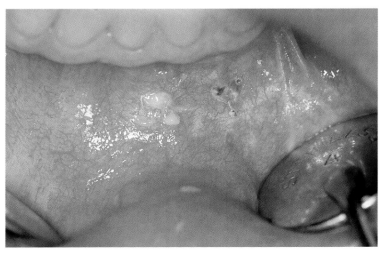
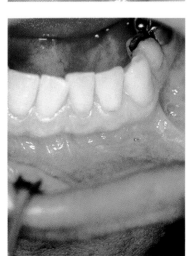

Erbium YAG Laser

Indications: Blood-rich lesions, such as circumscribed hemangiomas or vascular malformations. Treatment for scars of the skin. Treatment of dental hard substance. Primarily thermo-mechanical effects.

Application: Superficial application
Focused laser
Energy: 100 – 500 mJ
Pulse frequency: 1 – 4 Hz
Intervention duration: continuous

The erbium YAG laser can also be used for painless preparation of cavities and for osteotomy.

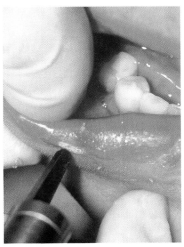
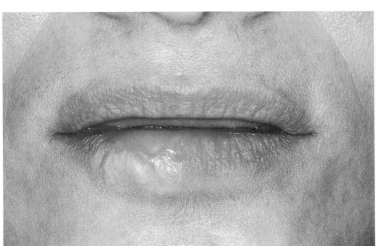

926 Indication
Condition following numerous attempts to correct scar formation on the right corner of the mouth in a 45-year-old female.

Left: superficial removal. In the labial region, the objectionable scar is removed and evened using the erbium YAG laser with a small focus.

Ⓒ

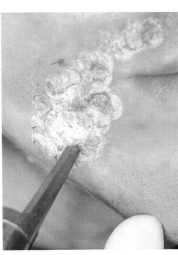
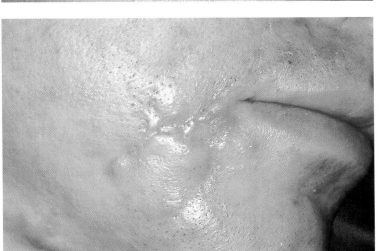

927 Evening out the scar
28-year-old male: Condition after severe skin burn and attempted plastic surgical correction on the right side of the face; note scarring and unevenness of contours.

Left: skin contouring. The very objectionable scar formation on the skin is treated and evened out using sweeping movement of the laser probe.

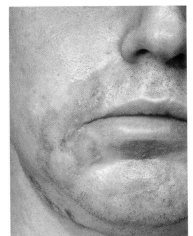
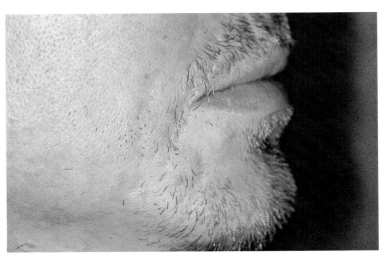

928 Later clinical result
Eight months postoperatively, the skin color is normal and the zone of scarring is hardly discernible.

Left: clinical course. Fourteen days after the laser surgical correction, the surgical site appears somewhat erythematous but the unevenness has been for the most part eliminated.

References

A

Ackermann, H.: Warum haben wir mit den Wurzelspitzenresektionen Mißerfolge? Vorschläge für ein vereinfachtes Verfahren, um einen einwandfreien Abschluß der Wurzel zu erhalten. Schweiz. Monatsschr. Zahnmed. 61: 821–836, 1951

Altner, H.: Physiologie des Geschmacks. In Schmidt, R. F.: Grundriß der Sinnesphysiologie. Springer, Berlin, S. 287–298, 1985

American Dental Association, American Heart Association: Preventing bacterial endocarditis. J. Am. Dent Assoc. 122: 87–92, 1991

Andrä, A.: Zur Diagnostik kieferchirurgischer Erkrankungen. Stomatol. DDR 39: 761–764, 1989

Andrä, A., Naumann, G.: Odontogene pyogene Infektionen. Barth, Leipzig 1991

Andreasen, J. O.: Traumatologie der Zähne. Schlüter, Hannover 1988

Andreasen, J. O.: Farbatlas der Replantation und Transplantation von Zähnen. Deutscher Ärzte-Verlag Köln 1993

Atac, M.: Nachuntersuchungsergebnisse der unilateralen Kiefergelenksfrakturen der Zürcher Klinik. Med. Diss, Zürich 1978

B

Bahr, F.: Einführung in die wissenschaftliche Akupunktur. Ohr-, Schädel- und Körperakupunktur. Bahr, München 1989

Barbakow, F., Imfeld, T.: Richtlinien bei der Replantation bleibender Zähne I und II. Quintessenz 31: 29–34, 41–45, 1980

Barco, C. T.: Prevention of infective endocarditis: a review of the medical and dental literature. J. Periodontol. 62: 510–523, 1991

Bartoshuk, L.: Genetic and pathological taste variation: What can we learn from animal models and human disease? Ciba Foundation Symposium 179: 251–267, 1993

Bartoshuk, L. M., Beauchamp G. K.: Chemical senses. Annu. Rev. psychol. 45: 419–449, 1994

Bauer, G., Donath, K., Dumbach, J., Sitzmann, F., Spitzer, W. J.: Vergleich verschiedener Ca-Phosphat-Keramiken zum Knochenersatz. Z. Zahnärztl. Implantol. 3: 101–106, 1987

Bauer, G., Donath, K., Dumbach, J., Kroha, E., Sitzmann, F., Spitzer, W. J.: Reaktion des Knochens auf Kalziumphosphatkeramiken unterschiedlicher Zusammensetzungen. Z. Zahnärztl. Implantol. 5: 263–266, 1989

Baum, B. J.: Salivary gland function during aging. Gerodontics 2: 61–64, 1986

Baumann, M.: Apikale, zystische Aufhellungen: ein Vergleich zwischen Röntgenbild und Histologie. Schweiz. Monatsschr. Zahnmed. 83: 1459–1467, 1973

Baumann, M.: Langzeiterfahrungen mit der Marsupialisation großer Unterkieferzysten zur Mundhöhle. Schweiz. Monatsschr. Zahnmed. 86: 1280–1293, 1976a

Baumann, M.: Die ambulant durchgeführte partielle Vestibulumplastik mit sekundärer Epithelisation. Schweiz. Monatsschr. Zahnmed. 86: 17–28, 1976b

Baumann, M.: Probeexzision wie und wann? Schweiz. Monatsschr. Zahnmed. 88: 39–43, 1978

Baumann, M., Pajarola, G.: Experiences on the sequela of maxillary sinusitis following closure of the causative oro-antral fistula. J. Maxillofac. Surg. 3: 164–169, 1975

Baurmash, H. D.: Marsupialization for treatment of oral ranula: a second look at the procedure. J. Oral Maxillofac. Surg. 50: 1274–1279, 1992

Beck-Mannagetta, J., Necek, D., Grasserbauer, M.: Zahnärztliche Aspekte der solitären Kieferhöhlen-Aspergillose: eine klinische, mikroanalytische und experimentelle Untersuchung. Z. Stomatol. 83: 283–315, 1986

Becker, R.: Pyogene Infektionen im Kieferbereich beim Kind. Dtsch. Zahnärztl. Z. 23: 1295–1302, 1968

Becker, R.: Verschiedene Methoden der Zystenoperation. Indikation und Ergebnisse. ZWR 80: 106–112, 1971

Becker, R.: Die Nachblutung nach zahnärztlich-chirurgischen Eingriffen in der Mundhöhle. Dtsch. Zahnärztl. Z. 29: 655–659, 1974

Bereiter, H., Melcher, G. A., Gautier, E., Huggler, H. A.: Erfahrungen mit Bio-Oss, einem bovinen Apatit, bei verschiedenen klinischen Indikationsbereichen. Hefte Unfallheilkunde 216, 1991

Bernimoulin, J-P., Lange, D. E.: Freie Gingivatransplantate — klinische Aspekte und Zytologie ihrer Einheilung. Dtsch. Zahnärztl. Z. 27: 357–364, 1972

Berthold, H.: Antibakterielle Chemotherapie. Schweiz. Monatsschr. Zahnmed. 103: 307–314, 1993

Berthold, H., Burkhardt, A.: Nichtdentogene Kieferzysten. Schweiz. Monatsschr. Zahnmed. 99: 1174–1178, 1989

Berthold, H., Hirt, H. P., Schramm-Scherer, B.: Wurzelspitzenresektion und transdentale Fixation, Fehler und Komplikationen. Schweiz. Monatsschr. Zahnmed. 102: 713–718, 1992

Bhaskar, S. N.: Periapical lesions — types, incidence and clinical features. Oral Surg. Oral Med. Oral Pathol. 21: 657–671, 1966

Bolz, U., Kalweit, K.: Vergleichende Untersuchungen zur Wärmeentwicklung mit innengekühlten und konventionellen Knochenbohrern und -fräsen. Dtsch. Zahnärztl. Z. 31: 959, 1976

Bork, K., Hoede, N., Korting, G. W.: Mundschleimhaut und Lippenkrankheiten, 2. Aufl. Schattauer, Stuttgart 1993

Bössmann, K., Bönning, J.: Die Empfehlung des Deutschen Arbeitskreises für Hygiene in der Zahnarztpraxis. DAHZ, Kiel/Norderstedt 1989

Briseño, B., Willershausen, B., Sonnabend, E.: Einfluß verschiedener Wurzelfüllmaterialien auf Gingivafibroblastenkulturen. Schweiz. Monatsschr. Zahnmed. 101: 294–298, 1991

Brøndum, N., Jensen, V. J.: Recurrence of keratocysts and decompression treatment: a long-term follow-up of forty-four cases. Oral Surg. Oral Med. Oral Pathol. 72: 265–269, 1991

Brosch, F.: Die Zysten des Kiefer-Gesichtsbereichs. In Häupl, K., Meyer, W., Schuchardt, K.: Die Zahn-, Mund- und Kieferheilkunde, Bd. III/1. Urban & Schwarzenberg, München, S. 411–456, 1957

Bull, H. G., Lentrodt, J., Zentner, C.: Technik und Ergebnisse der chirurgisch-kieferorthopädischen Einordnung verlagerter und retinierter Eckzähne. Fortschr. Kiefer. Gesichtschir. 21: 101–105, 1976

Buser, D.: Die Vestibulumplastik mit freien Schleimhauttransplantaten bei Implantaten im zahnlosen Unterkiefer. Schweiz. Monatsschr. Zahnmed. 97: 766–772, 1987

Buser, D., Berthold, H.: Knochendefektfüllung im Kieferbereich mit Kollagenvlies. Dtsch. Z. Mund-, Kiefer- u. Gesichtschir. 10: 191–198, 1986

Buser, D., Hotz, P.: Komplikationen bei der Überfüllung von Wurzelkanälen. Schweiz. Monatsschr. Zahnmed. 100: 1185–1191, 1990

C

Cerbo, R., Martucci, N., Agnoli, A.: Committee of the International Headache Society. Classification and diagnostic criteria for headache disorders, cranial neuralgias and facial pain. Cephalgia 8, Suppl. 7: 1—96, 1988

Ciancio, S. G.: Current status of indices of gingivitis. Review J. clin. Periodontol. 13: 375—378, 381—382, 1986

Clark, M. S., Seldin, R. D.: Cystectomy or marsupialisation: criteria for treatment. Quarterly NDA 38: 61, 1980

Cohen, L.: Mucoceles of the oral cavity. Oral Surg. Oral Med. Oral Pathol. 19: 365—372, 1965

Collings, V. B.: Human taste response as afunction of locus of stimulation on the tongue and soft palate. Perception and psychophysics 16: 169—174, 1974

Converse, J. M.: Complications in treatment of fractures. In Kazanjian, V. H., Converse, J. M.: Surgical Treatment of Facial Injuries. Williams & Wilkins, Baltimore, p. 235, 1974

D

Dahmer, H., Dahmer, J.: Gesprächsführung — eine praktische Anleitung, 3. Aufl. Thieme, Stuttgart 1992

Dahmer, J.: Anamnese und Befund. 7. Aufl. Thieme, Stuttgart 1994

Dajani, A. S., Bisno, A. L., Chung, K. J., et al: Prevention of bacterial endocarditis. JAMA 264: 2919—2922, 1990

Daniel, A.: Les incisions en chirurgie buccale. Schweiz. Monatsschr. Zahnmed. 87: 1228—1249, 1977

Davis, Ch. L.: Medical factors affecting treatment planning. In Fonseca, R. J., Davis, W. H.: Reconstructive Preprosthetic Oral and Maxillofacial Surgery, 2nd ed. Saunders, Philadelphia, pp. 127—134, 1995

Dean, O. T.: Surgery for the denture patient. J. Am. Dent. Assoc. 23: 2124—2128, 1936

De Foer, Ch., Fossion, E., Vaillant, J. M.: Sinus aspergillosis. J. Craniomaxillofac. Surg. 18: 33—40, 1990

Donath, K.: WHO-Klassifikation der odontogenen Zysten. Dtsch. Z. Mund. Kiefer. Gesichtschir. 4: 191—197, 1980

Draf, W.: Klinisch-experimentelle Untersuchungen zur Pathogenese, Diagnostik und Therapie der chronisch entzündlichen Kieferhöhlenerkrankungen unter Verwertung der direkten Beobachtung durch Sinuskopie. Med. Habil., Mainz 1974

Düker, J.: Konventionelle Röntgendiagnostik beim Mittelgesichtstrauma. Fortschr. Kiefer. Gesichtschir. 36: 18—21, 1991

Dumbach, J., Spitzer, W. J.: Knochenersatz mit pyrolisiertem xenogenen Knochen. Dtsch. Zahnärztl. Z. 43: 45—48, 1988

E

Edlan, A., Mejchar, B.: Plastic surgery of the vestibulum in periodontal therapy. Int. Dent. J. 13: 593—596, 1963

Egyedi, P., Beyazit, E.: Marsupialisation of large cysts of the maxillas into the maxillary sinus and/or nose. a follow-up investigation. In Kay, L. W.: Oral Surgery: Transactions of the 4th International Conference on Oral Surgery. Munksgaard, Kopenhagen, pp. 81—84, 1973

Ehrl, P. A.: Die Wurzelspitzenresektion mit orthograder Wurzelfüllung. In Chirurgische Zahnerhaltung. Hanser, München, S. 29—39, 1990

F

Fast, Th. B.: Physical evaluation and monitoring devices in dental practice. Gen. Dent. 41: 242—245, 1993

FDI: A revision of technical report No. 10. Recommendations for hygiene in dental practice, including treatment for the infectious patient. Int. Dent. J. 37: 142—145, 1987

Feifel, H., Riediger, D., Gustorf-Aeckerle, R., Claus, C.: Die hochauflösende Computertomographie in der Diagnostik verlagerter unterer Weisheitszähne unter besonderer Berücksichtigung der Strahlenbelastung. Dtsch. Z. Mund. Kiefer. Gesichtschir. 15: 226-231, 1991

Fischer, W.: Hygiene in der Zahnarztpraxis. Gesundheitsdirektion Kanton Zürich, Zürich 1991

Fischer-Brandies, E., Dielert, E.: Knochenersatzwerkstoff Hydroxylapatit. Zahnarzt 30: 567—583, 1986

Fleming, P., Feigal, R. J., Kaplan, E. L., Liljemark, W. F., Little, J. W.: The development of penicillinresistant oral streptococci after repeated penicillin prophylaxis. Oral Surg. Oral Med. Oral Pathol. 70: 440—444, 1990

Fowler, C. B., Brannon, R. B.: The paradental cyst: a clinicopathologic study of six new cases and review of the literature. J. oral Maxillofac. Surg. 47: 243—248, 1989

Frenkel, G..: Klinik und Therapie retinierter Zähne. In Frenkel, G., Aderhold, L., Leilich, G., Raetzke, P.: Die ambulante Chirurgie des Zahnarztes. Hanser, München, S. 121—158, 1989a

Frenkel, G.: Die Mund-Antrumverbindung und ihre Behandlung. In Frenkel, G., Aderhold, L., Leilich, G., Raetzke, P.: Die ambulante Chirurgie des Zahnarztes. Hanser, München, S. 159—174, 1989b

Frerich, B., Cornelius, C. P., Wiethölter, H.: Critical time of exposure of the rabbit inferior alveolar nerve to Carnoy's solution. J. Oral Maxillofac. Surg. 52: 599—606, 1994

Freyberger, P.: Die Radix relicta aus der Sicht des zahnärztlichen Sachverständigen. ZWR 80: 243—245, 1971

Friedman, S.: Retrograde approaches in endodontic therapy. Endod. Dent. Traumatol. 7: 97—107, 1991

Fuchsberger, A.: Verschiedene Bohrwerkzeuge zur spanenden Knochenbearbeitung im Vergleich. Z. Zahnärztl. Implantol. 3 267—281, 1987

Fuchsjäger, E.: Konzept zur Versorgung nachblutungsgefährdeter Patienten nach Zahnextraktionen. Z. Stomatol. 81: 179—184, 1984

G

Gabka, J.: Zur Diagnostik der Zysten des Kiefer-Gesichtsbereiches. Zahnmed. Bild 1: 126—130, 1960

Galloway, R. H., Gross, P. D., Thompson, S. H., Patterson, A. L.: Pathogenesis and treatment of ranula. J. Oral Maxillofac. Surg. 47: 299—302, 1989

Ganss, C., Hochban, W., Kielbassa, A. M., Umstadt, H. E.: Prognosis of third molar eruption. Oral Surg. Oral Med. Oral Pathol. 76: 688—693, 1993

Gersema, L., Baker, K.: Use of Corticosteroids in oral surgery. J. Oral. Maxillofac. Surg. 50: 270—277, 1992

Ghanremani, M., Arndt, R.: Instrumentenkunde in der zahnärztlichen Chirurgie. Thieme, Stuttgart 1994

Glanzmann, Ch., Grätz, K. W.: Radionecrosis of the mandibula: a retrospective analysis of the incidence and risk factors. Radiother. Oncol. 36: 94—100, 1995

Grätz, K. W.: Eine neue Klassifikation zur Einteilung von Unterkieferfrakturen. Med. Diss., Basel 1985

Grätz, K. W.: Die fortgeleitete phlegmonöse Mediastinitis bei eitrigen Infektionen von Unterkiefer und Oropharynx. Schriftenr. Ges. Kiefer. Gesichtschir. 2: 51—55, 1989

Greenspan, D., Greenspan, J. S., Pindborg, J. J., Schiødt, M.: AIDS, Konsequenzen für die zahnärztl. Praxis. Deutscher Ärzte-Verlag, Köln 1987

Grunder, U., Strub, J. R.: Die Problematik der Temperaturerhöhung beim Bearbeiten des Knochens mit rotierenden Instrumenten — eine Literaturübersicht. Schweiz. Monatsschr. Zahnmed. 96: 956—969, 1986

H

Halse, A., Molven, O., Grung, B.: Follow-up after periapical surgery: the value of the one-year control. Endod. Dent. Traumatol. 7: 246—250, 1991

Hammarström, L., Blomlöf, L., Feiglin, B., Andersson, L., Lindskog, S.: Replantation of teeth and antibiotic treatment. Endod. Dent. Traumatol. 2: 51—57, 1986

Hardt, N.: Behandlung von Kiefer- und Gesichtsschädelverletzungen im Wandel der Zeit. Swiss. Dent. 7: 40—49, 1986

Hardt, N.: Osteomyelitis: Szintigraphie. Schweiz. Monatsschr. Zahnmed. 101: 319–326, 1991

Hardt, N., Paulus, G.W.: Langzeiterfahrungen mit autologen Schleimhauttransplantaten bei Vestibulumplastiken im Oberkiefer. Schweiz. Monatsschr. Zahnheilk. 93: 1129–1135, 1983

Hardt, N., Von Arx, T.: Unterkieferfrakturen im Kindesalter. Schweiz. Monatsschr. Zahnmed. 99: 808–816, 1989a

Hardt, N., Von Arx, T.: Odontogene Keratozyste. Schweiz. Monatsschr. Zahnmed. 100: 980–985, 1990, 1989b

Hartmann, H.P., Jakob, O.: Die rechtliche Verantwortung des Zahnarztes bei lebensbedrohenden Zwischenfällen. Schweiz. Monatsschr. Zahnmed. 90: 305–314, 1980

Hausamen, J.E.: Kryochirurgie von Leukoplakien der Mundhöhlenschleimhaut. Dtsch. Zahnärztl. Z. 28: 1032–1036, 1973

Hausamen, J.E.: The basis, technique and indication for cryosurgery in tumors of the oral cavity and face. J. Maxillofac. Surg. 3: 41–49, 1975

Heeg, P., Setz, J.: Praxishygiene. Probleme und Lösungen. Thieme, Stuttgart 1994

Heimdahl, A., Hall, G., Hedeberg, M. et al: Detection and quantitation by lysis – filtration of bacteremia after different oral surgical procedures. J. Clin Microbiol 28: 2205–2209, 1990

Heusser, E.: Kauunfälle, Vorzustände, Spätfolgen/Rückfälle, UVG-Privatassekuranz. Schweiz. Monatsschr. Zahnmed. 97: 882–884, 1987

Hickel, R.: Wurzelfüllmaterialien – insbesondere für die retrograde Wurzelfüllung. In Chirurgische Zahnerhaltung. Hanser, München, S. 41–60, 1990

Hjørting-Hansen, E.: Studies on implantation of anorganic bone in cystic jaw lesions. Munksgaard, Copenhagen, 1970

Hochstein, H.J.: Rosenthals spezielle Mund-, Kiefer- und Gesichtschirurgie. 4. Aufl. Barth, Leipzig 1991

Holtgrave, E., Spiessl, B.: Die osteoplastische Behandlung großer Kieferzysten. Schweiz. Monatsschr. Zahnmed. 85: 585–597, 1975

Hotz, P.R.: Zahnunfälle: Unfälle an bleibenden Zähnen im jugendlichen Gebiß. Schweiz. Monatsschr. Zahnmed. 100: 849–858, 1990

Hotz, R.: Orthodontie in der täglichen Praxis, 4. Aufl. Huber, Bern 1970

Howe, G.L.: Minor oral surgery. Wright, Bristol, p. 89–116, 1971

Huch, R.: Die schwangere Patientin in der zahnärztlichen Praxis. Schweiz. Monatsschr. Zahnmed. 98: 1237–1245, 1988

I

Ilgenstein, B., Berthold, H., Beck, E.A.: Hämostasestörungen. Schweiz. Monatsschr. Zahnmed. 97: 473–477, 1987

Ingersoll, B.D.: Psychologische Aspekte der Zahnheilkunde. Quintessenz, Berlin, 1987

Isler, H.: Die Behandlung der Kopfschmerzen. Schweiz. Med. Wochenschr. 114: 1174–1180, 1984

J

Jaquiéry, C., Burkart, F.: Beeinflußbarkeit von Herzschrittmachern durch elektrische Geräte. Schweiz. Monatsschr. Zahnmed. 103: 987–992, 1993

Jacquiéry, C. Pajarola, G.F., Lambrecht, J.Th., Sailer, H.F.: Die Entfernung unterer retinierter Weisheitszähne (I). Schweiz. Monatsschr. Zahnmed. 104: 1517–1520, 1994

Jenni, M., Schürch, E. jr., Geering, A.H.: Schnellerfassung von Funktionsstörungen. Symptomtrias zur Schnellerfassung behandlungsbedürftiger Funktionsstörungen des Kausystems. Schweiz. Monatsschr. Zahnmed. 98: 1251–1252, 1988

Joho, J.-P., Schatz, J.-P.: Autotransplantation et planification orthodontique. Schweiz. Monatsschr. Zahnmed. 100: 174–187, 1990

Jokinen, M.A.: Bacteremia following dental extractions and its prophylaxis. Suom. Hammaslääk. Toim. 66: 69–100, 1970

K

Kamboozia, A.H., Punnia-Moorthy, A.: The fate of teeth in mandibular fracture lines. Int. J. Oral Maxillofac. Surg. 22: 97–101, 1993

Kanzler, L.: Die operative Entfernung unterer Weisheitszähne mit offener Nachbehandlung: eine bewährte und sichere Methode. Med. Diss., Zürich 1993

Kazanjian, V.H., Converse, J.M.: The Surgical Treatment of Facial Injuries. Williams & Wilkins, Baltimore 1949

Killey, H.C.: Fractures of the mandible, 2nd ed. Wright, Bristol, p. 32, 1971

Kirschner, H., Meyer, W.: Entwicklung einer Innenkühlung für chirurgische Bohrer. Dtsch. Zahnärztl. Z. 30: 436–438, 1975

Kirschner, H., Burkard, W., Pfütz, E., Pohl, Y., Obijou, C.: Frontzahntrauma: Aufbewahrung und Behandlung des verunfallten Zahnes. Schweiz. Monatsschr. Zahnmed. 102: 209–214, 1992

Kitsugi, T., Yamamuro, T., Nakamura, T. et al.: Four calcium phosphate ceramics as bone substitutes for non-weight-bearing. Biomaterials 14: 216–224, 1993

Klammt, J.: Zysten des Kieferknochens, Barth, Leipzig 1976

Klemmer, R.: Offene und halbgeschlossene Nachbehandlung nach operativer Entfernung unterer Weisheitszähne im Vergleich. Med. Diss., Zürich 1993

Köle, H.: Zur Spätbehandlung der Protrusion. DZZ 9: 275–278, 1959

König, J., Kocher, Th., Plagmann, H.-Ch.: Wechselwirkung zwischen Parodontitis und Pulpitis und ihre Auswirkungen auf die Therapie bei kombiniert endodontal-parodontalen Läsionen. Parodontologie 5: 93–102, 1994

Kristen, K., Singer, R.: Therapie und Prognose der Luxationsfrakturen des Kiefergelenks beim Jugendlichen. Fortschr. Kiefer. Gesichtschir. 21: 314–315, 1976

Krogh-Poulsen, W.G.: Examination, diagnosis, treatment. In Schwartz, L., Chayes, Ch.M.: Facial Pain and Mandibular Dysfunktion. Saunders, Philadelphia pp 249–280, 1968

Kunz, M.: Resultate der mit Hypomochlion behandelten Kieferköpfchenfrakturen. Med. Diss., Zürich 1985

Künzler, A., Sailer, H.F.: Erfahrungen mit der Verpflanzung von Kunsthaar als Ersatz für Kopfhaare und Barthaar. Fortschr. Kiefer. Gesichtschir. 34: 85–87, 1985

L

Lambrecht, J. Th.: Odontogene Kieferhöhlenerkrankungen. Fortschr. Kiefer. Gesichtschir. 40: 106–113, 1995

Lang, N.P., Adler, R., Joss, A., Nyman, S.: Absence of bleeding on probing: an indicator of periodontal stability. J. clin. Periodontol. 17: 714–721, 1990

Langer, B., Langer, L.: Subepithelial connective tissue graft technique for root coverage. J. Periodontol 56: 715–720, 1985

Lauer, G., Englerth, H., Schilli, W.: Die Narbe als Resultat der Wundheilung im Gesichtsbereich. Dtsch. Zahnärztl. Z. 50: 63–66, 1995

Lautenbach, E.: Zahn – Mund – Kiefer: Therapien, Materialien, Rezepte. Karger, Basel 1990

Le Clerc, G.C., Girard, C.: Un nouveau procédé de butée dans le traitement chirurgicale de la luxation récidivante de la mâchoire inférieure. Mém. Acad. Chir. 69: 457–459, 1943

Lehnert, S., Lehmann, J.: Klinische und röntgenologische Untersuchungen zur Frage der Sinusitis maxillaris nach Eröffnung der Kieferhöhle bei Zahnextraktion. Dtsch. Zahnärztl. Z. 22: 201–205, 1967

Lehnhardt, E.: HNO-Heilkunde für Zahnmediziner, 2. Aufl. Thieme, Stuttgart 1992

Lentrodt, J., Höltje, W.J.: Indikation zur operativen bzw. konservativen Versorgung von Unterkieferfrakturen. Fortschr. Kiefer- u. Gesichtschir. 19: 65–68, 1975

Lin, L.M., Pascon, E.A., Skribner, J., Gängler, P., Langeland, K.: Clinical, radiographic, and histologic study of endodontic treatment failures. Oral Surg. Oral Med. Oral Pathol. 11: 603–611, 1991

Lombardi, T., Budtz-Jørgensen, E.: Die zahnärztliche Untersuchung beim Betagten. Schweiz. Monatsschr. Zahnmed. 102: 1359–1363, 1992

Luhr, H.G.: Die Kompressionsosteosynthese bei Frakturen des zahnlosen Unterkiefers. Med. Habil., Hamburg 1969

Luhr, H.G.: A micro-system for cranio-maxillofacial skeletal fixation. J. Craniomaxillofac. Surg. 16: 312–314, 1988

Lütscher, D.: Erfahrungen mit der Kryochirurgie bei Mundschleimhauterkrankungen. Med. Diss., Zürich 1984

M

Machtens, E., Heuser, L.: Prinzipielles und abgestuftes Vorgehen in der Röntgendiagnostik bei Mittelgesichtstrauma in Abhängigkeit vom Schweregrad und von der Lokalisation. Fortschr. Kiefer- u. Gesichtschir. 36: 21–25, 1991

Mäglin, B.: Notfälle aus der zahnärztlichen Chirurgie. Schweiz. Monatsschr. Zahnmed. 84: 964–976, 1974

Maienfisch, A.: Langzeiterfahrungen mit der Wurzelspitzenresektion. Med. Diss., Zürich 1980

Makek, M., Sailer, H. F.: Speicheldrüseninfarkte – eine diagnostische Falle für Pathologen und Kliniker. Schweiz. Monatsschr. Zahnmed. 95: 113-123, 1985

Mandel, I. D.: The functions of saliva. J. Dent. Res. 66: 623. 627, 1987

Marinello, C. P., Kundert, E., Andreoni, C.: Die Bedeutung der periimplantären Nachsorge für Zahnarzt und Patient. Implantologie 1: 43–57, 1993

Marker, P., Eckerdal, A., Smith-Sivertsen, Ch.: Incompletely erupted third molars in the line of mandibular fractures. Oral Surg. Oral Med. Oral Pathol. 78: 426–431, 1994

Mashberg, A., Samit, A.: Early detection, diagnosis and management of oral and oropharyngeal cancer. CA Cancer J. Clin. 39: 67–88, 1989

Meier, E., Berthold, H., Zbinden, A.: Problem- und Risikopatienten. Schweiz. Monatsschr. Zahnmed. 104: 615–620, 1994

Mitchell, D. F., Standish, S. M., Fast, Th. B.: Oral Diagnosis, Oral Medicine. Lea & Fibiger, Philadelphia 1971

Mittermeier, C., Riede, U. N., Härle, F.: Präkanzerose der Mundhöhle. Hoechst, Frankfurt/Main 1980

Möbius, E.: Kieferzysten und Nebenhöhlen. Dtsch. Zahnärztl. Z. 5: 397–399, 1950

Mombelli, A., Buser, D., Lang, N. P., Berthold, H.: Suspected periodontopathogens in erupting third molar sites of periodontally healthy individuals. J. Clin. Periodontol. 17: 48–54, 1990

Mörmann, W., Bernimmoulin, J. P., Schmid, M. O.: Fluoreszein angiography of free gingival autografts. J. clin. Periodontol. 2: 177–189, 1975

Mörmann, W., Schaer, F. P.: Orale Schleimhauttransplantation mit dem Mucotom. Schweiz. Monatsschr. Zahnmed. 87: 656–666, 1977

Morris, A. L., Bohannan, H. M., Casello, D. P.: The Dental Specialities in General Practice. Saunders, Philadelphia 1983

Morse, D. R., Bhambhani, S. M.: A dentist's dilemma: nonsurgical endodontic therapy or periapical surgery for teeth with apparent pulpal pathosis and an associated periapical radiolucent lesion. Oral Surg. Oral Med. Oral Pathol. 70: 333–340, 1990

Mounce, R. E.: Risk management in after-hours care. Gen. Dent. 38: 350–356, 1990

Mühlemann, H. R.: Parodontale Gesichtspunkte in der zahnärztlichen Chirurgie. Schweiz. Monatsschr. Zahnmed. 73: 106–121, 1963

Mühlemann, H. R., Son, S.: Gingival sulcus bleeding: a leading symptom in initial gingivitis. Helv. Odont. Acta 15: 107–113, 1971

Müller, U.: Allergische Reaktionen. Schweiz. Monatsschr. Zahnmed. 98: 1224–1229, 1988

Müller, W.: In Zahn-, Mund-, Kieferheilkunde, Bd. 2, Spezielle Chirurgie. Replantation oder Transplantation von Zähnen. Thieme, Stuttgart, S. 42–48, 1990

N

Nair, P. N. R., Pajarola, G. F.: Raducular cysts: types and incidence among human apical periodontitis lesions. In press: Oral Surg. Oral Med. Oral Pathol. 1995

Nair, P. N. R., Schroeder, H. E.: Pathogenese periapikaler Läsionen. Schweiz. Monatsschr. Zahnmed. 93: 935–952, 1983

Neal, D. C., Wagner, W. F., Alpert, B.: Morbidity associated with teeth in the line of mandibular fractures. J. Oral Surg. 36: 859–862, 1978

Negm, M. M.: Microleakage associated with retrofilling of the apical two thirds with amalgam. Oral Surg. Oral Med. Oral Pathol. 70: 498–501, 1990

Neidhart, A.: Die Mundvorhofplastik mit sekundärer Epithelisierung am Oberkiefer: Entwicklung, Methodik, Ergebnisse. Med. Diss., Zürich 1963

Neumann, R.: Führer durch die operative Zahnheilkunde. Berlinische Verlagsanstalt, Berlin 1929

Nielsen, P. M., Berthold, H., Burkhardt, A.: Die odontogene Keratozyste. Retrospektive Untersuchung zur Klinik, Radiologie, Pathohistologie und Therapie. Schweiz. Monatsschr. Zahnmed. 96: 577–587, 1986

O

Oatis, G. W., Huggins, R., Yorty, J. S.: Oral surgery. Dent. Clin. North Am. 30: 583–601, 1986

Obwegeser, H. L.: Über eine einfache Methode der freihändigen Drahtschienung von Kieferbrüchen. Österr. Z. Stomatol 49: 652–670, 1952

Obwegeser, H. L.: Surgical preparation of the maxilla for prosthesis. J. Oral Surg. Anesth. Hosp. Dent. Serv. 22: 127–134, 1964

Obwegeser, H. L.: Zur Indikation für die einzelnen Methoden der Vestibulumplastik und Mundbodenplastik. Fortschr. Kiefer. Gesichtschir. 10: 1–8, 1965

Obwegeser, H. L.: Bewährtes und Neues in der präprothetischen Chirurgie. Schweiz. Monatsschr. Zahnmed. 97: 223–225, 1987

Obwegeser, H. L., Aarnes, K.: Zur Luxation des Discus articularis des Kiefergelenkes. Schweiz. Monatsschr. Zahnmed. 83: 67–70, 1973

Obwegeser, H. L., Sailer, H. F.: Experiences with intraoral resection and immediate reconstruction in cases of radio-osteomyelitis of the mandible. J. Maxillofac. Surg. 6: 257–265, 1978

Obwegeser, H. L., Steinhäuser, E.: Ein neues Gerät zur Vitalitätsprüfung der Zähne mit Kohlensäureschnee. Schweiz. Monatsschr. Zahnmed. 73: 1001–1012, 1963

Obwegeser, H. L., Tschamer, H.: Bakteriologische Resektionskontrollen nach desinfektionsloser einzeitiger Wurzelfüllung einkanaliger Gangränzähne. Dtsch. Zahn. Mund. Kieferheilkd. 26: 103–116, 1957

Obwegeser, J. A., Riegler, H., Mossböck, R.: Die Aktinomykose des Kiefer-Gesichtsbereiches. Zahnärztl. Prax. 40: 122–124, 1989

Olech, E.: Fracture lines in mandibule. Dent. Radiogr. Photogr. 28: 21–26, 1955

Ollerenshaw, R., Rose, S.: Sialography – a valuable diagnostic method. Dent. Radiogr. Photogr. 29: 37–46, 1956

Olson, R. A., Fonseca, R. J., Zeitler, D. L., Osbon, D. B.: Fractures of the mandibule: a review of 580 cases. J. Oral Maxillofac. Surg. 40: 23–28, 1982

Ørstavic, D.: Radiographic evaluation of apical periodontitis and endodontic treatment results: a computer approach. Int. Dent. J. 41: 89–98, 1991

Osborn, J. F.: Hydroxylapatitkeramik – Granulate und ihre Systematik. ZM 77: 840–848, 852, 1987

P

Pajarola, G. F., Sailer, H. F.: Operative Entfernung unterer Weisheitszähne. Schweiz. Monatsschr. Zahnmed. 104: 1202–1209, 1994

Pajarola, G. F., Grätz, K. W., Sailer, H. F., Eichmann, A., Makek, M.: Erkennung und Behandlung von Mundschleimhauterkrankungen (I). Schweiz. Monatsschr. Zahnmed. 105: 788–794, 1995

Pajarola, G. F., Jaquiéry, C., Sailer, H. F., Lambrecht, J. Th.: Die Entfernung unterer retinierter Weisheitszähne (II). Schweiz. Monatsschr. Zahnmed. 104: 1520–1534, 1994

Pallasch, T. J., Slots, J.: Antibiotic prophylaxis for medical-risk patients. J. Periodontol. 62: 227–231, 1991

Pantschev, A., Carlsson, A.-P., Andersson, L.: Retrograde root filling with EBA cement or amalgam. Oral Surg. Oral Med. Oral Pathol. 78: 101–104, 1994

Partsch, C.: Über Kieferzysten. Dtsch. Mschr. Zahnheilk. 32: 271–304, 1892

Partsch, C.: Erkrankungen der Hartgebilde des Mundes. In Partsch, C., Bruhn, C., Kantorowicz, A.: Handbuch der Zahnheilkunde, Bd. I. Bergmann, Wiesbaden, S. 273–299, 1917a

Partsch, C.: Erkrankungen der Hartgebilde des Mundes. In Partsch, C., Bruhn, C., Kantorowicz, A.: Handbuch der Zahnheilkunde, Bd. I. Bergmann, Wiesbaden, S. 300–302, 1917b

Partsch, C., Kunert, A.: Über Wurzelresektion. Dtsch. Mschr. Zahnheilk. 17: 348–367, 1899

Paulsen, G., Reimann, G. P.: Frakturierte Radix im Canalis mandibulae. Quintessenz 30: 19–22, 1979

Pedersen, G. W.: Surgical removal of teeth. In Pedersen, G. W.: Oral Surgery. Saunders, Philadelphia, pp 47–82, 1988

Perko, M.: Das Ernährungsproblem nach kieferchirurgischen Operationen oder Verletzungen im Kieferbereich. Schweiz. Monatsschr. Zahnmed. 76: 396–402, 1966

Pichler, H.: Zur Frage der Wurzelspitzenresektion. Z. Stomatol. 19: 15–20, 1921

Pindborg, J. J.: Atlas of Diseases of the Oral Mucosa, 5th ed. Munksgaard, Kopenhagen 1992

Pindborg, J. J.: Farbatlas der Mundschleimhauterkrankungen, 5. Aufl. Deutscher Ärzte-Verlag, Köln 1993

Pindborg, J. J., Hjørting-Hansen, E.: Atlas of Diseases of the Jaws. Munksgaard, Kopenhagen 1974

Pindborg, J. J., Kramer, I. R. H.: Histological Typing of Odontogenic Tumors, Jaw Cysts and Allied Lesions. World Health Organisation, Geneva, 1971

R

Rahn, R.: Endokarditis-Risiko bei zahnärztlich-chirurgischen Eingriffen. Zahnärztl. Praxis 40: 48–51, 1989

Rajasuo, A., Murtomaa, H., Meurman, J. H.: Comparison of clinical status of third molars in young men in 1949 and in 1990. Oral Surg. Oral Med. Oral Pathol. 76: 694–698, 1993

Raschein, R.: Die rechtliche Stellung des Zahnarztes. Schweiz. Monatsschr. Zahnmed. 101: 1033-1036, 1991

Rateitschak, K. H., Rateitschak, E., Wolf, H. F.: Parodontologie. Farbatlanten der Zahnmedizin, Bd.1. 3. Aufl., Stuttgart, Thieme 1996

Rehrmann, A.: Eine Methode zur Schließung von Kieferhöhlenperforationen. Dtsch. Zahnärztl. Wschr. 39: 1136–1138, 1936

Rehrmann, A.: Zur Frage der chirurgischen Wurzelfüllung und ihre Verbesserung durch Verwendung eines neuen Normbesteckes. Zahnärztl. Rundschau 60: 118–124, 1951

Reuter, I.: Röntgendiagnostik des unteren Weisheitszahnes. Dtsch. Zahnärztl. Z. 48: 94–99, 1993

Richter, M., Fiore-Donno, G., Kuffer, R.: Contribution à l'étude des kératokystes odontogènes. Schweiz. Monatsschr. Zahnmed. 85: 487–506, 1975

Ringeling, H.: Handlungsfähigkeit – Leidensfähigkeit – Medizin und Menschenbild. Schweiz. Monatsschr. Zahnmed. 95: 900–910, 1985

Robinson, H. B. G.: Oral Malignancies. The dentist's responsibility. Dent. Radiogr. Photogr. 21: 1–7, 1948

Robinson, H. B. G., Koch, W. E., Kolas, S.: Radiographic interpretation of oral cysts. Dent. Radiogr. Photogr. 29: 61–68, 1956

Roth, H., Müller, W., Spiessl, B.: Zur Behandlung großvolumiger Knochendefekte im Kieferbereich mit Hydroxylapatit-Granulat. Schweiz. Monatsschr. Zahnmed. 94: 222–227, 1984

Roth, P., Grätz, K. W., Sailer, H. F.: Syndrome de Gorlin-Goltz. Schriftenr. Schweiz. Ges. Kiefer. Gesichtschir. 2: 68–71, 1989

Rothlin, M., Babotai, I.: Der herzkranke Patient in der zahnärztlichen Praxis. Schweiz. Monatsschr. Zahnmed. 98: 1219–2121, 1988

Rowe, N. L., Williams, J. L.: Maxillofacial Injuries, Vol. I–II. Churchill Livingston, Edinburg, 1985

Rud, J., Andreasen, J. O., Möller Jensen, J. E.: A follow-up study of 1000 cases treated by endodontic surgery. Int. J. Oral Surg. 1: 215–228, 1972

Rud, J., Andreasen, J. O., Möller Jensen, J. E.: Radiographic criteria for the assessement of healing after endodontic surgery. Int. J. Oral Surg. 1: 195–214, 1972

Russell, J. H.: In St. Clair, F.G.: Familial Medical Quotations. Saunders, Boston, p. 97b, 1968

S

Sailer, H. F.: Behandlungsergebnisse bei Osteomyelitis und Radioosteomyelitis mandibulae nach Unterkieferresektion und gleichzeitiger Rekonstruktion. Proceedings, 3rd Congress Europ. Ass. Max. Fac. Surg., London 1976

Sailer, H. F.: Zur Wahl der Therapie der Präkanzerosen und Malignome im Kiefer-Gesichtsbereich: Chirurgie, Radiotherapie, Chemotherapie, Immunotherapie. Schweiz. Monatsschr. Zahnmed. 87: 1181–1196, 1977

Sailer, H. F.: Transplantation of Lyophilized Cartilage in Maxillo-facial Surgery. Experimental Foundations an Clinical Success. Karger, Basel 1983

Sailer, H. F.: Longterm results after implantation of different lyophilised bones & cartilage for reconstruction in craniofacial surgery. In Montoya, A.G.: Craniofacial Surgery, 4. Monduzzi, Bologna, p. 69-77, 1992

Sailer, H. F., Antonini, N.: Ergebnisse der Le Clerc-Operation bei habitueller Kiefergelenk- und Diskusluxationen. Fortschr. Kiefer- u. Gesichtschir. 25: 43–45, 1980

Sailer, H. F., Grätz, K. W.: Konzept der Behandlung schwerer Mittelgesichtsfrakturen beim Bezahnten und Unbezahnten. Fortschr. Kiefer- u. Gesichtschir. 36: 52–54, 1991

Sailer, H. F., Kolb, E.: Application of purified bone morphogenetic protein (BMP) in cranio-maxillifacial surgery. BMP in compromised surgical reconstructions using titanium implants. J. craniomaxillofac. Surg. 22: 2–11, 1994

Sailer, H. F., Kolb, E.: Application of purified bone morphogenetic protein (BMP) preparations in cranio-maxillo-facial surgery. J. craniomaxillofac. Surg. 22: 191–199, 1994

Sailer, H. F., Makek, M. S.: Blutbildende Knochenherde als Ursache zystoider Kieferläsionen, Schweiz. Monatsschr. Zahnmed. 95: 183–192, 1985

Schädle, C., Matter-Grütter, C.: Neue Methode zur Deckung freier Zahnhälse. Schweiz. Monatsschr. Zahnmed. 103: 1301–1306, 1993

Scharffetter, K. C., Balz-Hermann, C., Lagrange, W., Koberg, W., Mittermayer, Ch.: Proliferation kinetics-study of the growth of keratocysts. J. Craniomaxfac. Surg. 17: 226–233, 1989

Schettler, G., Greten, H.: Innere Medizin, Bd. I/II., 8. Aufl. Thieme, Stuttgart 1990

Scheunemann, H., Hausamen, J. E.: Gutachterliche Erfahrungen bei Verletzung des Nervus lingualis in Verbindung mit zahnärztlich-chirurgischen Eingriffen. Dtsch. Zahnärztl. Z. 35: 196–198, 1980

Schijatschky, M. M.: Lebensbedrohende Zwischenfälle in der zahnärztlichen Praxis. Quintessenz, Berlin 1992

Schlegel, K. A., Janson, O., Heumann, Ch., Toutenburg, H.: Attached Gingiva und Periimplantitis. Z. Zahnärztl. Implantol. 10: 212–218, 1994

Schmallenbach, H.-J., Austermann, K.-H.: Neue Aspekte zur Ätiologie und Morphologie der Nasolabialzysten. Fortschr. Kiefer. Gesichtschir. 21: 107–109, 1976

Schmelzle, R., Schwenzer, N., Ullmann, U., Mautsch, W.: Die Kontamination von Operationswunden im Mund-, Kiefe r- u. Gesichtsbereich mit Mikroorganismen. Dtsch. Zahnärztl. Z. 33: 785–787, 1978

Schmid-Meier, E.: Anamnese und Befunderhebung bei Kiefergelenkserkrankungen. Schweiz. Monatsschr. Zahnmed. 90: 897–904, 1980

Schmid-Meier, E.: Zahntransplantationen. In Stöckli, P. W., Ben Zur, E.: Zahnmedizin bei Kindern und Jugendlichen, 3. Aufl. Thieme, Stuttgart, S. 301–302, 1994

Schmidseder, R.; Lambrecht, J. Th.: Untersuchungen zur zweizeitig konservativ-chirurgischen Therapie der chronischen Sinusitis maxillaris bei Mund-Antrum-Fisteln unter Verwendung der Sinuskopie. Dtsch. Z. Mund-Kiefer-Gesichts. Chir. 2: 178–182, 1978

Schmidt, L. P., Hardt, N., Makek, M.: Die kalzifizierende odontogene Zyste (COC). Swiss. Dent. 14: 16–18, 1993

Schmidt, R. F.,: Grundriß der Sinnesphysiologie. Springer, Berlin 1985

Schmidt, W., Luhr, H. G.: Technik und Ergebnisse der funktionellen Frühbehandlung von Kollumfrakturen bei gleichzeitigem Vorliegen von Unterkieferkörperfrakturen. Fortschr. Kiefer. Gesichtschir. 21: 317–321, 1976

Schmitt, W., Weber, H. J., Jahn, D.: Thermische Untersuchungen beim Bohren in kortikalem Knochen unter Verwendung verschiedener Kühlsysteme. Dtsch. Zahnärztl. Z. 43: 802–805, 1988

Schmoker, R., Bronz, G., Knutti, D.: Die funktionsstabile Versorgung der Unterkieferfraktur: Indikation, Zugang, Osteosynthesemittel, Komplikationen. Schweiz. Monatsschr. Zahnmed. 93: 513–522, 1983

Schmoker, R., Rüfenacht, D., von Allmen, G., Bronz, G.: Die iatrogene Läsion des N. lingualis als Komplikation bei der operativen Weisheitszahnentfernung. Schweiz. Monatsschr. Zahnmed. 92: 916–921, 1982

Schmutziger, P.: Konservativ-chirurgische Behandlung von Kieferzysten. Schweiz. Monatsschr. Zahnmed. 61: 702–703, 1951

Schotland, C., Stula, D., Lévy, A., Spiessl, B.: Hirnabszess nach dentogenem Infekt. Schweiz. Monatsschr. Zahnmed. 89: 325–329, 1979

Schroeder, H. E.: Pathobiologie oraler Strukturen, 2. Aufl. Karger, Basel 1991

Schroeder, H. E.: Orale Strukturbiologie, 4. Aufl. Thieme, Stuttgart 1992

Schroeder, K.: Probleme der zivilrechtlichen Haftung des freipraktizierenden Zahnarztes. Schulthess, Zürich 1982

Schroll, K.: Ergebnisse der Zystenoperationen im Ober- und Unterkiefer. Fortschr. Kiefer. Gesichtschir. 21: 105–107, 1976

Schuchardt, K.: Die Epidermistransplantation bei der Mundvorhofplastik. Dtsch. Zahnärztl. Z. 7: 364–369, 1952

Schuchardt, K.: Zur Methodik des Verschlusses von Defekten im Alveolarfortsatz zahnloser Oberkiefer. Dtsch. Zahn. Mund. Kieferheilkd. 17: 366-369, 1953

Schuchardt, K.: Grundsätzliches zur Versorgung von kombinierten Weichteil-Knochenverletzungen im Gesichts-Kieferbereich. Fortschr. Kiefer. Gesichtschir. 11: 25–33, 1966

Schulte, W.: Die Knochenregeneration nach der Ausschälung großer Kieferzysten und ihre Konsequenzen für die Operationstechnik. Dtsch. Zahn. Mund. Kieferheilk. 45: 177–206, 1965

Schultz, H.: Die Würde des Patienten: ein Rechtsproblem? Schweiz. Monatsschr. Zahnmed. 90: 1107–1115, 1980

Schultze-Mosgau, S., Neukam, F. W., Berten, J. L., Eulzer, C.: Die autogene Zahntransplantation im Rahmen des orthodontischen Lückenschlusses bei Zahnnichtanlagen. Dtsch. Z. Mund. Kiefer. Gesichtschir. 18: 165–170, 1994

Schwenzer, N., Wüstenfeld, E.: Zur Klinik und Histologie freier Hauttransplantate in der Mundhöhle. Dtsch. Zahnärztl. Z. 25: 1049–1060, 1970

Schwimmer, A. M., Aydin, F., Morrison, S. N.: Squamous cell carcinoma arising in residual odontogenic cyst. Oral Surg. Oral Med. Oral Pathol. 72: 218–221, 1991

Shafer, W. G., Hine, M. K., Levy, B. M.: A Textbook of Oral Pathology, 3rd ed. Saunders, Philadelphia 1974

Shetty, V., Freymiller, E.: Teeth in the line of fracture: a review. J. Oral Maxillofac Surg 47: 1303–1306, 1989

Skouteris, Ch. A., Sotereanos, G. C.: Plunging ranula. J. Oral Maxillofac. Surg. 45: 1068-1072, 1987

Smee, G., Bolanos, O. R., Morse, D. R., Furst, M. L., Yesilsoy, C.: A comparative leakage study of P-30 resin bonded ceramic, Teflon, Amalgam and IRM as retrofilling seals. J. Endod. 13: 117–121, 1987

Sonis, S. T., Fazio, R. C., Fang, L.: Principles and practice of oral medicine. Saunders, Philadelphia S. 360–369, 1995

Spiekermann, H.: Implantologie. Farbatlanten der Zahnmedizin, Bd. 10. Thieme, Stuttgart 1994.

Spiessl, B.: Funktionsstabile Osteosynthese bei Unterkieferfrakturen – Problematik und Technik. Fortschr. Kiefer. Gesichtschir. 19: 68–71, 1975

Spiessl, B.: Trauma als Notfallsituation. Schweiz. Monatsschr. Zahnmed. 84: 915–933, 1974

Stefani, M.: Rezidivhäufigkeit von odontogenen Keratozysten nach Marsupialisation. Med. Diss., Zürich 1994

Steiner, J. E.: Beobachtung von Heilungsprozessen nach Zystenoperationen. Dtsch. Zahnärzteblatt 15: 404–409, 1961

Stöckli, P. W., Ben Zur, E. D.: Zahnmedizin bei Kindern und Jugendlichen, 3. Aufl. Thieme, Stuttgart 1994

Stoelinga, P. J. W., Bronkhorst, F. B.: The incidence, multiple presentation an recurrence of aggressive cysts of the jaws. J. Cranio-Max.-Fac. Surg. 16: 184–195, 1988

Strassburg, M., Knolle, G.: Farbatlas und Lehrbuch der Mundschleimhauterkrankungen, 3. Aufl. Quintessenz, Berlin 1991

Strobl, V., Traugott, D., Norer, B.: Dentoalveoläre Verletzungen im Oberkiefer. Fortschr. Kiefer. Gesichtschir. 36: 145–148, 1991

Strub, J. R., Kopp, F. R.: Das freie Schleimhauttransplantat. Genäht versus geklebt. Schweiz. Monatsschr. Zahnmed. 90: 1028–1036, 1980

T

Takenoshita, Y., Ishibashi, H., Oka, M.: Comparison of functional recovery after nonsurgical and surgical treatment of condylar fractures. J. Oral Maxillofac. Surg. 48: 1191-1195, 1990

Tetsch, P., Wagner, W.: Die operative Weisheitszahnentfernung. Hanser, München 1982

Toller, P.: Origin and growth of cysts of the jaws. Ann. R. Coll. Surg. Engl. 40: 306–336, 1967

Trauner, P., Obwegeser, H. L.: Zur Operationstechnik bei der Progenie und anderen Unterkieferanomalien. Dtsch. Zahn. Mund, Kieferheilkd. 23: 1–26, 1955

V

Van den Akker, H. P., Bays, R. A., Becker, A. E.: Plunging or cervical ranula. J. Maxillofac. Surg. 6: 286–293, 1978

Van der Waal, I.: Kiefererkrankungen – Diagnose und Therapie. Deutscher Ärzte-Verlag, Köln, S. 113–234, 1993

Van Waues, H., Gnoinski, W., Ben Zur, E.: Die Draht-/Kompositschiene. Schweiz. Monatsschr. Zahnmed. 97: 629–636, 1987

Velvart, P., Reimann, Chr.: Sensibilitätstestung. Schweiz. Monatsschr. Zahnmed. 98: 517–523, 1988

Ventä, I.: Predictive model for impaction of lower third molars. Oral Surg. Oral Med. Oral Pathol. 76: 699–703, 1993

Von Arx, T.: Mesiodens. Schweiz. Monatsschr. Zahnmed. 100: 433–442, 1990

Von Arx, T.: Traumatologie im Milchgebiß, I und II. Schweiz. Monatsschr. Zahnmed. 100: 1195–1206, 1990 und 101: 57–70, 1991

Von Wowern, N., Nielsen, H. O.: The fate of impacted lower third molars after the Age of 20. Int. J. Oral Maxillofac. Surg. 18: 277–280, 1989

Voorsmit, R. A. C. A.: The art of treating keratocysts: fixation bevore enucleation. Autumn Meeting of the British Assoc. of Oral and Maxillofacial Surgeons, London 1990

Voorsmit, R. A. C. A., Stoelinga, P. J. W., van Haelst, U. I. G. M.: The management of keratocysts. J. Maxillofac. Surg. 9: 228–236, 1981

W

Wagner, J. D., Moore, D. L.: Preoperative laboratory testing for the oral and maxillofacial surgery patient. J. Oral Maxillofac. Surg. 49: 177–182, 1991

Walder, H.: Der ärztliche Kunstfehler aus strafrechtlicher Sicht. Schweiz. Ärztez. 62: 3470–3474, 1981

Walder, H.: Die Aufklärungspflicht des Zahnarztes aus forensischer Sicht. Schweiz. Monatsschr. Zahnmed. 95: 889–894, 1985

Wassmund, M.: Lehrbuch der praktischen Chirurgie des Mundes und der Kiefer, Bd. 1–2. Barth, Leipzig 1935–1939

Wiehl, P.: Orale Physiotherapie – eine zusätzliche Hilfe für Myoarthropathie-Patienten. Schweiz. Monatsschr. Zahnmed. 93: 235–247, 1983

Wiehl, P., Guggenheim, B.: Hygienegerechtes Praxiskonzept I und II. Schweiz. Monatsschr. Zahnmed. 103: 179–181 und 1127–1140, 1993

Windecker-Gétaz, I., Richter, M., Gremion, G., Zabala, I., Samson, J., Piletta-Zanin, S., Belser, U.: Algies faciales et troubles de la fonction masticatrice. Schweiz. Monatsschr. Zahnmed. 103: 1573–1584, 1993

Winter, L.: A textbook of exodontia: exodontia, oral surgery and anesthesiea. 5th ed. Mosby, St. Louis 1943

Wolfe, S. A., Baker, St.: Facial Fractures. Thieme, New York 1993

Work, W. P., Batsakis, J. G.: Classification of salivary gland diseases. Otolaryngol. Clin. North Am. 10: 287–296, 1977

Wüthrich, S.: Integritätsentschädigung. Schweiz. Monatsschr. Zahnmed. 97: 880, 1987

Y

Yaremchuk, M. J., Gruss, J. S., Manson, P. N.: Rigid Fixation of the Craniomaxillofacial Skeleton. Butterworth-Heinemann. Boston 1992

Z

Zander, A., Buddeberg, C., Frei, R.: Befunderhebung und Therapieplanung bei Patienten mit mandibulärer Dysfunktion. Schweiz. Monatsschr. Zahnmed. 92: 497–514, 1982

Zetzmann, D., Berthold, H., Buser, D.: Die Defektfüllung großvolumiger Knochenhöhlen im Kieferbereich mit Kollagenvlies. Schweiz. Monatsschr. Zahnmed. 92: 119–126, 1982

Zimmerli, Ph., Hardt, N., Altermatt, H. J.: Kieferhöhlenoperation. Aspergillose der Kieferhöhle durch Wurzelfüllmaterial. Schweiz. Monatsschr. Zahnmed. 98: 527–530, 1988

Zimmermann, M., Nentwig, G. H.: Die Therapie des Postextraktionssyndroms mit Taurolin. Schweiz. Monatsschr. Zahnmed. 102: 1327–1332, 1992

Zou, Z. J., Wu, W. T., Sun, G. X., Zhu, X. P., Zhang, K. H., Wu, Q. G., Su, L. D., Lin, J. X.: Remodelling of the temporomandibular joint after conservative treatment of condylar fractures. Dentomaxillofac. Radiol. 16: 91–98, 1987

Index

Note: page numbers in *italics* refer to figures

This book is to be returned on or before
the last date stamped below.